CRASH COURSE
Psychiatry

Isabel Benson

02066845@student.gla.ac.uk

Other titles in the Crash Course series

There are 23 books in the Crash Course series in two ranges: Basic Science and Clinical. Each book follows the same format, with concise text, clear illustrations and helpful learning features including access to online USMLE test questions.

Basic Science titles

Pathology
Nervous System
Renal and Urinary Systems
Gastrointestinal System
Respiratory System
Endocrine and Reproductive Systems
Metabolism and Nutrition
Pharmacology
Immunology
Musculoskeletal System
Cardiovascular System
Cell Biology and Genetics
Anatomy

Clinical titles

Surgery
Cardiology
History and Examination
Internal Medicine
Neurology
Gastroenterology
OBGYN
Psychiatry
Pediatrics

Forthcoming:
Imaging

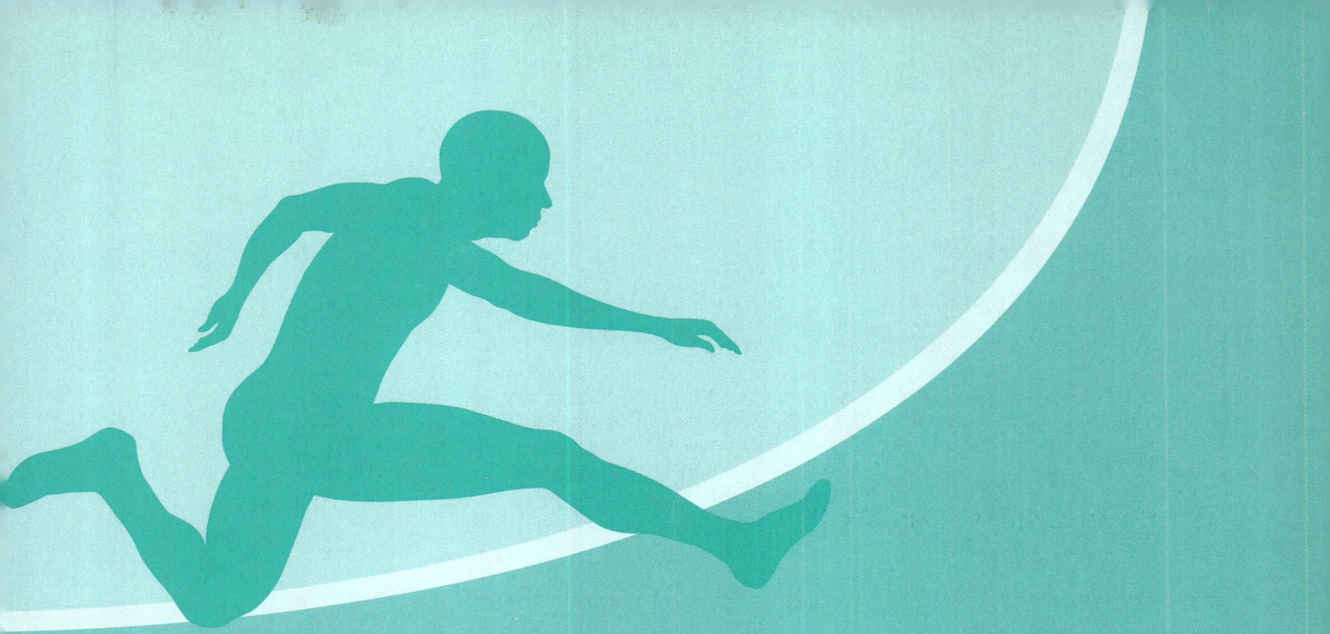

Psychiatry

Jonathan Birnkrant, MD
Child and Adolescent Psychiatry
Pediatrics
Providence, Rhode Island

Andrea Carlsen, MD
Private Practice
Shelter Island, New York

UK edition authors
Alasdair D. Cameron, Darren Bloye, and Simon Davies

UK series editor
Daniel Horton-Szar

MOSBY
ELSEVIER

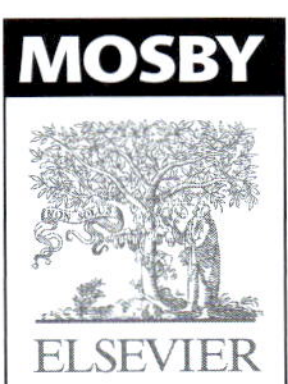

Isabel

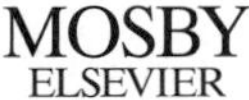

1600 John F. Kennedy Blvd.
Suite 1800
Philadelphia, PA 19103-2899

CRASH COURSE: PSYCHIATRY

ISBN-13: 978-0-323-04832-3
ISBN-10: 0-323-04832-3

Notice

Knowledge and best practice in this field are constantly changing. As new research and experience broaden our knowledge, changes in practice, treatment and drug therapy may become necessary or appropriate. Readers are advised to check the most current information provided (i) on procedures featured or (ii) by the manufacturer of each product to be administered, to verify the recommended dose or formula, the method and duration of administration, and contraindications. It is the responsibility of the practitioner, relying on their own experience and knowledge of the patient, to make diagnoses, to determine dosages and the best treatment for each individual patient, and to take all appropriate safety precautions. To the fullest extent of the law, neither the Publisher nor the Authors assumes any liability for any injury and/or damage to persons or property arising out or related to any use of the material contained in this book.

The Publisher

Adapted from Crash Course: Psychiatry, 2e by Alasdair D. Cameron
ISBN: 0-7234-3340-2. © 2004, Elsevier Science Limited

Library of Congress Cataloging-in-Publication Data
Birnkrant, Jonathan.
Crash course psychiatry/Jonathan Birnkrant, Andrea Carlsen.—1st American ed.
p. ; cm.—(Crash course)
Includes index.
ISBN 978-0-323-04832-3
1. Psychiatry—Outlines, syllabi, etc. I. Carlsen, Andrea. II. Title. III. Series.
[DNLM: 1. Mental Disorders. 2. Diagnosis, Differential. 3. Psychiatry—methods. WM 140 B619c 2007]
RC457.2.B57 2007
616.89—dc22 2006037541

Commissioning Editor: Alex Stibbe
Developmental Editor: Stan Ward
Project Manager: David Saltzberg
Design: Andy Chapman
Cover Design: Antbits Illustration
Illustration Manager: Mick Ruddy

Printed in China

Last digit is the print number:
9 8 7 6 5 4 3 2 1

Preface

The field of psychiatry offers many opportunities and challenges. Among these are appreciating the subtleties of patient presentation as well as the nuances of diagnosis and treatment. In order for students to accomplish these goals, they need to understand basic concepts of the discipline. In *Crash Course Psychiatry*, we have attempted to clarify these basic concepts as well as to convey the breadth and depth of this unique and fascinating field.

The book is divided into three parts. In Part I, 'The Patient Presents With,' each chapter begins with a patient vignette and then explains the clinical features and differential diagnoses associated with this clinical presentation. Part II, 'Diseases and Disorders,' further explains each of the disorders presented in Part I by systematically describing the disease, including its etiology, epidemiology, assessment, treatment, and prognosis. Part III, 'Assessment and Therapy,' provides a comprehensive explanation of the initial psychiatric interview and the diagnostic formulations in the *Diagnostic and Statistical Manual of Mental Disorders*, 4th edn., Text Revision (DSM-IV-TR) as well as an in-depth discussion of therapies and pharmacologic interventions.

Furthermore, in order to provide a more realistic test-taking experience that closely approximates the conditions for the now computerized USMLE, this edition of *Crash Course Psychiatry* provides convenient web-based multiple choice questions for self assessment.

Psychiatric disorders are found in all disciplines of medicine. We believe this book will provide a foundation not only for future psychiatrists but also for all future physicians as they manage the mental health issues of their patients.

Dedication

To my parents, Dr. and Mrs. Andrew Carlsen, and to Max (The Maximum).
AC

To Andrea, your love, support and friendship are gifts from the most beautiful, caring and intelligent woman there is. Thank you is not enough.
JB

Acknowledgments

In this U.S. edition of the *Crash Course Psychiatry*, we would like to acknowledge the U.K. authors for bringing this book to fruition. Furthermore, we would like to acknowledge the many people at Elsevier who have come together to make this U.S. edition a reality – in particular, Alex Stibbe, Stan Ward, and Kate Dimock.

Contents

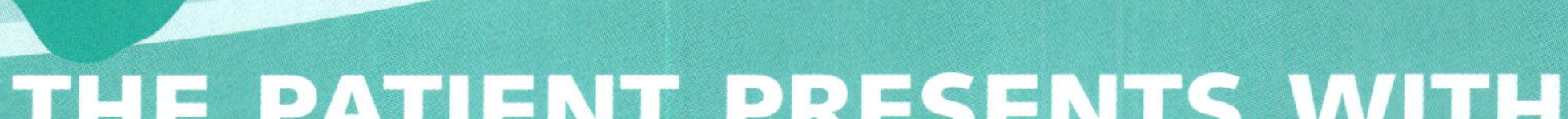

THE PATIENT PRESENTS WITH

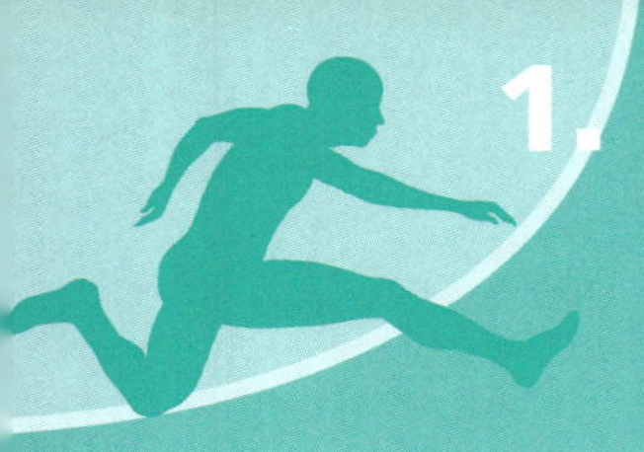

1. The Patient with Low Mood

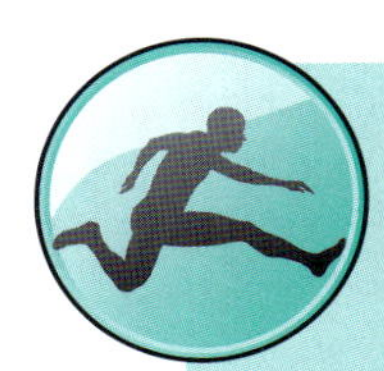

Mrs LM, a 32-year-old married homemaker with two children aged 4 and 6 years, presented to her family doctor stating that she felt persistently unhappy and had been crying repeatedly over the past few weeks. She had no previous psychiatric history or significant medical history, and her only regular medication was oral contraception. She had moved to the area 3 years earlier when her husband was promoted and, at first, appeared to have integrated well into the neighborhood by involving herself in the organization of a toddlers' group. Unfortunately, the group had dissolved a few months before when her co-organizer and only close confidante had moved away. Deprived of her most important social outlet, Mrs LM found herself increasingly dominated by her young children. Although usually an outgoing person, she noticed that her motivation to keep in touch with other mothers from the group had started to dwindle. At the same time, she started feeling persistently weary even though her work schedule had not increased, and often awakened 2–3 hours earlier in the morning. Although her appetite had not increased, she had turned to food for "comfort" and had gained over 14 lb in weight. Mrs LM also candidly admitted that she was drinking more alcohol than usual. She described feeling incompetent because she was always miserable and had become too tired to look after the children. She felt guilty for burdening her husband and started crying when talking about her loss of interest in sex and her feelings of unattractiveness. Mrs LM maintained that no aspect of her life gave her pleasure and, when asked specifically by her doctor, admitted that she had started to wonder whether her children and husband would be better off without her.

(For a discussion of the case study see the end of the chapter)

Feeling sad or upset is a normal part of the human condition; thus, a patient presenting with emotional suffering does not necessarily warrant a psychiatric diagnosis or require treatment. However, most psychiatrists agree that when patients present with a certain number of key *depressive features*, they are likely suffering from some form of psychiatric issue that will require, and usually respond to, specific kinds of treatment.

Definitions and clinical features

Whereas feelings describe a short-lived emotional experience, *mood* refers to a patient's *sustained, subjectively experienced emotional state over a period of time*. Patients are described as having a depressed mood when they report feeling depressed, sad, dejected, despondent, "down in the dumps," miserable, "blue," or "heavy-hearted." They are unable to lift themselves out of this mood, and its severity is often out of proportion to the stressors in their surrounding social environment.

The term *affect* is used by psychiatrists to describe the *observed, external expression of emotion* as perceived by another person. The range of affect (i.e., the range of emotional expression) can be described in a number of ways. For example, a *blunted* affect indicates a significant reduction in the normal intensity of emotional expression as evidenced by a monotonous voice and minimal facial expression (see Ch. 26). The affect may be incongruous with the patient's subjectively reported mood (e.g., the smiling patient who reports feeling miserable).

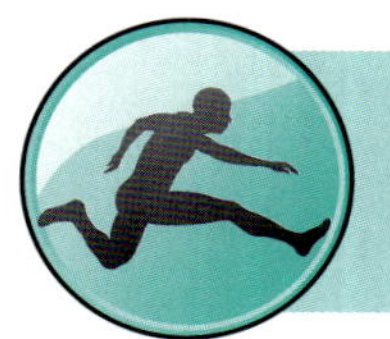

Remember the distinction between the terms "mood" and "affect"; they are not the same.

The DSM-IV-TR classification system requires two key features in a major depressive episode: a *persistently depressed mood* or *anhedonia* (loss of pleasure or interest). At least one of these features, in combination with four other symptoms, must be present for a minimum of **2 weeks** in order to qualify as this diagnosis.

These symptoms must cause clinically significant impairment in multiple areas of functioning, including social, occupational, and family. The symptoms must not be secondary to a medical condition, substance abuse, or bereavement.

In addition to a depressed mood, the constellation of these symptoms can best be remembered by the mnemonic **SIGE CAPS**:

1. **S**leep (insomnia or hypersomnia)
2. **I**nterest (loss of pleasure or interest in activities)
3. **G**uilt (feelings of worthlessness or inappropriate guilt)
4. **E**nergy (decreased)
5. **C**oncentration (decreased)
6. **A**ppetite (increased or decreased)
7. **P**sychomotor agitation or retardation
8. **S**uicidal ideation.

The 10th revision of the *International Statistical Classification of Diseases and Mental Health Problems* (ICD-10) is a comprehensive classification system of medical and psychiatric disorders. It is used throughout the world to describe various diseases. However, the DSM-IV is used in the US and will be referred to in this text.

These symptoms are described as follows:

Sleep disruption

Patients may experience changes in their normal sleep pattern. During a depressive episode, they may get off to sleep at their normal time, wake at least 2 hours earlier than usual and then find it impossible to get back to sleep again. Further disturbances of sleep in depression include difficulty falling asleep (initial insomnia), frequent awakening during the night, or excessive sleep (hypersomnia).

Loss of interest or pleasure in activities that are normally enjoyable

Anhedonia means an inability to derive pleasure or excitement from any activities. This key symptom in depression is also associated with the related concept of having a markedly reduced interest in previously enjoyable activities.

Guilt

Depressed patients often have guilty preoccupations about minor past failings. This guilt is often inappropriate and out of proportion to the original "offense." Patients often have guilty thoughts about the very act of developing the depressed mood itself.

Energy

The patient describes fatigue or loss of energy every day.

Reduced concentration and attention

Depressed patients report difficulty in sustaining attention while doing previously manageable tasks. They often appear easily distracted and may complain of memory difficulties.

Marked loss of appetite and weight loss

Depressed patients may experience a significant decrease in appetite. In addition to loss of appetite, a loss of 5% body weight in the past month is an important biologic symptom. Note that the reversed biologic features of overeating and oversleeping can also occur and are sometimes referred to as *atypical depressive symptoms*.

Psychomotor retardation or agitation

The term "psychomotor" is used to describe a patient's motor activity as a reflection of concurrent mental processes. Psychomotor changes in depression include retardation (slow, monotonous speech; long pauses before answering

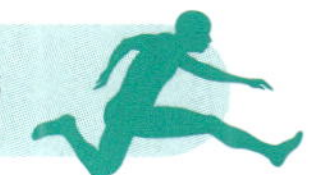

questions or muteness; leaden body movements and limited facial expression, i.e., blunted affect) and agitation (inability to sit still; fidgeting, pacing or hand-wringing; rubbing or scratching skin or clothes). Note that psychomotor changes must be severe enough to be observable by others, not just the subjective experience of the patient.

Suicide or self-harm

Depressed patients frequently have thoughts of death and harming themselves. In severe cases suicidal ideation may lead to an actual suicide attempt. At these times, patients may believe that they face insurmountable difficulties or must escape a relentlessly painful emotional state. Self-harm is discussed fully in Chapter 3.

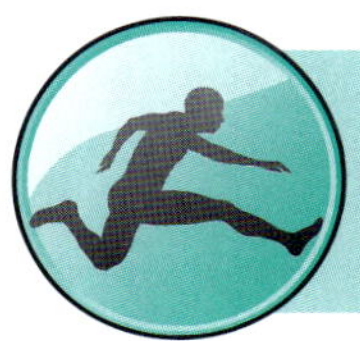

Know the biologic symptoms of depression; they are often asked for in exams.

It is always crucial to assess the risk of suicide in patients who present with low mood. Chapter 3 will help you in this regard.

There are six specific subtypes that may be used to describe major depressive disorder (MDD):

1. ***MDD with psychotic features:*** In severe depressive episodes, patients may suffer from the psychotic symptoms of delusions and hallucinations (see Ch. 4). Delusions and hallucinations can be further classified as "mood congruent" or "mood incongruent." These terms indicate whether the content of the psychotic symptoms is *consistent* with the patient's mood. Delusions and hallucinations in depression are most often mood congruent and may involve an irrational conviction of guilt or sin, or the belief that parts of the body are dead or wasting away. Hallucinations may take the form of accusatory or defamatory voices criticizing the patient (auditory hallucination) or the smell of rotting flesh (olfactory hallucination). Once psychotic symptoms appear, they tend to be present in each subsequent depressive episode.
2. ***MDD with melancholic features:*** In this type of depression, patients experience a loss of pleasure or a lack of reactivity to things that they used to enjoy. In addition, three or more of the following symptoms must be present: a depressed mood, depression that is worse in the morning, early morning awakening (at least 2 hours before the usual time), marked psychomotor retardation or agitation, significant anorexia or weight loss, excessive or inappropriate guilt.
3. ***MDD with atypical features:*** Patients with this type of depression will display mood reactivity (mood brightens in response to actual or potential positive events) as well as two or more of the following symptoms: significant weight gain or an increase in appetite, hypersomnia, leaden paralysis, a pattern of interpersonal rejection sensitivity. There is a younger age of onset for the first depressive episode, more severe motor retardation, and more frequent comorbidities of panic disorder, substance abuse, and somatization disorder. Patients have a more chronic course and are more likely to receive a diagnosis of bipolar disorder and/or have a seasonal pattern to their depression.
4. ***MDD with postpartum onset:*** In this case, the major depressive episode occurs within 4 weeks postpartum (i.e., 4 weeks after giving birth). See Chapter 20 for details.
5. ***MDD with a seasonal pattern:*** The onset of these depressive episodes consistently coincides with certain times of the year, usually fall and winter.
6. ***MDD with catatonic features:*** In this subtype, at least two of the following symptoms must be present: motoric immobility (such as waxy flexibility or stupor), excessive motor activity that appears purposeless, extreme negativism (rigid posture, resistance to commands, mutism), unusual involuntary movements (bizarre postures, stereotypical movements, grimacing), and echolalia or echopraxia. It is important to be aware that catatonic symptoms are a behavioral syndrome seen in several

disorders, including mood disorders and schizophrenia, as well as medical and neurologic disorders. Therefore, these symptoms do not imply a specific diagnosis.

Differential diagnosis of low mood

Careful history taking and examination should reveal whether the patient presenting with low mood is suffering from a primary mood disorder, or whether their depression is secondary to a medical condition, psychoactive substance or other psychiatric condition. Figure 1.1 presents the differential diagnosis. An algorithm for the diagnosis of mood disorders is presented in Chapter 2.

Mood (affective) disorders

Depressive episode

The DSM-IV-TR has set out certain diagnostic guidelines for diagnosing a depressive episode (Fig. 1.2). The minimum duration of the episode is 2 weeks, and five or more symptoms must be present during this time period. At least one of the symptoms is either (1) depressed mood or (2) loss of interest or pleasure (anhedonia) A depressive episode can be graded mild, moderate, or severe, depending on the number and severity of symptoms. A depressive episode occurring with hallucinations, delusions, or a catatonic stupor is always coded as *severe with psychotic features*.

Differential diagnosis of low mood

Mood disorders
- Depressive episode
- Recurrent depressive disorder
- Dysthymia
- Bipolar affective disorder
- Cyclothymia

Schizoaffective disorder

Secondary to a general medical condition

Secondary to psychoactive substance use (including alcohol)

Secondary to other psychiatric disorders
- Psychotic disorders
- Anxiety disorders
- Adjustment disorder (including bereavement)
- Eating disorders
- Personality disorders
- Dementia

Fig. 1.1 Differential diagnosis for patient presenting with low mood.

Recurrent depressive disorder

Many patients will have several depressive episodes in their lifetime. Recurrent depressive disorder is diagnosed when a patient has another depressive episode after the first, regardless of the time lapse between episodes.

Dysthymia

In this type of depression, the patient experiences a mildly depressed mood for at least 2 years. This disorder usually has its onset in early adulthood and typically persists throughout the patient's life with variable periods of wellness in between. The patient's mood is seldom severe enough to satisfy the formal criteria for a depressive episode and does not present with discrete episodes as in genuine *recurrent depressive disorder*. Sometimes dysthymia has its onset in later adult life, often after a discrete depressive episode, and is usually associated with bereavement or some other serious stress. Note that patients may develop a depressive episode on a baseline mood of dysthymia (so-called *double depression*).

Bipolar affective disorder/cyclothymia

Unipolar depression means that the patient's mood is either depressed or normal. When patients suffer from episodes of either depressed or elevated mood, the disorder is termed *bipolar*, as the mood is considered to deviate from normal to either a depressed or elated (manic) state. When this instability of mood involves only mild elation and depression it is termed cyclothymia. Bipolar illness and cyclothymia are presented in Chapter 2.

Schizoaffective disorder

A diagnosis of schizoaffective disorder can be made when patients present with both mood (depression or mania) symptoms and psychotic symptoms within the same episode of illness. It is important that these symptoms occur simultaneously or at least within a few days of each other. As you can imagine, this is a difficult diagnosis to establish, as it is not uncommon to have psychotic symptoms in a severe episode of depression (*depressive episode with psychotic features*); likewise, depressive

Major depressive episode

A. Five (or more) of the following symptoms have been present during the same 2-week period and represent a change from previous functioning; at least one of the symptoms is either (1) depressed mood or (2) loss of interest or pleasure.

Note: Do not include symptoms that are clearly due to a general medical condition, or mood-incongruent delusions or hallucinations.

(1) depressed mood most of the day, nearly every day, as indicated by either subjective report (e.g., feels sad or empty) or observation made by others (e.g., appears tearful)

Note: In children and adolescents, can be irritable mood.

(2) markedly diminished interest or pleasure in all, or almost all, activities most of the day, nearly every day (as indicated by either subjective account or observation made by others)
(3) significant weight loss when not dieting or weight gain (e.g., a change of more than 5% of body weight in a month), or decrease or increase in appetite nearly every day

Note: In children, consider failure to make expected weight gains.

(4) insomnia or hypersomnia nearly every day
(5) psychomotor agitation or retardation nearly every day (observable by others, not merely subjective feelings of restlessness or being slowed down)
(6) fatigue or loss of energy nearly every day
(7) feelings of worthlessness or excessive or inappropriate guilt (which may be delusional) nearly every day (not merely self-reproach or guilt about being sick)
(8) diminished ability to think or concentrate, or indecisiveness, nearly every day (either by subjective account or as observed by others)
(9) recurrent thoughts of death (not just fear of dying), recurrent suicidal ideation without a specific plan, or a suicide attempt or a specific plan for committing suicide

B. The symptoms do not meet criteria for a Mixed Episode.
C. The symptoms cause clinically significant distress or impairment in social, occupational, or other important areas of functioning.
D. The symptoms are not due to the direct physiological effects of a substance (e.g., a drug of abuse, a medication) or a general medical condition (e.g., hypothyroidism).
E. The symptoms are not better accounted for by bereavement, i.e., after the loss of a loved one, the symptoms persist for longer than 2 months or are characterized by marked functional impairment, morbid preoccupation with worthlessness, suicidal ideation, psychotic symptoms, or psychomotor retardation.

Fig. 1.2 DSM-IV-TR criteria for depressive episode.

symptoms often occur in patients with schizophrenia. Schizoaffective disorder is discussed in more detail in Chapter 4.

Depression secondary to psychiatric or general medical disorders or to psychoactive substances

The mood disorders as described above are considered primary; however, depressive symptoms are nonspecific and can occur secondary to a range of other conditions. For example, a patient who has schizophrenia, an anxiety disorder, a personality disorder, an eating disorder, or dementia may experience depression as a consequence. These depressive symptoms may even meet the criteria for a depressive episode.

General medical conditions that may produce depression through a presumed direct depressant effect are listed in Figure 1.3. Note that any medical condition that causes a significant degree of suffering may cause secondary depression indirectly for "psychological reasons."

Both prescribed (Fig. 1.4) and illicit drugs can be etiologically responsible for symptoms of depression. For example, reserpine, an antihypertensive agent, is thought to produce depression through depletion of presynaptic catecholamine stores. Remember that alcohol is the psychoactive substance most associated with substance-induced depression.

Low mood may be one of several symptoms that appear when a patient has had to adapt to a

General medical conditions causing low mood			
Neurological	**Endocrine**	**Infections**	**Others**
Multiple sclerosis Parkinson's disease Huntington's disease Spinal cord injury Stroke (especially left anterior infarcts) Head injury Cerebral tumors	Cushing's disease Addison's disease Thyroid disorders (especially hypothyroidism) Parathyroid disorders Menstrual cycle-related	Hepatitis Infectious mononucleosis Herpes simplex Brucellosis Typhoid HIV/AIDS Syphilis	Malignancies (especially pancreatic cancer) Systemic lupus erythematosus Rheumatoid arthritis Renal failure Porphyria Vitamin deficiencies (e.g., niacin) Chronic pain states

Fig. 1.3 General medical conditions causing low mood.

Prescribed drugs causing low mood				
Antihypertensives	**Steroids**	**Neurologic drugs**	**Analgesics**	**Psychiatric**
Beta-blockers Methyldopa Reserpine	Corticosteroids Oral contraceptives	L-dopa Carbamazepine Phenytoin Benzodiazepines	Opiates Ibuprofen Indometacin	Antipsychotics (phenothiazines, butyrophenones)

Fig. 1.4 Prescribed drugs causing low mood.

significant change in life (e.g., divorce, retirement). When it can be confidently assumed that the symptoms would not have arisen without the stress due to the life event, the diagnosis of Adjustment disorder is made. Bereavement is a form of adjustment reaction and is discussed in more detail in Chapter 7.

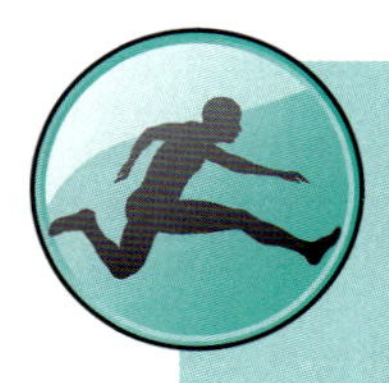

A basic physical examination, including a thorough neurologic and endocrine system examination, should be performed on all patients with depression.

Assessment

Clinical

The following questions might be helpful in eliciting the key symptoms of depression:

- Have you been cheerful or quite low in mood or spirits lately?
- Do you find that you no longer enjoy things the way you used to?
- Do you find yourself often feeling very tired or worn out?
- How do you see things turning out in the future?
- Sometimes when people are depressed they have a poor sex drive. Has this happened to you?

Special investigations

Social

- Collateral information from family doctor, community mental health team, family.
- Consider interviewing immediate family if disturbed interpersonal family dynamics are suspected.

Psychological

- Patient may be asked to keep a mood diary.
- Self-report inventories for quantitative ratings of mood, such as the Beck Depression Inventory (BDI).

Physical

Physical investigations are performed to (1) exclude possible medical or substance-related causes of depression; (2) establish baseline values before administering treatment that may alter blood chemistry (e.g., antidepressants may cause hyponatremia, lithium may cause hypothyroidism); and (3) assess renal and liver functioning, which may affect the elimination of medication.

- Complete blood count: check for anemia (low hemoglobin), infection (elevated white count), and a high mean cell volume (MCV; a marker of high alcohol intake)
- Urea and electrolytes (renal function)
- Liver function tests and gamma-glutamyl transpeptidase (γGT) (also a marker for high alcohol intake)
- Thyroid function tests and calcium
- Erythrocyte sedimentation rate (ESR).

If indicated:

- Vitamin B_{12} and folate (if deficiencies suspected)
- Urine drug screen (if drug use is suspected)
- An ECG should be done in patients with cardiac problems, as tricyclic antidepressants and lithium may prolong the QT interval and have the potential to cause lethal ventricular arrhythmia
- Serologic tests for syphilis if indicated (e.g., VDRL)
- EEG (if epileptic focus or other intracranial pathology is suspected).

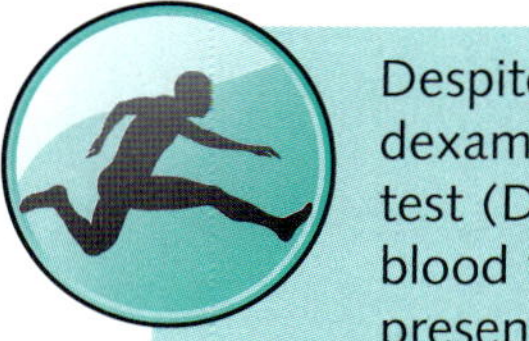

Despite much research on the dexamethasone suppression test (DST), there is no reliable blood test to indicate the presence of depression. However, one biologic finding that is strongly associated with depression is a reduction in the latency (time to onset after falling asleep) of rapid eye movement (REM) sleep.

Discussion of case study

Mrs LM meets the criteria for a depressive episode, at least moderate in severity. She has had the two core symptoms of depression for longer than 2 weeks: depressed mood and loss of interest or pleasure. The family doctor has also elicited associated depressive symptoms of disturbed sleep, feelings of incompetence (reduced self-esteem), and guilt and possible thoughts of self-harm. Mrs LM also has somatic symptoms of loss of interest or pleasure, early morning awakening, and loss of libido. As this is a first episode, the diagnosis of recurrent depressive disorder is not appropriate. Dysthymia is not a suitable diagnosis as the period of low mood is far too short, the severity of the present episode too great, and the deterioration in functioning too marked. There appear to be no instances of elated mood or increased energy, which goes against a diagnosis of bipolar affective disorder or cyclothymia.

In order to grade the severity of the depression (and possibly the presence of a somatic syndrome) it would be useful to inquire about all the cognitive, biologic, suicidal, and psychotic components of depression. In all cases of suspected depression it is imperative to inquire about thoughts and or plans of suicide or self-harm (see Ch. 3 for a full discussion). It is also important to rule out secondary causes of depression; these include general medical conditions (Fig. 1.3), psychoactive substance use (Fig. 1.4), and other psychiatric conditions. Mrs LM admitted to using increased quantities of alcohol. Patients often use alcohol as a form of self-medication to alleviate feelings of dysphoria. However, alcohol can aggravate and in some cases even cause depressive symptoms. Mrs LM's use of oral contraception long before the onset of her depressive symptoms suggests that it is unlikely that this prescribed drug is causing her depression.

Now go to Chapter 13 to read about the mood disorders and their management.

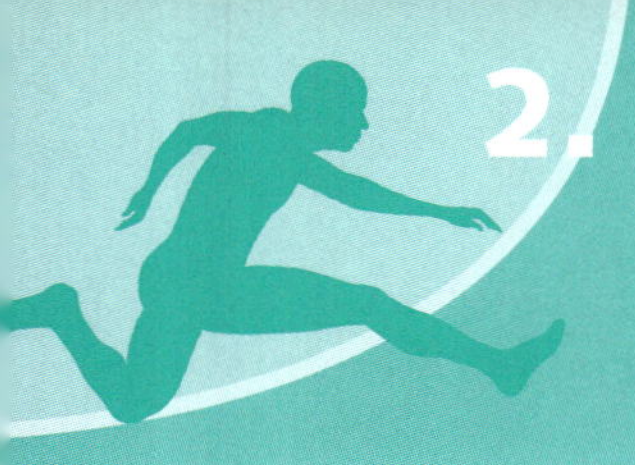

2. The Patient with Elevated or Irritable Mood

Mr EM is a 37-year-old freelance writer with no psychiatric history other than a period of depression 2 years ago. He had progressively needed less sleep over the previous 2 weeks and had not slept at all for 48 hours. Recently, he had started taking on increasing amounts of work and seemed to thrive on this due to an "inexhaustible source of boundless energy." He told his wife and all his friends that he had a new lease of life, as he was "happier than ever." Mrs EM became concerned when he developed lofty ideas that he was a world expert in his field and would talk incessantly for hours about elaborate and complicated writing schemes. Mr EM's behavior had become markedly uncharacteristic over the past day or two, when he started making sexually inappropriate comments to his neighbor's wife and presented her with reams of poetry which he had spent the night writing. When Mrs EM suggested that he visit their primary care physician (PCP), Mr EM became verbally aggressive, saying that she was trying to bring him down because she was threatened by his "irresistible sex appeal and wit." Mrs EM was unable to reason with him and noticed that he struggled to keep to the point of the conversation, often bringing up issues that seemed completely irrelevant. The PCP noted that, other than a recent bout of flu, Mr EM had no medical problems and was not using any prescribed medication.

(For a discussion of the case study see the end of the chapter)

Just as spells of feeling sad and miserable are quite normal to the human experience, so too are periods where we feel elated, excited, and full of energy. Although an irritable or elevated mood is not in itself pathologic, it can be when grossly and persistently so, and when associated with other manic psychopathology.

Definitions and clinical features

In Chapter 1 we observed how a disturbance in mood, in addition to various other cognitive, biologic, and psychotic symptoms, all contribute to the recognition of a *depressive episode*. A similar approach is taken to *hypomanic* and *manic episodes*; these occur on the opposite pole of the mood disorder spectrum to depression.

Mood

The hallmark of a manic episode is an elevated or irritable mood. When their mood is elevated, manic patients often enjoy the experience and might describe themselves as feeling "high," "on top of the world," "fantastic," or "euphoric." This mood has an infectious quality, although those who know the patient well clearly see it as deviation from normal. Some patients tend to become extremely irritable or suspicious when manic and do not enjoy the experience at all. They have a low frustration tolerance and any thwarting of their plans can lead to a rapid escalation in anger or even delusions of persecution. Some patients alternate rapidly between manic and depressive symptoms from day to day or even hour to hour; this is termed *rapid cycling*.

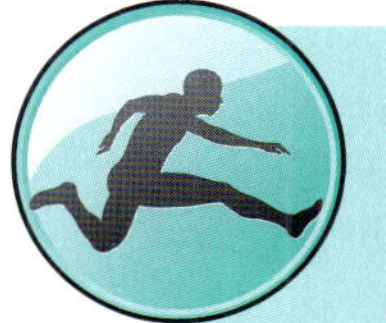

Most patients with mania experience irritability (80%), depressed mood (72%), and labile or fluctuating mood (69%) just as often as euphoria (71%) – *prevalence in parentheses.*

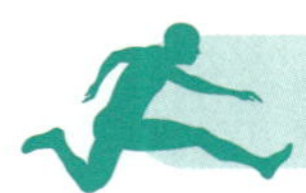

Biologic symptoms

Decreased need for sleep

This is a very important early warning sign of mania or hypomania. Sleep disturbance can range from only needing a few hours sleep a night to a manic patient going for days on end with no sleep at all.

Increased energy

This initially results in an increase in goal-directed activity and, when coupled with impaired judgment, can have disastrous consequences (e.g., patients may instigate numerous risky business ventures, go on excessive spending sprees, or engage in reckless promiscuity that is unusual for them). However, in severe episodes actions can become repetitive, stereotyped, and apparently purposeless, even progressing to a psychotic state in the extreme case. If left untreated, excessive overactivity can lead to physical exhaustion and sometimes even death. On mental status examination, increased energy can be seen as *psychomotor agitation*: the patient is unable to sit still, frequently stands up, paces around the room, and gesticulates expansively.

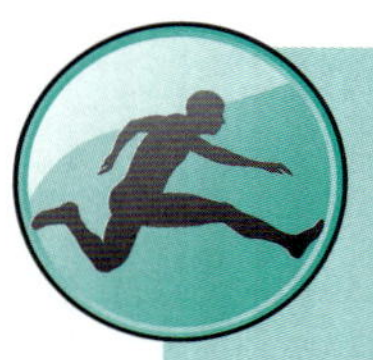

In patients with mania, 98% have pressured speech; 87% have psychomotor agitation; 81% have decreased need for sleep; and 57% have sexual disinhibition.

Cognitive symptoms

Elevated sense of self-esteem or grandiosity

Hypomanic patients may overestimate their abilities and social or financial status. In severe cases, manic patients may have delusions of grandeur (see later).

Poor concentration

Manic patients may find it difficult to maintain their focus on any one thing as they struggle to filter out irrelevant external stimuli (background noise, other objects, or people in the room), consequently making them highly distractible.

Accelerated thinking

A manic patient may subjectively experience their thoughts or ideas racing even faster than they can articulate them. When thoughts are rapidly associating in this way in a stream of connected concepts it is termed *flight of ideas*. When patients have an irrepressible need to express these thoughts verbally, making them difficult to interrupt, it is termed *pressured speech*. Some hypomanic patients express themselves by incessant letter writing, poetry, doodling, or artwork.

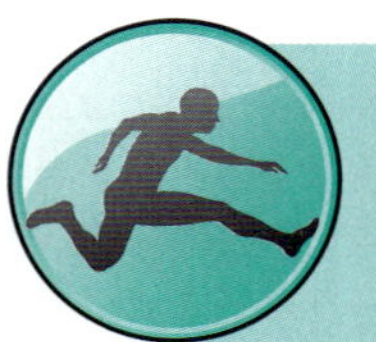

Grandiosity (78%), racing thoughts (71%), and distractibility (68%) are the most common nonpsychotic cognitive disturbances in patients with mania – *prevalence in parentheses.*

Impaired judgment and insight

This is typical of manic illness and sometimes results in costly indiscretions that patients may later regret. Lack of insight into their illness can be a difficult barrier to overcome when trying to engage patients in essential treatment.

Psychotic symptoms

Psychotic symptoms are far more common in manic than depressive episodes and include disorders of *thought process*, *thought content*, and *perception*.

Disordered thought process

Disordered thought process (see Ch. 4) commonly occurs in schizophrenia but is regularly seen in manic episodes with psychotic features and to a lesser degree in psychotic forms of unipolar depression. The most common disruptions to thought process in mania are circumstantiality, tangentiality, and flight of ideas. However, signs of thought disorder most typical to schizophrenia can also be seen in manic episodes (e.g., loosening of association, neologisms, and thought blocking).

Circumstantiality and tangentiality

Circumstantial (overinclusive) speech means speech that is delayed in reaching its final goal because of the overinclusion of details and unnecessary asides and diversions. However, the speaker, if allowed to finish, does eventually connect the original starting point to the desired destination. Circumstantiality

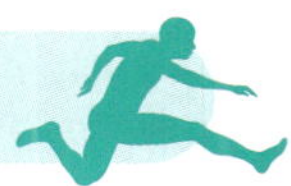

can also be found in normal people – most families have at least one person who takes for ever to finish a story! *Tangential speech*, on the other hand, is more indicative of psychopathology and sees the speaker diverting from the initial train of thought but never returning to the original point, jumping tangentially from one topic to the next.

Flight of ideas

As described above, this occurs when thinking is markedly accelerated, resulting in a stream of connected concepts. The link between concepts can be as in normal communication, where one idea follows directly on from the next; through a pun or clang association; or through some vague idea that is not part of the original goal of speech (e.g., "I need to go to bed now. Have you ever smelt my bed of roses? Ah, but a rose by any other name would smell just as sweet!"). Even though manic patients may appear to be talking absolute gibberish, a written transcript of their speech will usually reveal that their ideas are related in some, albeit obscure, way.

As patients become increasingly manic, their associations tend to loosen as they find it increasingly difficult to link their thoughts. Eventually they start approaching the incoherent thought disorder of the schizophrenic patient, who exhibits *loosening of association* (the ideas appear to be unrelated and idiosyncratically connected), *word salad* (incomprehensible connections of thought), and *neologisms* (new words created through the combination or condensation of other words), where ideas are very loosely or not at all related (see Ch. 4). Flight of ideas is regarded as a psychotic phenomenon when speech is practically incomprehensible.

Secondary delusions

Secondary delusions are those that develop *in response* to another psychopathological state – in this case, abnormal mood. Inherent in this definition is the implication that it is *understandable* how the delusion originated when one examines the patient's mental state. This is in contrast to primary delusions, which develop spontaneously from no pre-existing pathologic mental state, thus making their genesis completely *beyond understanding*. Primary delusions are almost exclusively seen in patients with schizophrenia (see Ch. 4). Patients with elated mood therefore, will typically present with *grandiose delusions* in which they believe they have special importance or unusual powers. *Persecutory delusions* are also common, especially in patients with an irritable mood, and often feature them believing that others are trying to take advantage of their exalted status. When the content of delusions matches the mood of the patient, the delusions are termed *mood congruent*. Very often, patients with elevated mood may have overvalued ideas as opposed to true delusions, which are important to distinguish, as the former are not regarded as psychotic in nature (see Ch. 4).

Disordered perception

Some hypomanic patients may describe subtle distortions of perception. These are not psychotic symptoms and mainly include altered intensity of perception such that sounds seem louder (hyperacusis) or colors seem brighter and more vivid (visual hyperesthesia). Psychotic perceptual features develop when manic patients experience hallucinations. This is usually in the form of voices encouraging or exciting them.

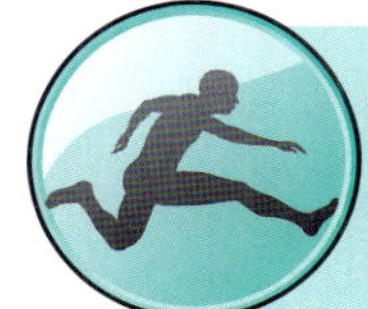

Phenomenologic studies have shown that, in patients with bipolar affective disorder, at least two-thirds reported experiencing psychotic symptoms during a manic episode, and up to one-third reported experiencing psychotic symptoms during a depressive episode.

Differential diagnosis of elevated or irritable mood

Like depression, an elevated or irritable mood can be secondary to a medical condition, psychoactive substance use, or other psychiatric disorder. These will have to be excluded before a primary mood disorder can be diagnosed. Figure 2.1 shows the differential diagnosis for patients presenting with elevated or irritable mood.

Mood (affective) disorders

Bipolar affective disorder

If a patient has had at least one hypomanic, manic, or mixed affective episode in association with any kind of past mood episode (hypomanic, manic, depressive, mixed), then *bipolar affective disorder* is the correct diagnosis. Most patients who experience hypomanic or manic episodes also experience depressive episodes, hence the commonly used term "manic-depression." However, patients who only suffer from manic or hypomanic episodes with no intervening depressive episodes are also classified as having bipolar affective disorder, even though their mood does not swing to the depressive pole. It is good practice to record the nature of the current episode in a patient with longstanding bipolar affective disorder (e.g., *"bipolar affective disorder, current episode manic without psychotic features."*)

Differential diagnosis for patient presenting with elevated or irritable mood

Mood disorders
- Bipolar affective disorder (hypomania, mania, mixed affective episode)
- Cyclothymia
- Depression (may present with irritable mood)

Secondary to a general medical condition

Secondary to psychoactive substance use

Psychotic disorders
- Schizoaffective disorder (may be similar to mania with psychotic features)
- Schizophrenia

Personality disorders

Delirium/dementia

Fig. 2.1 Differential diagnosis for patient presenting with elevated or irritable mood.

Cyclothymia

Cyclothymia is analogous to dysthymia (see Ch. 1) in that it usually begins in early adulthood and follows a chronic course with intermittent periods of wellness in between. It is characterized by an instability of mood resulting in alternating periods of mild elation and mild depression, none of which are sufficiently severe or long enough to meet the criteria for either a hypomanic or a depressive episode. DSM-IV-TR requires a minimum of 2 years of this type of mood disorder to diagnose cyclothymia.

Depression

There are two scenarios where a patient with a primary depressive disorder may present with an elevated or irritable mood. An "agitated depression" can present with a prominent irritable mood, which, when coupled with psychomotor agitation, can be difficult to distinguish from a manic episode. Secondly, depressed patients who are responding to antidepressants or electroconvulsive therapy (ECT) may experience a transient period of elevated mood.

Manic episodes secondary to a general medical condition or psychoactive substance use

A medical or psychoactive substance cause of mania should always be sought for and ruled out. Figure 2.3 lists the medical and substance-related causes of mania. The medical condition or substance use should predate the development of

DSM-IV-TR distinguishing features of hypomania and mania

Features	Hypomania	Mania without psychotic features	Mania with psychotic features
Mood	Mildly elevated or irritable mood – greater than cyclothymia	Greatly elevated or irritable mood	Severely elevated or suspicious mood accompanied by delusions, hallucinations, incomprehensible pressure of speech or psychotic state
Duration	Several days	1 week	1 week
Psychosocial functioning	Considerable interference with work or social activity but disruption is not complete or severe	Disrupts work and social activities completely	Disrupts work and social activities completely. Associated with violent excitement, dehydration, and self-neglect

Fig. 2.2 DSM-IV-TR distinguishing features of hypomania and mania.

the mood disorder and symptoms should resolve with treatment of the condition or abstinence from the offending substance. Absence of previous manic episodes or a family history of bipolar affective disorder also supports this diagnosis.

Psychotic disorders

Schizoaffective disorder

See Chapters 1 and 4. This can be very difficult to distinguish from a manic episode with psychotic features.

Schizophrenia

Patients with schizophrenia can present with an excited, suspicious, or agitated mood and therefore can be difficult to distinguish from manic patients with psychotic symptoms. Figure 2.4 compares relevant features that might act as clues to the correct diagnosis.

Personality disorders

Psychiatrists often see patients with disorders of personality who present with features in common with hypomania, e.g. impulsivity, displays of temper, and lability of mood in borderline personality disorder. However, personality disorders involve stable and enduring behavior patterns, unlike the more discrete episodes of bipolar affective disorder, which are characterized by a distinct, demarcated deterioration in psychosocial functioning.

Delirium/dementia

See Chapter 9.

Medical and substance causes of mania	
Medical conditions	**Substances**
Cerebral neoplasms, infarcts, trauma, infection (including HIV)	Amphetamines
Cushing's disease	Anticholinergics
Huntington's disease	Antidepressants
Hyperthyroidism	Antiviral drugs
Multiple sclerosis	Antimalarials
Renal failure	Captopril
Systemic lupus erythematosus	Cimetidine
Temporal lobe epilepsy	Cocaine
Vitamin B_{12} and niacin deficiency (pellagra)	Corticosteroids
	Hallucinogens
	L-dopa

Fig. 2.3 Medical and substance causes of mania.

Assessment

Clinical

The following questions might be helpful in eliciting the key symptoms of mania/hypomania:

- Have you been feeling particularly happy or on top of the world lately?
- Do you sometimes feel as though you have too much energy compared to people around you?
- Do you find yourself needing less sleep but not getting tired?
- Have you had any new interests or exciting ideas lately?
- Have you noticed your thoughts racing in your head?
- Do you have any special abilities or powers?

Schizophrenia		
Psychopathology	**Mania**	**Schizophrenia**
Thought form	Circumstantiality, tangentiality, flight of ideas	Loosening of association, neologisms, thought blocking
Delusions	Most often mood congruent (grandiose delusions or persecutory delusions)	Delusions unrelated to mood, bizarre delusions, thought insertion, withdrawal, broadcast
Speech	Pressured speech, difficult to interrupt	Speech is often hesitant or halting
Biologic symptoms	Significantly reduced need for sleep, increased physical and mental energy	Sleep less disturbed, less hyperactive
Psychomotor function	Agitation	Agitation, catatonic symptoms, or negative symptoms

Fig. 2.4 Psychopathologic distinctions between mania and schizophrenia (these are guidelines only; typically psychotic symptoms can occur in mania and vice-versa).

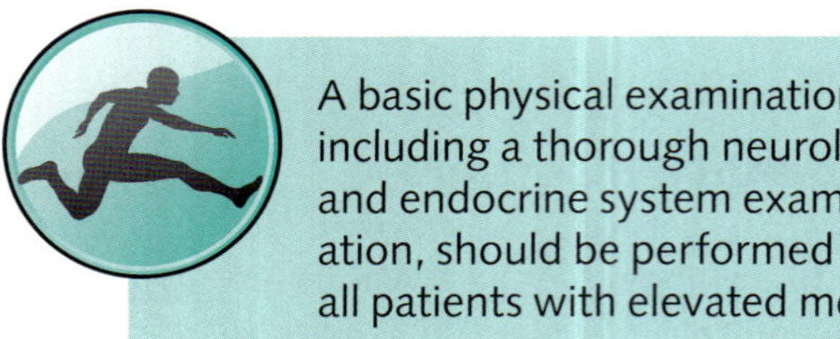

A basic physical examination, including a thorough neurologic and endocrine system examination, should be performed on all patients with elevated mood.

Special investigations

As for the depressive disorders, social, psychological, and physical investigations are normally performed on manic patients mainly to establish the diagnosis and to rule out an organic or substance-related cause (see Fig. 2.3). The Young Mania Rating Scale, a self-report inventory, is a useful screening tool for bipolar affective disorder.

Algorithm for the diagnosis of mood disorders

See Figure 2.5.

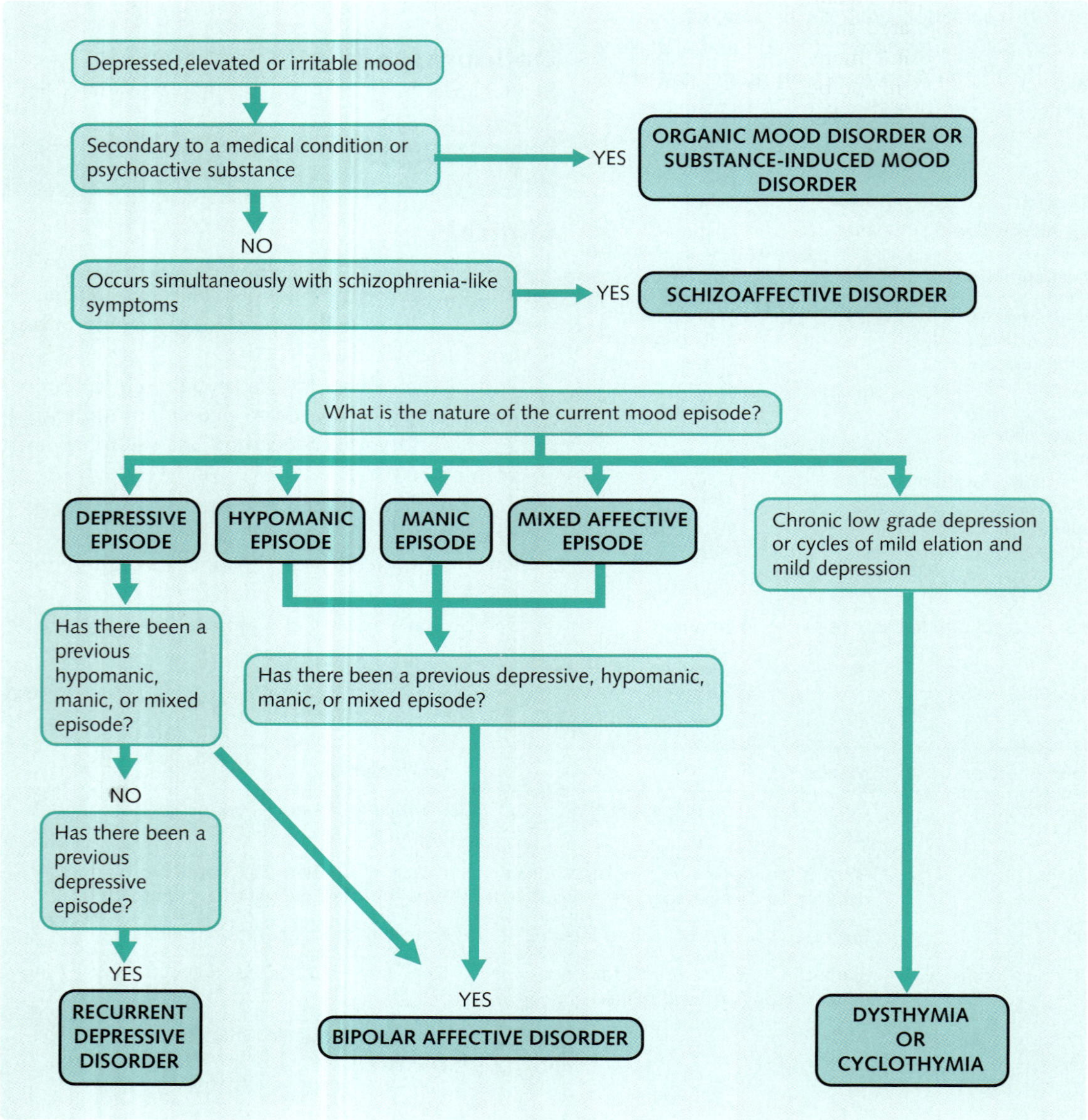

Depressed,elevated or irritable mood

Secondary to a medical condition or psychoactive substance → YES → ORGANIC MOOD DISORDER OR SUBSTANCE-INDUCED MOOD DISORDER

NO

Occurs simultaneously with schizophrenia-like symptoms → YES → SCHIZOAFFECTIVE DISORDER

What is the nature of the current mood episode?

DEPRESSIVE EPISODE

HYPOMANIC EPISODE

MANIC EPISODE

MIXED AFFECTIVE EPISODE

Chronic low grade depression or cycles of mild elation and mild depression

Has there been a previous hypomanic, manic, or mixed episode?

Has there been a previous depressive, hypomanic, manic, or mixed episode?

NO

Has there been a previous depressive episode?

YES

RECURRENT DEPRESSIVE DISORDER

YES

BIPOLAR AFFECTIVE DISORDER

DYSTHYMIA OR CYCLOTHYMIA

Fig. 2.5 Algorithm for the diagnosis of mood disorders.

Discussion of case study

Mr EM appears to be suffering from a *manic episode with psychotic features*. He has an elated mood and has developed the grandiose delusion that he is a world expert secondary to this mood (mood-congruent psychotic symptom); note also the rapid switch to irritable mood when confronted. Biologic symptoms include the reduced need for sleep and increased mental and physical energy with overactivity. Cognitive symptoms include elevated sense of self-importance, poor concentration, accelerated thinking with pressure of speech, and impaired judgment and insight. The episode is classified as manic because of the severe impairment in social and probably work functioning.

The past psychiatric history is extremely important in this case. A previous mood episode (hypomanic, manic, depressive, mixed) is required in order to make the diagnosis of bipolar affective disorder. Mr EM had a period of depression 2 years prior to developing this manic episode. If that episode was a genuine depressive episode, then the correct diagnosis would be: *bipolar affective disorder, current episode manic with psychotic features*. Previous psychotic episodes should add schizoaffective disorder and schizophrenia to the differential diagnosis.

Now go to Chapter 13 to read about the mood disorders and their management.

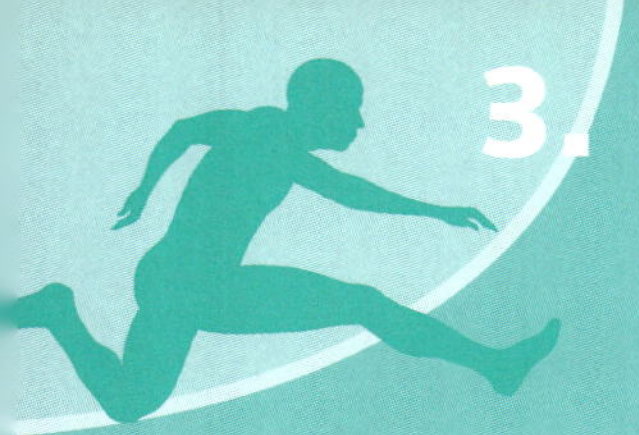

3. The Patient with Suicide or Self-Harm Intent

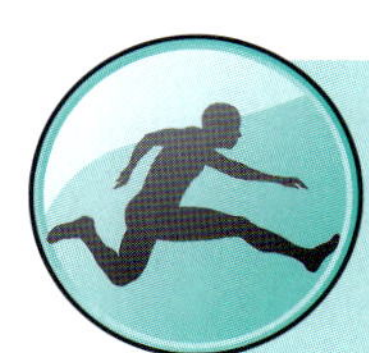

At 1:30 a.m. the psychiatry resident receives a call from the emergency department of an inner city hospital. He is asked for his opinion on Mr SA, a 28-year-old unemployed, recently divorced man, who has been brought in by his landlord. The landlord had dropped by to discuss rent that was overdue, only to find the door unlocked and Mr SA asleep on his bed with an empty bottle of acetaminophen tablets and several empty cans of beer littered around the bedroom floor. He also found a hastily scribbled suicide note addressed to Mr SA's children on the bedside table. Mr SA was easily roused but was upset to have been found and initially refused the landlord's persistent pleas that they should go along to the hospital. Only when he was violently sick did he finally agree. The resident reports that, other than the smell of alcohol on his breath, Mr SA's medical examination was normal. Special investigations revealed acetaminophen in his blood, but not at a sufficiently high level to require medical admission. The resident is concerned because Mr SA is ambivalent about a possible further suicide attempt, saying that his life is a failure and that there is nothing worth living for. Before coming to see the patient, the psychiatrist on call proceeds to ask the resident some routine questions.

(For a discussion of the case study see the end of the chapter)

While any psychiatric illness can present with self-harm or suicide intent, many patients who attempt suicide or self-harm are not previously known to mental health services. Assessments of patients who have self-harmed are very often made by nonpsychiatric personnel. It is vital that primary care clinicians are able to detect and manage any underlying mental illness and have a sound approach to assessing and managing risk.

Definitions and clinical features

Self-injurious behavior is the blanket term used to mean any intentional act done in the knowledge that it is potentially harmful. Self-injurious behavior can take the form of self-poisoning (overdosing) or self-injury (cutting, slashing, burning). The motives for self-injurious behavior are vast and include emotional relief, self-punishment, attention seeking, and can even be a form of self-help by way of channeling an intolerable emotional experience into a discrete physical sensation. *Suicide* is the act of intentionally and successfully ending one's own life.

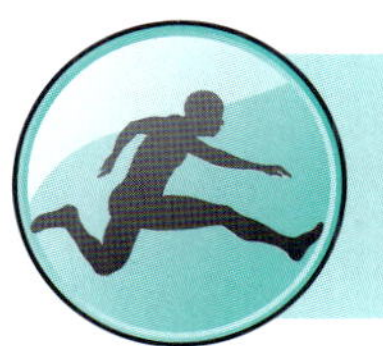

Suicide ranks as the eighth leading cause of death for Americans aged 10 and older.

Assessment of the patient who has attempted suicide

Patients who present with self-harm have a 100-fold greater chance of completing suicide in the following year than the general population and therefore need to be assessed comprehensively. Unfortunately, psychiatry has some way to go before we are able to reliably predict the risk of someone attempting suicide. However, numerous studies have shown that certain epidemiologic and clinical variables are more prevalent among those who have completed suicide (see later) and it is important to bear these risk factors in mind when assessing a patient's risk. Remember, however, that determining suicide risk is extremely difficult, even for experienced psychiatrists, and that no patient questionnaire or suicide risk scoring system has been shown to be better than thorough clinical assessment. A thorough risk assessment should include a full psychiatric history (see Ch. 26) with specific focus on:

1. Risk factors
2. Suicide intent
3. Mental state examination
4. Current social support.

Suicide risk factors

Figure 3.1 summarizes the most important epidemiological and clinical risk factors for suicide.

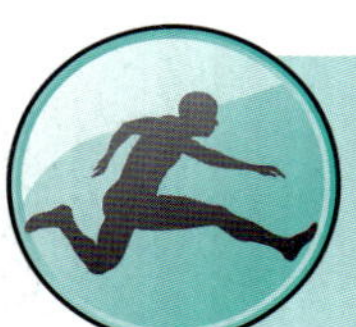

Make sure you know the risk factors for suicide well; they are often asked for in exams!

Risk factors for suicide

Epidemiological factors:
- Men more likely to complete suicide (although women are more likely to attempt it)
- Divorced > widowed > single
- Unemployed or retired
- Living alone, social isolation

Clinical factors:
- Psychiatric illness (see Fig. 3.2)
- Previous deliberate self-harm
- Alcohol dependence
- Physical illness (especially terminal illness, and debilitating or chronically painful conditions)
- Family history of depression, alcohol dependence, or suicide
- Recent adverse life events (especially bereavement)

Fig. 3.1 Risk factors for suicide.

Psychiatric illness

About 90% of patients who commit suicide have a diagnosable psychiatric disorder. However, a 5-year study showed that only one-quarter of suicides in England, Wales, Scotland and Northern Ireland had been in contact with the mental health services in the year before death.

It is important to note that patients who have recently been discharged from a psychiatric hospital are a very high-risk group for suicide, particularly in the first 1–2 weeks following discharge. Figure 3.2 summarizes the most important psychiatric conditions associated with suicide.

Association between psychiatric disorders and suicide

Psychiatric disorder	Comments
Depression	Most common psychiatric disorder (50–80% of completed suicides) Lifetime risk of suicide is 15%
Schizophrenia	Risk greatest in severe illness with delusions Lifetime risk of suicide is 10% High risk: young, intelligent, unemployed males with good insight and relapsing illness
Alcohol dependence	Lifetime risk of suicide is 3–4% High risk: elderly males, poor work record, social isolation, previous suicide attempt Often have comorbid depression
Personality disorders: antisocial and borderline personality disorders	High risk: labile mood, impulsive, aggressive, alcohol and substance abuse
Organic brain disease (dementia, delirium, epilepsy, head injury)	5% of all completed suicides
Anxiety and eating disorders	Increased risk

Fig. 3.2 Association between psychiatric disorders and suicide.

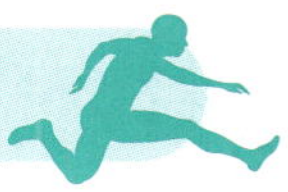

Not only is alcohol a psychoactive depressant, but it also impairs judgment and leads to disinhibition, which increases the likelihood of suicidal thoughts being acted upon. The lifetime risk of suicide in problem drinkers is about 3–4%, which is 60–120 times greater than the normal population.

Physical illness

Any disabling medical condition may predispose to or precipitate a suicide attempt. Many patients have comorbid depression that potentially will respond well to treatment; however, some patients do not have a mental illness and have made a "rational" decision to die (very rare). Most common examples are:

- Chronic illnesses (AIDS, renal failure on hemodialysis)
- Central nervous system diseases (epilepsy, multiple sclerosis, Huntington's disease)
- Cancers (genitals, breast, or gastrointestinal)
- Endocrine and metabolic conditions (Cushing's disease, porphyria).

Recent adverse life events

Stressful life events are more common in the 6 months prior to a suicide attempt. These stressors may include relationship break-ups, personal or family health problems, legal prosecution, financial difficulties, or problems at home.

Suicidal ideation

Suicidal ideation describes the thoughts and wishes of wanting to die. The seriousness or intensity of this wish is determined by the following:

The attempt was planned in advance

A lethal suicide attempt usually involves days or weeks of planning the method and location of suicide. It is rarely an impulsive, spur-of-the-moment idea (the exception is the psychotic patient who impulsively responds to hallucinations or delusions). Planning is strongly suggested by the evidence of *final acts*. These include the making of a will or the leaving of a suicide note.

Precautions were taken to avoid discovery or rescue

For example, a patient might check into a hotel room in a distant town or ensure that no friends or family will be visiting over the ensuing hours or days.

A dangerous method was used

Violent methods (hanging, jumping from heights, firearm use, electrocution) are more suggestive of lethal intent than overdosing. That said, use of an apparently ineffective method (e.g., taking six acetaminophen tablets) might reflect lack of knowledge of the lethal dose needed rather than a lack of intent to die. Therefore, it should be ascertained whether the method used was seen as dangerous from the patient's perspective.

No help was sought after the act

Patients who immediately regret their action and seek help are less at risk than those who simply wait to die. Contrast Mr SA in the case study above with an adolescent who takes a mouthful of pills, then runs downstairs to reveal to his/her parents what he/she has done.

Mental state examination

This should be done in a calm, quiet and confidential setting, preferably when the patient has had a chance to rest and is not under the influence of drugs or alcohol. This might seem too obvious a point were it not for the unfortunate reality that patients are often referred for a psychiatric assessment while still drowsy from an overdose of sleeping pills. Check specifically for:

- Current mood state. Is the suicide attempt regretted or is there ongoing suicidal ideation? Cognitive features of hopelessness and worthlessness are associated with higher risk of suicide.
- Delirium or psychosis (particularly command hallucinations) may predispose the patient to impulsive and unpredictable behavior.
- It is also useful to ascertain whether there are protective factors that would stop a patient from attempting suicide again. For example, a mother may have ongoing suicidal ideation, yet be adamant that she would not desert or frighten her children again.

- Undiagnosed mental illness, especially depression, schizophrenia, alcohol dependence and personality disorders. Remember that so-called "rational" suicide is rare in Western countries.

The following questions might be helpful when asking about suicidal ideation:

- Have you been feeling that life isn't worth living?
- Do you sometimes feel like you would like to end it all?
- Have you actually given some thought as to how you might do it?
- How close do you think you are to going through with your plans?
- Do you currently have the means (rope, gun, pills) to carry out this plan?
- Is there anything that might stop you from attempting suicide?

A patient may appear to be at greater risk of imminent self-harm on mental state examination if they are tired, emotionally upset, or intoxicated.

Current social support

This is important to ascertain when deciding upon management. Does the patient have the resources and ability to cope if discharged? Patients with ongoing suicidal ideation can often be managed in the community if a strong social support network exists. It may be necessary to refer the at-risk patient for follow-up by the local community mental health team. Known psychiatric patients should be followed up by their outpatient providers (see Ch. 30). Always inform the patient's PCP of suicidal ideation or attempts.

Differential diagnosis

It is crucial to rule out a mental illness as a cause of a suicide attempt (see Fig. 3.2).

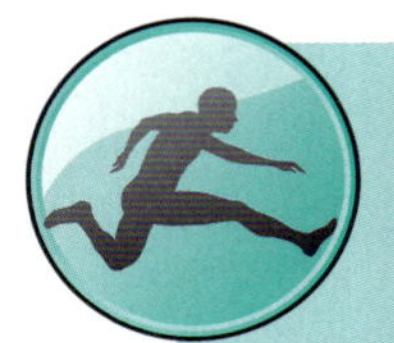

When assessing a patient who has engaged in self-injurious behavior it is crucial that clinicians appear nonjudgmental and empathic. Establishing a rapport with a challenging patient is a unique skill and should be a main priority.

Discussion of case study

Self-harm risk assessment

Mr SA's epidemiologic risk factors are that he is a young man, recently divorced, unemployed, and apparently living alone in social isolation. His clinical risk factors are that he may have alcohol use problems and has recently experienced adverse life events (divorce, financial difficulties). The evidence of final acts (suicide note) and the failure of Mr SA to seek help after the act suggest strong suicide intent. The fact that he would not have been discovered but for the landlord's timely arrival indicates a degree of forward planning, although his leaving of the door unlocked and his willingness to go to hospital after vomiting suggests some ambivalence. Mr SA had clearly consumed a significant degree of alcohol at the time of the overdose, which could have clouded his judgment and given him determination that he otherwise might not have had. On mental state examination, Mr SA has ongoing suicidal ideation and cognitive features of worthlessness and hopelessness, which are known to be associated with suicide.

Further management

More information is necessary. The psychiatrist should ask about all the epidemiological and clinical risk factors: past or current mental illness (is Mr SA known to the mental health services?); previous episodes of self-harm; alcohol or substance dependence; physical illness; family history of depression, alcohol dependence, or suicide; and other recent adverse life events. The resident has provided enough information about the lethality of the suicide attempt; however, the psychiatrist will want to know if there was any evidence of mental illness on mental state examination, especially depression. The psychiatrist will also be interested in Mr SA's current social support in order to try and help him formulate the most appropriate management plan.

As this is a complex risk assessment, the psychiatrist will probably have to reassess the patient himself, especially as regards detecting mental illness on mental state examination. The psychiatrist might ask the resident to keep Mr SA overnight, so that a mental state examination can be performed in the morning when he is refreshed and no longer under the influence of alcohol. A hospital admission or follow-up by a community mental health team seems to be the most likely outcome.

Now go to Chapters 13 and 18 to read about affective and personality disorders and their management.

4. The Psychotic Patient

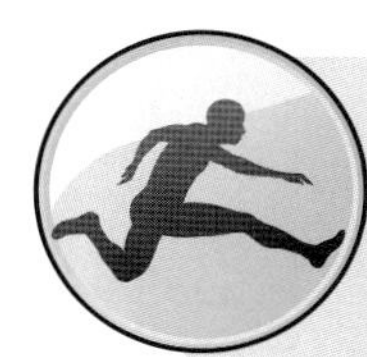

Mr PP, aged 23, was assessed by his primary care physician because his family had become concerned about his behavior. Over the past 6 months his college attendance had been uncharacteristically poor, and he had terminated his part-time work. He had also become increasingly reclusive by spending more time alone in his apartment, refusing to answer the door or see his friends. After some inappropriate suspiciousness, he allowed the PCP into his apartment and then disclosed that government scientists had started to perform experiments on him over the past year. These involved the insertion of an electrode into his brain that detected gamma rays transmitted from government headquarters, which issued him with commands and "planted" strange ideas in his head. When the PCP asked how he knew this, he replied that he heard the "men's voices" as "clear as day" and that they continually commented on what he was thinking. He explained that his suspicion that "all was not right" was confirmed when he heard the neighbor's dog barking in the middle of the night – at that point he knew "for certain" that he was being interfered with. Prompted by the PCP, Mr PP also mentioned that a man in his local bar knew of his plight and had sent him a "covert signal" when he overheard the man conversing about the dangers of nuclear experiments. He also admitted to "receiving coded information" from the radio whenever it was turned on. The PCP found no evidence of abnormal mood, incoherence of speech, or disturbed motor function. Mr PP denied use of illicit drugs and appeared physically well. After the PCP discussed the case with a psychiatrist, Mr PP was admitted to a psychiatric hospital. He agreed to a voluntary admission, as he was now afraid of staying alone at home.

(For a discussion of the case study see the end of the chapter)

The psychotic patient can present in many different ways. It is often very difficult to elicit and describe specific symptoms when a patient is speaking or behaving in a grossly disorganized or even frightening fashion. Therefore, it is important to approach the psychotic patient in a logical and systematic fashion as well as to have a good understanding of the psychopathology involved.

Definitions and clinical features

The term "psychotic" is classically used to describe a patient who has grossly impaired reality testing. This definition is not that clinically useful as "reality testing" encompasses almost all conscious processes and so any dysfunction can present in a number of ways. Probably the narrowest clinical definition of psychosis is simply: delusions and hallucinations. However, patients with schizophrenia and other psychotic disorders often have more symptoms than just delusions or hallucination (e.g., psychomotor abnormalities, mood/affect disturbance, cognitive deficits, and disorganization of thought and behavior).

There are many classifications that attempt to describe all the symptoms seen in schizophrenia and psychosis. So, in order to simplify matters it is useful to approach psychotic psychopathology using four somewhat interrelated parameters:

1. Perception
2. Thought disorder

3. Negative symptoms
4. Psychomotor function.

Perceptual disturbance

Perception is the process of making sense of the physical information we receive from our five sensory modalities.

Hallucinations are perceptions occurring in the absence of an external physical stimulus which have the following important characteristics:

- To the patient, the nature of a hallucination is exactly the same as a normal sensory experience i.e., it appears real. Therefore, patients often have little insight into their abnormal experience.
- They are experienced as external sensations from any one of the five sensory modalities (hearing, vision, smell, taste, touch) and should be distinguished from ideas, thoughts, image, or fantasy, which originate in the patient's own mind.
- They occur without an external stimulus and are not merely distortions of an existing physical stimulus (see illusions).

Illusions are misperceptions of real external stimuli (e.g., in a dark room, a dressing gown hanging on a bedroom wall is perceived as a person). Illusions often occur in normal people and are usually associated with inattention or strong emotion.

According to which sense organ they appear to arise from, hallucinations are classified as auditory, visual, olfactory, gustatory, or somatic. Special forms of hallucinations will also be discussed. See Figure 4.1 for an outline of the classification of hallucinations.

Auditory hallucinations

These are hallucinations of the hearing modality and are the most common type of hallucinations in clinical psychiatry. *Elementary hallucinations* are simple, unstructured sounds (e.g., whirring,

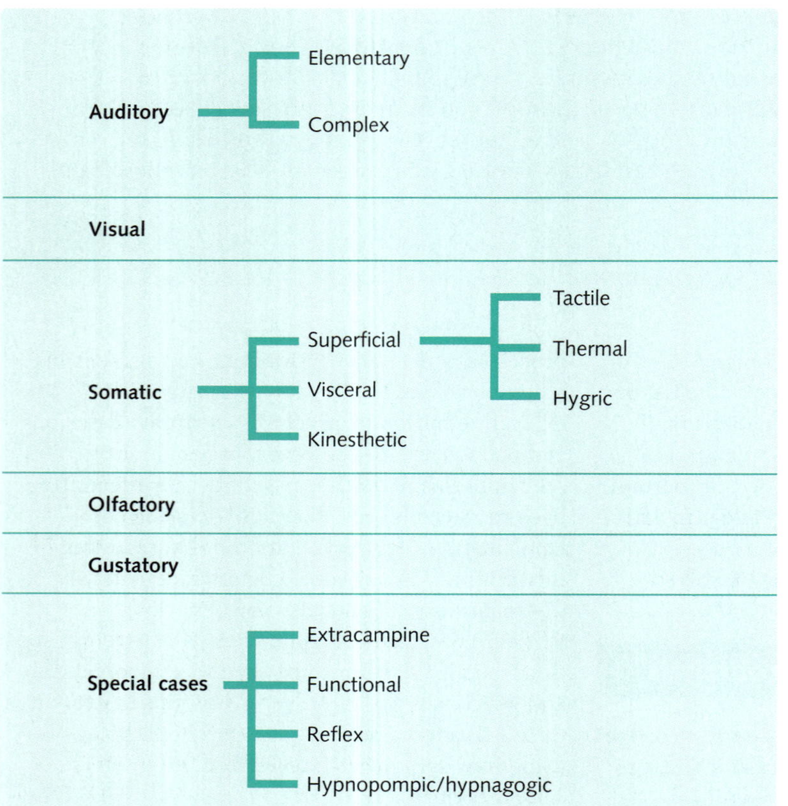

Fig. 4.1 Outline of classification of hallucinations.

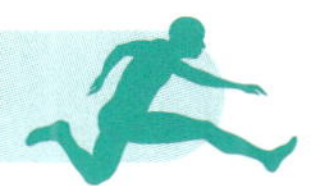

buzzing, whistling, or single words). This type of hallucination commonly occurs in acute organic states. Complex hallucinations occur as spoken phrases, sentences, or even dialogue.

Patients can experience auditory hallucinations in different ways. They may hear their own thoughts spoken aloud or echoed by a voice after they have thought them. They may hear a voice talking to them; this voice may be persecutory or highly critical or issue commands to the patient (*command hallucinations*). They may hear two or more voices discussing the patient among themselves, or one or more voices giving a *running commentary* on the patient's thoughts or actions.

Visual hallucinations

These are hallucinations of the visual modality and occur less frequently than auditory hallucinations in clinical psychiatry. They occur more commonly in organic brain disturbances (delirium, occipital lobe tumours, epilepsy, dementia) and in the context of psychoactive substance use (lysergic acid diethylamide [LSD], mescaline, gas- or glue-sniffing, alcoholic hallucinosis).

- An *autoscopic hallucination* is the experience of seeing an image of oneself in external space.
- The *Charles Bonnet syndrome* describes the condition in which patients experience complex visual hallucinations associated with no other psychiatric symptoms or impairment in consciousness. It usually occurs in the elderly and is associated with loss of vision.
- *Lilliputian hallucinations* are hallucinations of miniature people or animals.

Somatic hallucinations

These are hallucinations of bodily sensation and include *superficial*, *visceral*, and *kinesthetic* hallucinations.

Superficial hallucinations describe sensations on or just below the skin and may be:

- *Tactile:* experience of the skin being touched, pricked, or pinched. Formication is the unpleasant sensation of insects crawling on or just below the skin; it is commonly associated with long-term cocaine use (cocaine bugs) and alcohol withdrawal
- *Thermal:* false perception of heat or cold
- *Hygric:* false perception of a fluid (e.g., "I can feel water sloshing in my brain").

Visceral hallucinations describe false perceptions of the internal organs. Patients may be distressed by deep sensations of their organs throbbing, stretching, distending, or vibrating.

Kinesthetic hallucinations are false perceptions of joint or muscle sense. Patients may describe their limbs vibrating or being twisted. The fleeting but distressing sensation of free falling, just as one is about to fall asleep, is an example that most people have experienced (see *hypnagogic hallucinations* below).

Olfactory and gustatory hallucinations

These are the false perceptions of smell and taste. Note that they commonly occur together because the two senses are closely related. Remember that in patients with olfactory or gustatory hallucinations, it is important to rule out epilepsy (especially of the temporal lobe) and other organic brain diseases.

Special forms of hallucination

Hypnagogic hallucinations are false perceptions in any modality (usually auditory or visual) that occur as a person goes to sleep.

Hypnopompic hallucinations occur as a person awakens. These occur in normal people and are not indicative of psychopathology.

Extracampine hallucinations are false perceptions that occur outside the limits of a person's normal sensory field (e.g., a patient describes hearing voices from 100 miles away). Patients often give delusional explanations for this phenomenon.

A *functional hallucination* occurs when a normal sensory stimulus is required to precipitate a hallucination in that same sensory modality (e.g., voices that are only heard when the doorbell rings).

A *reflex hallucination* occurs when a normal sensory stimulus in one modality precipitates a hallucination in another (e.g., voices that are only heard whenever the lights are switched on).

Thought disorder

Describing the disturbance of a patient's thought content is one of the most challenging tasks facing clinicians. This problem is compounded by two factors. First, it is impossible to know what patients are actually thinking – thought content has to be inferred from their speech and behavior.

Second, the unfortunate situation has arisen where various authors in psychiatry have described different conceptual views of thought disorder, which has resulted in conflicting and confusing classification systems. It is probably not that important that you are able to classify and subgroup thought disorder, but rather that you have a clear understanding of the individual definitions you intend to use and are able to recognize them in the patients that you assess. In this regard, it is particularly helpful if you document and are able to cite examples of the patient's speech in his/her own words.

A simple classification divides thought disorders in two broad groups: *abnormal beliefs* and *disorganized thinking*.

Abnormal beliefs

Abnormal beliefs include *delusions* and *overvalued ideas*.

Delusions

A delusion is a false belief, held with extraordinary conviction, that is not accepted by other members of the patient's culture. It is important to understand the following characteristics of delusional thinking:

- To the patient, there is no difference between a delusional belief and a true belief – they are the same experience. Therefore, only an external observer can diagnose a delusion.
- The delusion is false because of faulty reasoning. A man's delusional belief that his wife is having an affair may actually be true (she may indeed be unfaithful), but it remains a delusion because the reason he gives for this belief is undoubtedly false. For example, she "must" be having an affair because she is part of a top-secret sexual conspiracy to prove that he is a homosexual.
- It is out of keeping with the patient's social and cultural background. It crucial to establish that the belief is not one likely to be held by that person's subcultural group (e.g., a belief in the imminent second coming of Christ may be appropriate for a member of a religious group but not for a formerly atheist, middle-aged businessman).

It is diagnostically significant to classify delusions as:

- Mood-congruent or mood-incongruent
- Bizarre or nonbizarre

according to the content of the delusion.

In mood-congruent delusions, the contents of the delusions are appropriate to the patient's mood and are commonly seen in depression or mania with psychotic features.

Bizarre delusions are those that are completely impossible (e.g., the belief that aliens have planted radioactive detonators in the patient's brain). They are considered to be characteristic of schizophrenia.

Figure 4.2 lists the classification of delusions by their *content*. It is important that you are able to label a delusion according to its content, so take some time to familiarize yourself with this table.

Note that the term "paranoid" refers to any delusions or ideas that are unduly self-referential – typically delusions or ideas of persecution, grandeur, or reference. It should not be used synonymously with the term persecutory; i.e., when a patient has a false belief that people are trying to harm him, do not say that he is paranoid; rather say that he has persecutory delusions.

Finally, beliefs that were previously held with delusional intensity but then become held with less conviction are termed *partial delusions*. This occurs when patients start recovering after receiving treatment.

Direct questioning about perceptual experience may alienate a nonpsychotic patient and raise undue suspicion in a psychotic patient. To maintain rapport with patients, begin these questions with a primer such as: "I am now going to ask you some questions that may seem a little strange but are routine questions that I ask all patients."

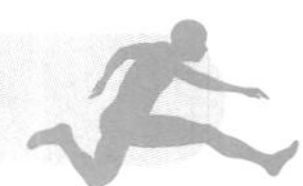

Content of delusions	
Classification	**Content**
Persecutory delusions	False belief that one is being harmed, threatened, cheated, harassed, or is a victim of a conspiracy
Grandiose delusions	False belief that one is exceptionally powerful (including having "mystical powers"), talented, or important
Delusions of reference	False belief that certain objects, people, or events have intense personal significance and refer specifically to oneself (e.g., believing that a television newsreader is talking directly about one)
Religious delusions	False belief pertaining to a religious theme, often grandiose in nature (e.g., believing that one is a special messenger from God)
Delusions of love (erotomania)	False belief that another person is in love with one (commoner in women). In one form, termed *de Clérambault syndrome*, a woman (usually) believes that a man, frequently older and of higher status, is in love with her
Delusion of infidelity (morbid jealousy, Othello syndrome)	False belief that one's lover has been unfaithful. Note that morbid jealousy may also take the form of an overvalued idea, that is, nonpsychotic jealousy
Delusions of misidentification	*Capgras syndrome*: belief that a familiar person has been replaced by an exact double – an impostor *Fregoli syndrome*: belief that a complete stranger is actually a familiar person already known to one
Nihilistic delusions (see Cotard's syndrome, p. 172)	False belief that oneself, others, or the world is nonexistent or about to end. In severe cases, negation is carried to the extreme, with patients claiming that nothing, including themselves, exists
Somatic delusions	False belief concerning one's body and its functioning, e.g., that one's bowels are rotting. Also called *hypochondriacal delusions* (to be distinguished from the overvalued ideas seen in hypochondriasis)
Delusions of infestation (Ekbom's syndrome)	False belief that one is infested with small but visible organisms. May also occur secondary to tactile hallucinations, e.g., formication (see text)
Delusions of control	False belief that one's thoughts, feelings, actions, or impulses are controlled or "made" by an external agency (e.g., believing that one was *made* to break a window by demons) Delusions of thought control include: *Thought insertion*: belief that thoughts or ideas are being implanted in one's head by an external agency *Thought withdrawal*: belief that one's thoughts or ideas are being extracted from one's head by an external agency *Thought broadcasting*: belief that one's thoughts are being diffused or broadcast to others such that they know what one is thinking

Fig. 4.2 Classification of delusions by content.

Overvalued ideas

An overvalued idea is a plausible belief that a patient becomes preoccupied with to an unreasonable extent. The key feature is that the pursuit of this idea causes considerable distress to the patient or those living around them – it is overvalued. Patients who hold overvalued ideas have usually had them for many years and typically have abnormalities of personality. They are distinguished from delusions by the lack of a gross abnormality in reasoning; these patients can often give fairly logical reasons for their beliefs. Overvalued ideas differ from obsessions and compulsions in that patients do not regard them as senseless or undesirable (i.e., they are ego-syntonic), whereas patients with obsessive-compulsive disorder recognize that their thoughts or behaviors are irrational or excessive (i.e., ego-dystonic; see Ch. 7). Typical disorders that feature overvalued ideas are anorexia nervosa, hypochondriasis, body dysmorphic disorder, paranoid personality disorder, and morbid jealousy (this can also take the form of a delusion).

Disorganized thinking

Many patients with delusions are able to communicate in a clear and coherent manner; although their beliefs may be false, their speech is organized. However, there is a subgroup of psychotic patients who speak in such a disorganized way that it becomes difficult to understand what they are saying. The coherency of patients with disorganized thinking varies from being mostly understandable in patients exhibiting circumstantial thinking to being completely incomprehensible in patients with a word salad phenomenon.

The following are important signs of disorganized thinking:

Circumstantial and tangential thinking

See Chapter 2.

Loosening of association

This is when the patient's train of thought shifts suddenly from one very loosely or unrelated idea to the next. In its worst form, speech becomes a mixture of incoherent words and phrases and is termed word salad. Loosening of association is characteristic of schizophrenia.

Neologisms and idiosyncratic word use

Neologisms are new words created by the patient, often combining syllables of other known words. Patients can also use recognized words idiosyncratically by attributing them with a nonrecognized meaning (metonyms).

Flight of ideas

See Chapter 2.

Thought blocking

This occurs when patients experience a sudden cessation of their flow of thought, often in mid-sentence (observed as sudden breaks in speech). Patients have no recall of what they were saying or thinking and thus continue talking about a different topic.

Perseveration

This is when patients unnecessarily repeat a word or phrase they have previously expressed. Palilalia describes the repetition of the last word of their sentence. Logoclonia describes the repetition of the last syllable of their last word. Perseveration is highly suggestive of organic brain disease.

Echolalia

This is when patients senselessly repeat words or phrases spoken around them by others – like a parrot.

Irrelevant answers

Patients give answers that are completely unrelated to the original question.

Negative symptoms

Some psychiatrists classify schizophrenic patients according to whether they exhibit predominantly positive or negative symptoms. Positive symptoms are those that are actively produced and include delusions, hallucinations, loosening of association, and bizarre speech or behavior. This is opposed to negative symptoms that indicate a clinical deficit, which include marked apathy, poverty of thought and speech, blunting of affect, social isolation, poor self-care, and cognitive deficits. Patients can have positive and negative symptoms simultaneously or, as often happens, develop a negative presentation after initially presenting with predominantly positive symptoms. Remember that patients with a depressed mood or those experiencing significant side effects from psychotropic medication may also present with negative symptoms.

Psychomotor function

Although a relatively rare phenomenon in industrialized countries, some psychotic patients will present with abnormalities of motor function. Motor system dysfunction in schizophrenia is, invariably, due to the extrapyramidal side effects of neuroleptic medication (see Ch. 27). However, psychotic patients can occasionally present with impressive motor signs that are not caused by psychiatric medication or a known organic brain disease. Although undoubtedly associated with the patient's abnormal mental state, the cause of this psychomotor dysfunction is far from clarified. The term *catatonia* literally means extreme muscular tone or rigidity; however, it commonly describes any excessive or decreased motor activity that is apparently purposeless and includes abnormalities of movement, tone, or position. Note that catatonic symptoms are not diagnostic of schizophrenia; they may also be caused by brain diseases, metabolic abnormalities, and psychoactive substances, and can

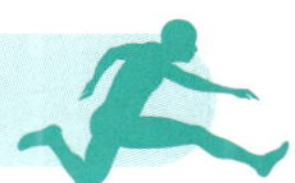

Motor symptoms in schizophrenia	
Catatonic rigidity	Maintaining a fixed position and rigidly resisting all attempts to be moved
Catatonic posturing	Adopting an unusual or bizarre position that is then maintained for some time
Catatonic negativism	A seemingly motiveless resistance to all instructions or attempts to be moved; patients may do the opposite of what is asked
Catatonic waxy flexibility (flexibilitas cerea)	Patients can be "molded" like wax into a position that is then maintained
Catatonic excitement	Agitated, excited, and seemingly purposeless motor activity, not influenced by external stimuli
Catatonic stupor	A presentation of *akinesis* (lack of voluntary movement), *mutism*, and *extreme unresponsiveness* in an otherwise alert patient (there may be slight clouding of consciousness)
Echopraxia	Patients senselessly repeat or imitate the actions of those around them. Associated with *echolalia* (see p. 30) – also occurs in patients with frontal lobe damage
Mannerisms	Apparently goal-directed movements (e.g., waving, saluting) that are performed repeatedly or at socially inappropriate times
Stereotypies	A complex movement that does not appear to be goal-directed (e.g., rocking to and fro, gyrating)

Fig. 4.3 Motor symptoms in schizophrenia.

also occur in mood disorders. Figure 4.3 describes the common motor symptoms seen in schizophrenia.

Differential diagnosis of the psychotic patient

Psychotic symptoms are nonspecific and are associated with many primary psychiatric illnesses. They can also present secondary to a general medical condition or psychoactive substance use. See Figure 4.4 for the differential diagnosis for the psychotic patient.

Differential diagnosis of the psychotic patient

Psychotic disorders
- Schizophrenia
- Schizophreniform disorder
- Schizoaffective disorder
- Delusional disorder
- Brief reactive psychosis

Mood disorders
- Depressive episode, severe, with psychotic features
- Manic episode with psychotic features

Secondary to a general medical condition
Secondary to psychoactive substance use
Dementia/delirium
Personality disorder (schizotypal, borderline, schizoid, paranoid)

Fig. 4.4 Differential diagnosis for the psychotic patient.

Psychotic disorders

Schizophrenia

There are no pathognomonic or singularly defining symptoms of schizophrenia; it is a syndrome characterized by a heterogeneous cluster of symptoms and signs. The DSM-IV-TR has set out diagnostic guidelines based on the most commonly occurring symptom groups, which have been discussed in the preceding section (Fig. 4.5). It is important to establish that there has been a clear and marked deterioration in the patient's social and work functioning.

In the 1970s, psychiatrists used Schneider's first-rank symptoms to make the diagnosis of schizophrenia. Kurt Schneider suggested that the presence of one or more first-rank symptoms in the absence of organic disease was of pragmatic value in making the diagnosis of schizophrenia. First-rank symptoms are still referred to, so you should familiarize yourself with them; they are presented in Figure 4.6.

Schizophrenia

A. *Characteristic symptoms:* Two (or more) of the following, each present for a significant portion of time during a 1-month period (or less if successfully treated):
   (1) delusions
   (2) hallucinations
   (3) disorganized speech (e.g., frequent derailment or incoherence)
   (4) grossly disorganized or catatonic behavior
   (5) negative symptoms, i.e., affective flattening, alogia, or avolition

   Note: Only one criterion A symptom is required if delusions are bizarre or hallucinations consist of a voice keeping up a running commentary on the person's behavior or thoughts, or two or more voices conversing with each other.

B. *Social/occupational dysfunction:* For a signifi cant portion of the time since the onset of the disturbance, one or more major areas of functioning such as work, interpersonal relations, or self-care are markedly below the level achieved prior to the onset (or when the onset is in childhood or adolescence, failure to achieve expected level of interpersonal, academic, or occupational achievement).
C. *Duration:* Continuous signs of the disturbance persist for at least 6 months. This 6-month period must include at least 1 month of symptoms (or less if successfully treated) that meet Criterion A (i.e., active-phase symptoms) and may include periods of prodromal or residual symptoms. During these prodromal or residual periods, the signs of the disturbance may be manifested by only negative symptoms or two or more symptoms listed in Criterion A present in an attenuated form (e.g., odd beliefs, unusual perceptual experiences).
D. *Schizoaffective and Mood Disorder exclusion:* Schizoaffective Disorder and Mood Disorder With Psychotic Features have been ruled out because either (1) no Major Depressive, Manic, or Mixed Episodes have occurred concurrently with the active-phase symptoms; or (2) if mood episodes have occurred during active-phase symptoms, their total duration has been brief relative to the duration of the active and residual periods.
E. *Substance/general medical condition exclusion:* The disturbance is not due to the direct physiological effects of a substance (e.g., a drug of abuse, a medication) or a general medical condition.
F. *Relationship to a Pervasive Developmental Disorder:* If there is a history of Autistic Disorder or another Pervasive Developmental Disorder, the additional diagnosis of Schizophrenia is made only if prominent delusions or hallucinations are also present for at least a month (or less if successfully treated).

Fig. 4.5 DSM-IV-TR diagnostic guidelines for schizophrenia.

Schneider's first-rank symptoms of schizophrenia

- Delusional perception
- Delusions of thought control: insertion, withdrawal, broadcast
- Delusions of control: passivity experiences of affect (feelings), impulse, volition and somatic passivity (influence controlling the body)
- Hallucinations: audible thoughts, voices arguing or discussing the patient, voices giving a running commentary

Fig. 4.6 Schneider's first-rank symptoms of schizophrenia.

Schizophrenia subtypes

Because of the differing presentations of schizophrenia, researchers have tried to identify schizophrenia subtypes. The importance of these subtypes is that they vary in their prognosis and treatment response. The DSM-IV-TR has coded the following subtypes, which are not necessarily exclusive:

- *Paranoid schizophrenia:* dominated by the presence of delusions and hallucinations (positive symptoms). Negative and catatonic symptoms as well as thought disorganization are not prominent. The prognosis is usually better and the onset of illness later than the other subtypes.
- *Disorganized schizophrenia:* characterized by thought disorganization, disturbed behavior, and inappropriate or flat affect. Delusions and hallucinations are fleeting or not prominent. Onset of illness is earlier (15–25 years of age) and the prognosis poorer than paranoid schizophrenia.
- *Catatonic schizophrenia*: a rare form characterized by one or more catatonic symptoms (see Fig. 4.3).
- *Residual schizophrenia:* 1 year of predominantly chronic negative symptoms, which must have been preceded by at least one clear cut psychotic episode in the past.

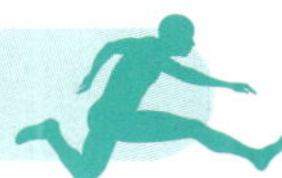

Schizophreniform disorder

Throughout the history of psychiatry, researchers have speculated on the possibility that some psychotic patients with schizophrenia-like symptoms might, in fact, have a separate psychotic illness with a different mode of onset, different time course, and, perhaps, better prognosis. This idea was born from the observation that some psychotic episodes had an abrupt onset (without a prodromal phase), seemed to be precipitated by an acute life stress, or had a duration of symptoms less than that usually observed in schizophrenia. The DSM-IV-TR makes provision for this presentation under the diagnoses of *schizophreniform disorder* and *brief psychotic disorder*.

Schizoaffective disorder

Schizoaffective disorder describes the presentation of both schizophrenic and mood (depressed or manic) symptoms that present in the same episode of illness, either simultaneously or within a few days of each other. The mood symptoms should meet the criteria for either a depressive or manic episode. In addition, the patient experiences psychotic symptoms (delusions or hallucinations) for at least 2 weeks when euthymic. Depending on the particular mood symptoms displayed, this disorder can be coded in the DSM-IV-TR as *schizoaffective disorder, manic type* or *schizoaffective disorder, depressed type*.

Delusional disorder

In this disorder, the development of a single or set of delusions for the period of at least 3 months is the most prominent or only symptom. It usually has its onset in middle age and expressed delusions may persist throughout the patient's life and include persecutory, grandiose, and hypochondriacal delusions. Typically schizophrenic delusions, like delusions of thought control or passivity, exclude this diagnosis. Hallucinations, if present, tend to be only fleeting and are not typically schizophrenic in nature; brief depressive symptoms may also be evident. Affect, speech, and behavior are all normal and these patients usually have well-preserved personal and social skills. Rarely, patients may present with an *induced delusional disorder* (folie à deux), which occurs when nonpsychotic patients with close emotional ties to another person suffering from delusions (usually a dominant figure) begin to share those delusional ideas themselves. The delusions in the nonpsychotic patient tend to resolve when the two are separated.

Mood (affective) disorders

Depressive episode, severe with psychotic features

See Chapter 1.

Manic episode with psychotic features

See Chapter 2.

Psychotic episodes secondary to a general medical condition or psychoactive substance use

A medical or psychoactive substance cause of psychosis should always be looked for and ruled out. Figure 4.7 lists the medical and substance-related causes of psychotic episodes. The medical condition or substance use should predate the development of the psychosis and symptoms should resolve with treatment of the condition or abstinence from the offending substance. Absence of previous psychotic episodes or a family history of schizophrenia also supports this diagnosis.

Delirium and dementia

Visual hallucinations and delusions are common in delirium and may also occur in dementia, particularly diffuse Lewy body dementia (see Chapter 9).

Personality disorder

Schizotypal personality disorder is characterized by eccentric behavior and peculiarities of thinking and appearance. Although there are no clear psychotic symptoms evident and its course resembles that of a personality disorder, the DSM-IV-TR actually describes schizotypal disorder in the chapter on psychotic disorders. This is because it is more prevalent among relatives of patients with schizophrenia and, occasionally, it progresses to overt schizophrenia. Borderline, paranoid, and schizoid personality disorders also share similar features to schizophrenia without displaying clear-cut psychotic symptoms. Personality disorders are discussed in greater detail in Chapter 11.

Medical conditions	Substances
Acute intermittent porphyria	Alcohol
Cerebral neoplasm, infarcts, trauma, infection (including HIV, CJD, neurosyphilis, herpes encephalitis)	Amphetamines
Endocrine (thyroid, parathyroid, adrenal disorders)	Anticholinergics
Epilepsy (especially temporal lobe epilepsy)	Antiparkinsonian drugs
Huntington's disease	Cocaine
Systemic lupus erythematosus	Corticosteroids
Vitamin B_{12}, niacin (pellagra) and thiamine deficiency (Wernicke's encephalopathy)	Hallucinogens
HIV: human immunodeficiency virus	Inhalants/solvents
CJD: Creutzfeldt-Jakob disease	Organophosphates
	Phencyclidine (PCP)

Fig. 4.7 Medical and substance-related causes of psychotic symptoms.

Algorithm for the diagnosis of psychotic disorders

See Figure 4.8.

Assessment

Clinical

The following questions may be helpful in eliciting psychotic phenomena on mental state examination:

Hallucinations

- Do you ever hear strange noises or voices when there is no one else about?
- Do you ever hear your own thoughts spoken aloud such that someone standing next to you might possibly hear them?
- Do you ever hear your thoughts echoed just after you have thought them? (*thought echo*)
- Do these voices talk directly to you or give you commands?
- Do these voices ever talk about you with each other or make comments about what you are doing?

Delusions

- Are you afraid that someone is trying to harm or poison you? *(persecutory delusions)*
- Have you noticed that people are doing or saying things that have a special meaning for you? *(delusions of reference)*
- Do you have any special abilities or powers? *(grandiose delusions)*
- Does it seem as though you are being controlled or influenced by some external force? *(delusions of control)*
- Are thoughts that don't belong to you being put into your head? *(thought insertion)*

A basic physical examination, including a thorough neurologic and endocrine system examination, should be performed on all patients with psychotic symptoms.

Special investigations

- It is important to obtain collateral information from the patient's family doctor, family and care coordinator (if they have one) to establish premorbid personality and functioning as well as pattern of deterioration.
- Lab work is obtained to:
  a. Exclude possible medical or substance-related causes of psychosis
  b. Establish baseline values before administering antipsychotics and other psychotropic drugs that may alter blood composition
  c. Assess renal and liver functioning, which may affect elimination of drugs that are likely to be taken long-term and possibly in depot form.

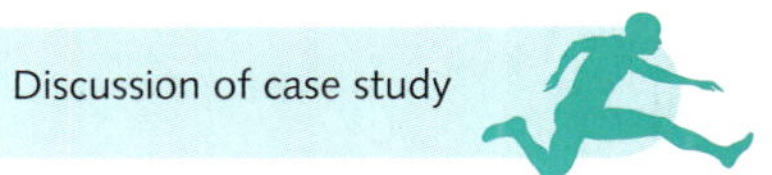

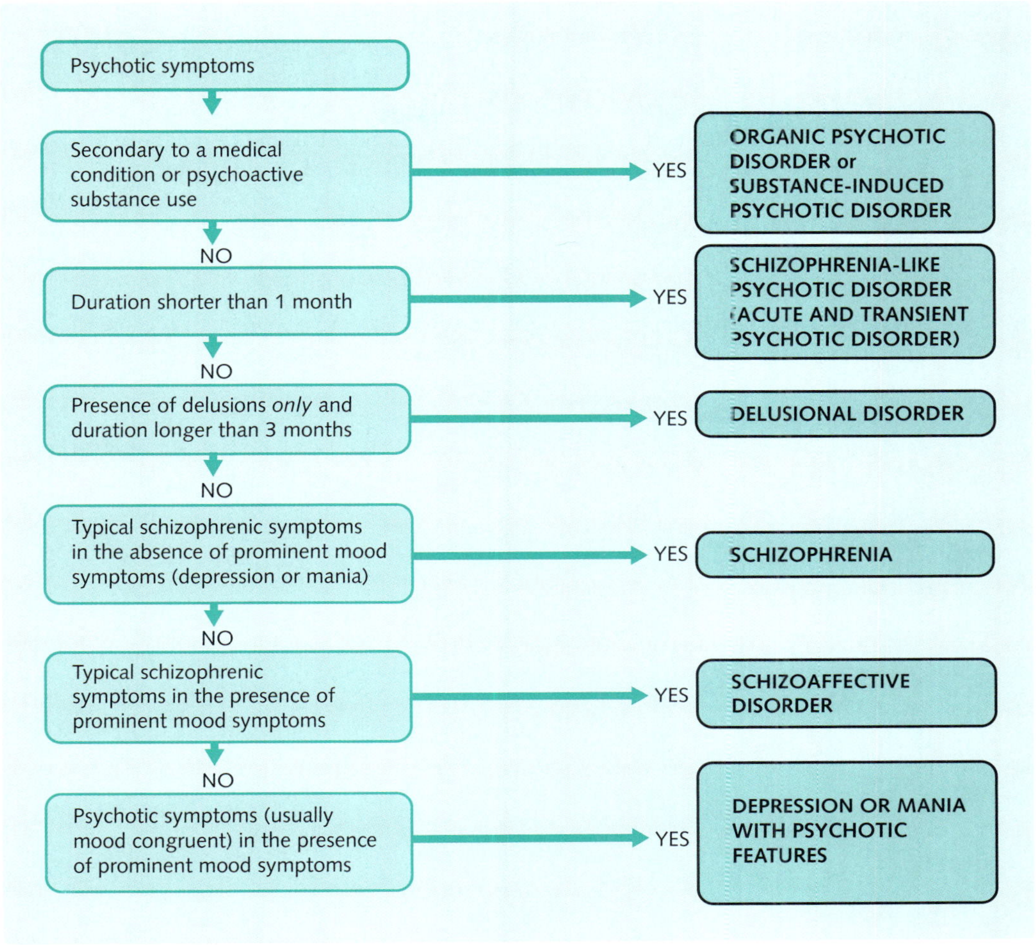

Psychotic symptoms

↓

Secondary to a medical condition or psychoactive substance use → YES → **ORGANIC PSYCHOTIC DISORDER or SUBSTANCE-INDUCED PSYCHOTIC DISORDER**

↓ NO

Duration shorter than 1 month → YES → **SCHIZOPHRENIA-LIKE PSYCHOTIC DISORDER (ACUTE AND TRANSIENT PSYCHOTIC DISORDER)**

↓ NO

Presence of delusions *only* and duration longer than 3 months → YES → **DELUSIONAL DISORDER**

↓ NO

Typical schizophrenic symptoms in the absence of prominent mood symptoms (depression or mania) → YES → **SCHIZOPHRENIA**

↓ NO

Typical schizophrenic symptoms in the presence of prominent mood symptoms → YES → **SCHIZOAFFECTIVE DISORDER**

↓ NO

Psychotic symptoms (usually mood congruent) in the presence of prominent mood symptoms → YES → **DEPRESSION OR MANIA WITH PSYCHOTIC FEATURES**

Fig. 4.8 Algorithm for the diagnosis of a patient presenting with psychotic symptoms.

- If the patient presents with a first episode of psychosis, a good basic screen consists of complete blood count (essential when starting clozapine), erythrocyte sedimentation rate, BUN and electrolytes, thyroid function, liver function tests, glucose, serum calcium, and VDRL if syphilis is suspected, and an HIV test.
- A urine drug screen should always be done because illicit drugs both cause and exacerbate a psychosis.
- An ECG should be done in patients with cardiac problems as many antipsychotics have the potential to prolong the QT interval and to cause lethal ventricular arrhythmia (rare).
- The use of a routine EEG or CT scan to help exclude an organic psychosis (e.g., temporal lobe epilepsy, brain tumor) varies between psychiatric units; they should always be considered in atypical cases, cases with treatment resistance, or patients with cognitive or neurologic abnormalities.

Discussion of case study

Mr PP meets the DSM-IV-TR criteria for *schizophrenia, paranoid subtype*. He has had a marked deterioration in his social and work functioning. He has *delusions of persecution* (believing he was a victim of government experiments), *thought control* (believing that ideas were being planted in his head [*thought insertion*]),

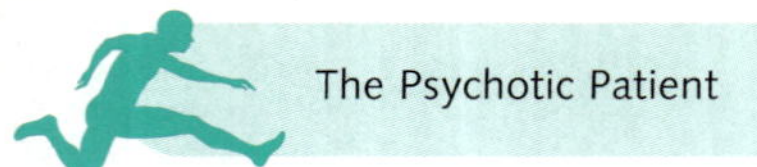

and *reference* (believing that the man in the local bar was referring specifically to him). His claim that he knew these things after hearing the neighbor's dog bark suggests *delusional perception*. He also has *person command hallucinations* and *running commentary hallucinations*. "Receiving coded information" from the radio might be a hallucination or a delusion of reference, depending on how Mr PP described this experience subjectively. Mr PP's description that "all was not right" could indicate the presence of a *delusional atmosphere* prior to the development of the full-blown delusions.

It is imperative that a *substance-induced psychotic disorder* or *psychotic disorder secondary to a medical condition* is excluded. It would be important to ascertain the duration of Mr PP's psychotic symptoms. It seems as though he has had schizophrenic symptoms for over a month. If the duration of symptoms had been less than month, it would be advisable to diagnose a schizophrenia-like psychotic disorder (e.g., *acute and transient psychotic disorder*). It is important to rule out a mood disorder with psychotic features. The presence of a mood episode associated with simultaneous schizophrenic symptoms would suggest a schizoaffective episode. Prominent hallucinations make a diagnosis of delusional disorder less likely.

Now go to Chapter 14 to read more about the psychotic disorders and their management.

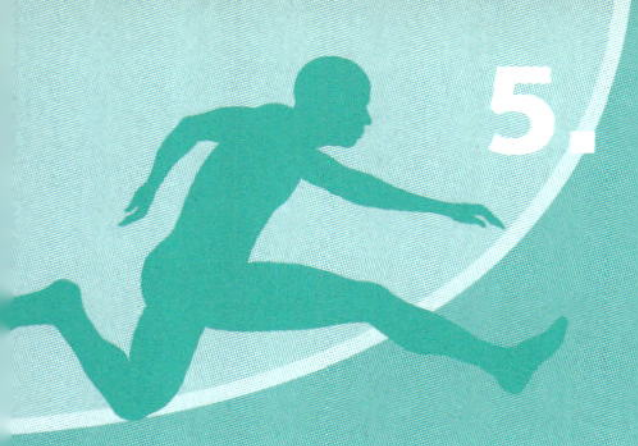

5. The Patient with Anxiety, Fear, or Avoidance

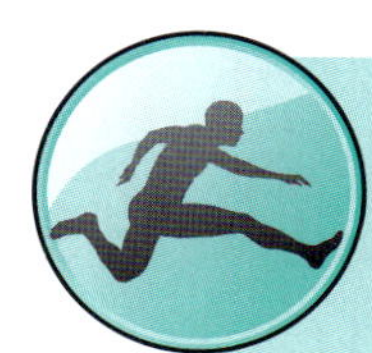

Mrs PA, a 32-year-old divorced interior designer, was referred to a consultant psychiatrist by her family doctor because of a 6-month history of sudden, dramatic anxiety attacks accompanied by heart palpitations, profuse sweating, dizziness, a choking sensation, and a fear that she was going to die. There appeared to be no logical reason for the attacks, and Mrs PA described them as coming on "out of the blue." They reached their maximum intensity within 2 minutes and seldom lasted longer than 15 minutes, occurring two to three times a week. Because of these attacks, which occurred in any situation and at any time of day, Mrs PA had stopped going into shops or crowded public places for fear of having an attack and not being able to escape to a safe place and appearing like a "blubbering idiot." She had started relying on her mother to accompany her on "absolutely necessary" household excursions "just in case" she had another attack. She hasn't worked for the past 3 months, as she was too frightened to visit potential clients' houses in the event that she had another attack. Mrs PA told the psychiatrist that she had almost become housebound and felt that she was "losing her mind." A full physical examination, routine blood tests (including complete blood count, BUN and electrolytes, fasting glucose, liver functions, thyroid functions, and calcium concentration), and an electrocardiogram (ECG) revealed no abnormalities.

(For a discussion of the case study see the end of the chapter)

Feelings of anxiety or fear are both common and essential to the human experience. It is the very uncomfortable nature of this experience that makes anxiety such an effective alerting and therefore harm-avoiding device. However, for the same reasons, when anxiety is excessive and unchecked it can create an extremely debilitating condition. To distinguish between normal and psychopathological anxiety it is important to observe the patient's level of functioning. The Yerkes–Dodson law states that the relationship between performance and anxiety has the shape of an inverted U: mild to moderate levels of anxiety improve performance, but high levels impair it. Figure 5.1 demonstrates the Yerkes–Dodson curve.

Definitions and clinical features

Both anxiety and fear are alerting signals that occur in response to a potential threat. Some authors suggest that *anxiety* occurs in response to threat that is unknown, internal, or vague (i.e., objectless), whereas *fear* occurs in response to a threat from a known, external, or definite object.

The experience of anxiety consists of two interrelated components: (1) *thoughts* of being apprehensive, nervous, or frightened, and (2) the awareness of a *physical reaction* to anxiety (autonomic or peripheral anxiety). Figure 5.2 summarizes the physical signs of anxiety. The experience of anxiety may lead to a change in behavior, particularly an *avoidance* of the real or imagined threat.

There are two patterns of pathologic anxiety:

1. *Generalized (free-floating) anxiety* does not occur in discrete episodes and tends to last for hours, days, or even longer and is of mild to moderate severity. It is not associated with a specific external threat or situation but is rather excessive worry or apprehension about many normal life events (e.g., job security, relationships, and responsibilities).

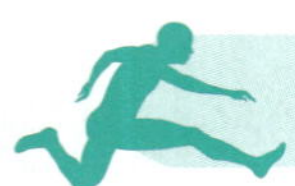
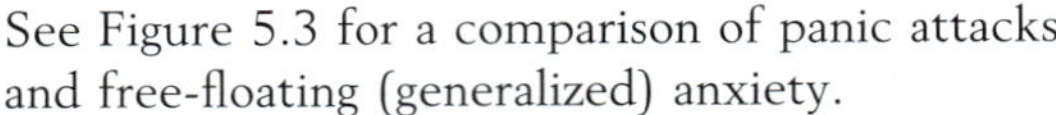

2. *Paroxysmal anxiety* has an abrupt onset, occurs in discrete episodes, and tends to be quite severe. In its severest form, paroxysmal anxiety presents as *panic attacks*. These are discrete episodes of short-lived (usually less than 1 hour), intense anxiety. They have an abrupt onset and rapidly build up to a peak level of anxiety. They are accompanied by strong autonomic symptoms (see Fig. 5.2), which may lead patients to believe that they are dying, having a heart attack, or going crazy – this increases their anxiety level and produces further physical symptoms, thereby creating a vicious cycle.

See Figure 5.3 for a comparison of panic attacks and free-floating (generalized) anxiety.

Paroxysmal anxiety can further be subdivided into episodes of anxiety that occur seemingly spontaneously, *without* a specific imagined or external threat (panic disorder) and those episodes that occur *in response* to a specific imagined or external threat. The phobic disorders are the most common cause of paroxysmal anxiety in response to a perceived threat.

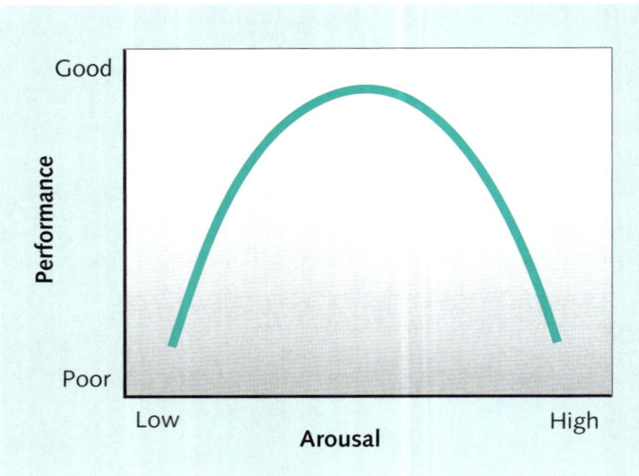

Fig. 5.1 Yerkes–Dodson law (1908).

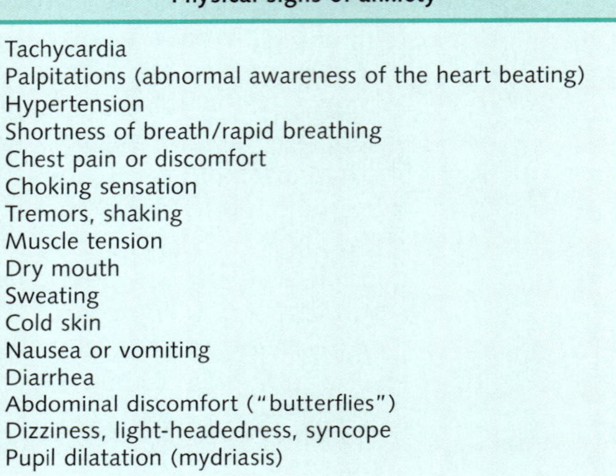
Physical signs of anxiety

Tachycardia
Palpitations (abnormal awareness of the heart beating)
Hypertension
Shortness of breath/rapid breathing
Chest pain or discomfort
Choking sensation
Tremors, shaking
Muscle tension
Dry mouth
Sweating
Cold skin
Nausea or vomiting
Diarrhea
Abdominal discomfort ("butterflies")
Dizziness, light-headedness, syncope
Pupil dilatation (mydriasis)

Fig. 5.2 Physical signs of anxiety.

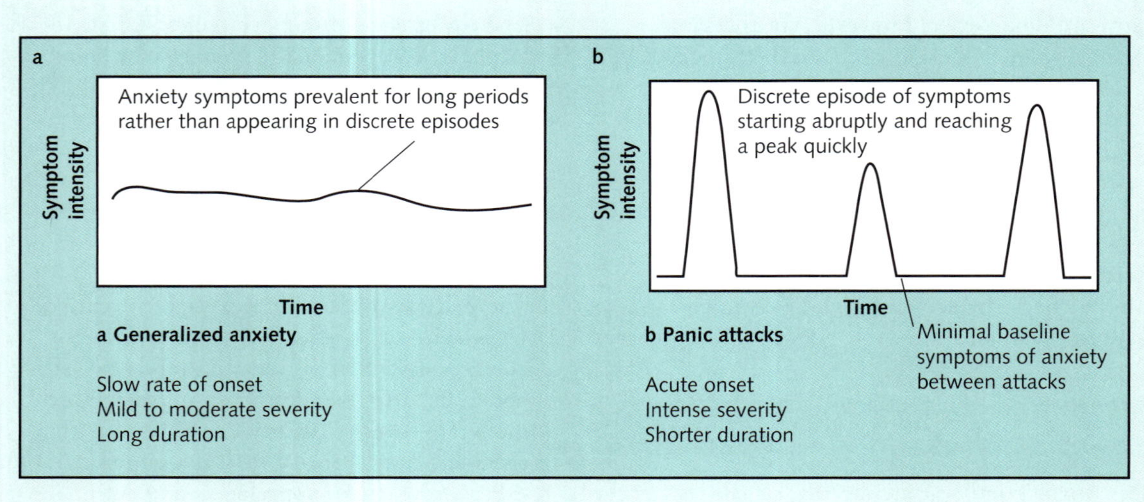

Fig. 5.3 Graphs comparing generalized (free-floating) anxiety (a) and panic attacks (b).

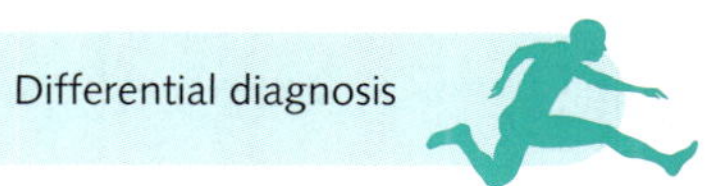

A *phobia* is an intense, irrational fear of an object, activity, or situation (e.g., flying, heights, animals, blood, public speaking). Although they may recognize that their fear is irrational, patients characteristically avoid the phobic stimulus or endure it with extreme distress. It is the degree of fear that is irrational in that the feared objects or situations are not inevitably dangerous and do not cause such severe anxiety in most other people. In severe cases, phobic anxiety may progress to frank panic attacks.

Differential diagnosis

When considering the differential diagnosis of anxiety you should determine:

- The *rate of onset*, *severity*, and *duration* of the anxiety, i.e., is the anxiety generalized or paroxysmal?
- Whether the anxiety is *in response* to a specific threat or whether it arises *spontaneously* (unprovoked)
- Whether the anxiety only occurs in the context of a *pre-existing psychiatric* or *medical condition*.

Figure 5.4 presents the differential diagnosis for patients presenting with anxiety.

Differential diagnosis for patients presenting with anxiety

Anxiety disorders:
- Phobic disorders
    - Social phobia
    - Specific phobia
- Nonsituational disorders
    - Generalized anxiety disorder
    - Panic disorder
- Reaction to stress
    - Acute stress disorder
    - Posttraumatic stress disorder
    - Adjustment disorder
- Obsessive-compulsive disorder

Secondary to other psychiatric disorders (especially depression and psychosis)
Secondary to a general medical condition
Secondary to psychoactive substance use (especially alcohol use)

Fig. 5.4 Differential diagnosis for patients presenting with anxiety.

Anxiety disorders

It is useful to consider the primary anxiety disorders under the headings: phobic disorders, nonsituational anxiety disorders, reaction to stress, and obsessive-compulsive disorder.

Nonsituational anxiety disorders

These disorders, unlike the phobic disorders, are characterized by primary anxiety symptoms that are not restricted to any specific situation or circumstance.

Generalized anxiety disorder

The key element of generalized anxiety disorder is long-standing, free-floating anxiety that is difficult to control. Patients describe excessive worry about minor matters and are apprehensive on most days for about 6 months. According to the DSM-IV-TR, the anxiety and worry are associated with three (or more) of the following six symptoms:

1. Restlessness or feeling on edge
2. Being easily fatigued
3. Difficulty concentrating or mind going blank
4. Irritability
5. Muscle tension
6. Sleep disturbance.

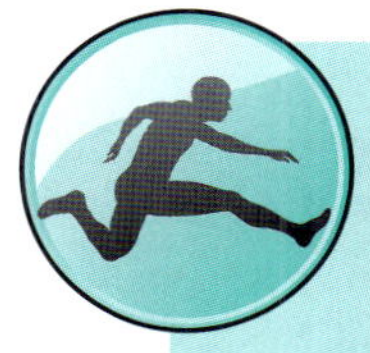

Blood–injection–injury phobias differ from others in that they are characterized by bradycardia and possibly syncope (vasovagal response), rather than tachycardia.

Panic disorder

Panic disorder is characterized by the presence of panic attacks that occur unpredictably and are not restricted to any particular situation (phobic disorders) or objective danger. Panic attacks are so distressing that patients commonly develop a fear of having further attacks; this is known as anticipatory anxiety. Except for anticipatory anxiety, patients are relatively free from anxiety symptoms between attacks.

In the DSM-IV-TR panic disorder occurs with or without agoraphobia.

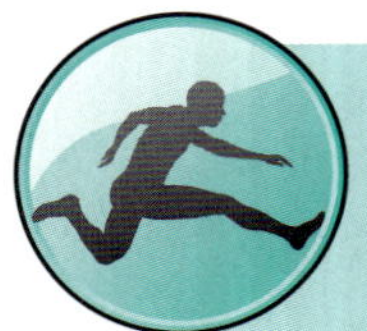

Panic attacks can occur spontaneously (unprovoked) or as an extreme response to a phobic stimulus.

Phobic disorders

Remember that:

- All phobic disorders are associated with a prominent *avoidance* of the feared situation.
- The situationally induced anxiety may be so severe as to take the form of a *panic attack*.

Agoraphobia

Agoraphobia literally means *fear of the marketplace* (i.e., fear of public places). In psychiatry today, it has a wider meaning that also includes a fear of entering crowded spaces (shops, trains, buses, elevators) where an immediate escape is difficult or in which help might not be available in the event of having a panic attack. At the worst extreme, patients may become housebound or refuse to leave the house unless accompanied by a close friend or relative.

There is a close relationship between agoraphobia and panic disorder that occurs when patients develop a fear of being in a place from where escape would be difficult in the event of having a panic attack. In fact, studies have shown that, in a clinical setting, up to 95% of patients presenting with agoraphobia have a current or past diagnosis of panic disorder. In the DSM-IV-TR you can code agoraphobia as agoraphobia *without history of panic disorder.*

Social phobia

Patients with social phobia fear social situations where they might be exposed to scrutiny by others, which might lead to humiliation or embarrassment. This fear might be limited to an isolated fear (e.g., public speaking, eating in public, fear of vomiting, or interacting with the opposite sex) or may involve almost all social activities outside the home.

Specific phobia

Specific (simple) phobias are restricted to clearly specific and discernible objects or situations (other than those covered in agoraphobia and social phobia). Examples from adult psychiatric samples in order of decreasing prevalence include:

- *Situational:* specific situations: public transportation, flying, driving, tunnels, bridges, elevators
- *Natural environment:* heights, storms, water, darkness
- *Blood–injection–injury:* seeing blood or an injury, fear of needles or an invasive medical procedure
- *Animal or insects* (e.g., spiders, dogs, mice)
- *Other:* fear of choking or vomiting, contracting an illness (e.g., AIDS), children's fear of costumed characters.

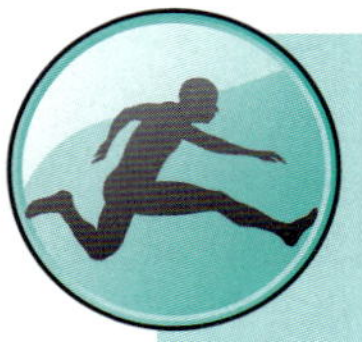

Patients with a phobic disorder may experience little anxiety in their daily living because they go to extreme lengths to avoid the phobic stimulus.

Reaction to stress and obsessive-compulsive disorder

The disorders associated with a reaction to stress and obsessive-compulsive disorder will be discussed in Chapters 6 and 7, respectively.

Other psychiatric conditions

Anxiety is a nonspecific symptom and can occur secondary to other psychiatric conditions. See Figure 5.5 for examples of psychiatric problems commonly associated with anxiety.

Note that depression and anxiety are inextricably intertwined. Not only can anxiety occur secondary to a depressive disorder and vice versa, but some authors have also suggested that the two disorders have a common etiology. About 65% of patients with anxiety also have depressive symptoms; therefore, when making a diagnosis, it is essential to decide which symptoms came first or are predominant and which are secondary. If symptoms of anxiety occur only in the context of a genuine depressive episode then depression takes precedence and should be diagnosed alone.

Anxiety secondary to a general medical condition or psychoactive substance use

A medical or psychoactive substance cause of anxiety should always be actively evaluated and

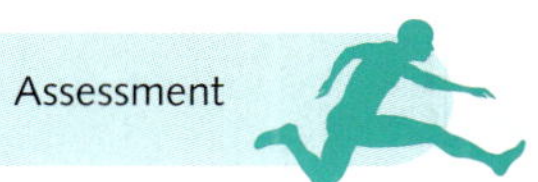

Examples of psychiatric problems commonly associated with anxiety	
Focus of anxiety	**Psychiatric problem**
Gaining weight	Eating disorder (see Ch. 12)
Having many physical complaints	Somatization disorder (see Ch. 8)
Having a serious illness	Hypochondriasis (see Ch. 8)
Fear of being poisoned or killed	Delusional beliefs in paranoid schizophrenia (see Ch. 4)
Ruminatory thoughts of guilt or worthlessness	Depression (see Ch. 1)
When having an obsessional thought or resisting a compulsion	Obsessive-compulsive disorder (see Ch. 7)

Fig. 5.5 Examples of psychiatric problems commonly associated with anxiety.

Medical conditions and substances that are associated with anxiety			
Medical conditions	**Substances**		
	Intoxication	**Withdrawal**	**Side effects of prescribed drugs**
Cerebral trauma Chronic obstructive airways disease Congestive cardiac failure Cushing's disease Hyperthyroidism Hypoglycemia Malignancies Pheochromocytoma Pulmonary embolism Temporal lope epilepsy Vitamin deficiencies	Alcohol Amphetamines Caffeine Cannabis Cocaine Hallucinogens Inhalants Phencyclidine	Alcohol Benzodiazepines Caffeine Cocaine Nicotine Other sedatives and hypnotics	Analgesics Anticholinergics Antidepressants (e.g., SSRIs and tricyclics in first 2 weeks of use) Antipsychotics Corticosteroids Sympathomimetics Thyroid hormones

Fig. 5.6 Medical conditions and substances that are associated with anxiety.

ruled out. Figure 5.6 lists the medical and substance-related causes of anxiety. The medical condition or substance use should predate the development of the anxiety and symptoms should resolve with treatment of the condition or abstinence from the offending substance. Absence of previous anxiety or a family history of anxiety disorder also supports this diagnosis.

Assessment

Clinical

The following questions may be helpful in eliciting anxiety symptoms on mental state examination:

- Do you sometimes wake up feeling anxious and dreading the day ahead? *(any form of anxiety)*
- Do you worry excessively about minor matters on most days of the week? *(generalized anxiety)*
- Have you ever been so frightened that your heart was pounding and you thought you might die? *(panic attack)*
- Do you avoid leaving the house alone because you are afraid of having a panic attack or being in a situation (like being in a crowded mall or on a train) from which escape will be difficult or embarrassing? *(panic disorder with agoraphobia)*
- Do you get anxious in social situations, like speaking in front of people or making conversation? *(social phobia)*
- Do some things or situations make you very scared? Do you avoid them? *(specific phobia)*

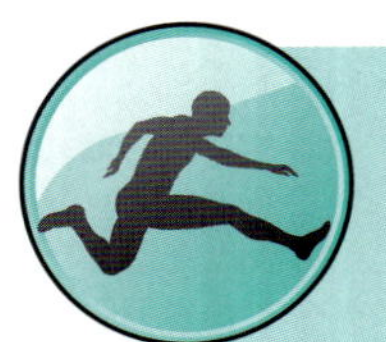

A basic physical examination, including a thorough neurologic and endocrine system examination, should be performed on all patients with symptoms of anxiety.

Special investigations

The anxiety disorders can only be diagnosed when the symptoms are not due to the direct effect of a substance or medical condition. This stipulation is particularly relevant when considering diagnoses of generalized anxiety disorder and panic disorder. It is impractical to test for each of the large number of drugs and organic conditions capable of producing anxiety symptoms (see Fig. 5.6). It is, however, important to exclude any disease or substance that may be implicated through any clues in the history (e.g., past medical history and drug history) and physical examination. For example, a patient with a rapid pulse and heat intolerance should have thyroid function tests in case thyrotoxicosis is causing the anxiety symptoms. The possibility of withdrawal syndromes (e.g., alcohol, benzodiazepines, opiates) causing anxiety symptoms should also be considered.

Discussion of case study

Repeated, unexpected episodes of short-lived intense anxiety of abrupt onset and rapidly building up to a peak level of anxiety associated with palpitations, sweating, dizziness, a choking sensation, and thoughts of being about to die, with no organic cause, suggest a diagnosis of *panic disorder*.

As is common in many patients with panic disorder, *agoraphobia* has developed as an additional problem as evidenced by a fear of going into situations from which escape might be difficult or humiliating. Mrs PA is showing the important sign of *avoidance* of the feared situation by refusing to go out unless it is essential and then only accompanied by her mother. Note that fear of having another panic attack indicates *anticipatory anxiety*; fear of having a panic attack in a situation from which escape will be difficult or humiliating, thus resulting in avoidance of those situations, indicates *agoraphobia* – Mrs PA has both.

It is important to rule out depression or other psychiatric conditions as well as medical conditions and psychoactive substance use.

Now go to Chapter 15 to read about the anxiety disorders and their management.

6. The Patient with a Reaction to a Stressful Event or Bereavement

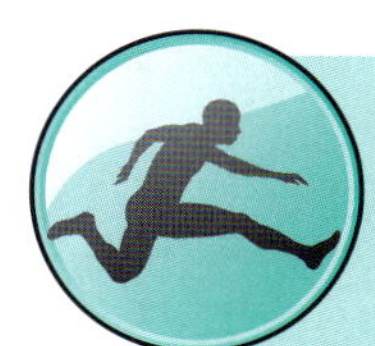

Mrs PT, a 28-year-old divorced woman, is referred by her psychiatrist to see a cognitive-behavioral psychotherapist. She was well until 3 months ago, working night shifts as a cleaner in an inner city office block. One evening, on her way to work, two large men cornered her alone at a secluded bus shelter. They pushed her violently to the ground and then proceeded to brutally rape her, threatening to "slit her throat" if she screamed. The men ran off when they heard someone approaching, leaving Mrs PT visibly shaken and with superficial cuts and bruises. She felt low in mood for a few days after the assault but attempted to carry on with her job and to forget that anything had ever happened. In the month that ensued, Mrs PT avoided all attempts by her family and friends to talk about the incident and became socially withdrawn, leaving the house only when she went to work. After a month, she started having nightmares about the incident and would wake up drenched in sweat. Her work colleagues noticed that she had become "jumpy and quick-tempered" and that sudden movements or noises easily startled her. She had also started avoiding public transportation and refused to watch any television for fear of seeing something that reminded her of the rape. Mrs PT finally sought professional help when, one night while at work, her supervisor found her lying on the floor screaming, "Leave me alone!" repeatedly, seemingly in a trance. Later Mrs PT recounted to her psychiatrist how she had "relived" the rape in her mind and how she could actually hear the voices of the men saying that they were going to kill her, just as they did on the specific night 3 months before. The psychiatrist noticed that Mrs PT could not recall certain important aspects of the trauma.

(For a discussion of the case study see the end of the chapter)

It is not unusual to have some psychological symptoms after a stressful or traumatic event or bereavement. However, in some cases, these symptoms may be in excess of those usually expected and, subsequently, impair a patient's functioning. It is important to be able to distinguish between a normal reaction to a difficult life event and a specific constellation of symptoms that denote psychiatric psychopathology deserving of clinical attention.

Definitions and clinical features

When assessing the patient who seemingly has had a pathologic response to a stressful event, it is important to explore two variables: (1) the nature and severity of the *life event* and (2) the nature and severity of the *patient's reaction* to the life event.

Nature and severity of the life event

Stress

A psychosocial stressor is the term used for any life event, condition, or circumstance that places a strain on a person's current coping skills. It is pivotal to remember that what constitutes stress is entirely dependent on the specific person's ability to adapt or respond to a life challenge. For example, one resilient medical student may breeze through an exam period without experiencing any stress, whereas another might feel under tremendous pressure because of a perceived or actual mismatch between individual ability and the demands of the situation. Also note that the same person's coping skills vary throughout his/her developmental life; the death of a distant relative may be far more stressful for a middle-aged man contemplating his own mortality than for an "invincible" adolescent.

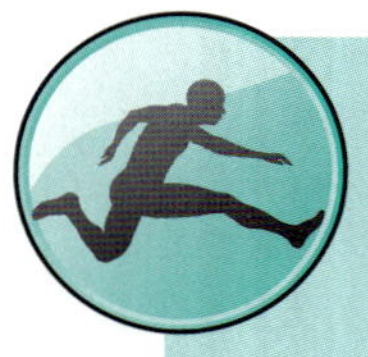

Remember that a seemingly innocuous life event may be a significant psychosocial stressor for a vulnerable patient (e.g., change of location for an elderly widow).

Traumatic stress

A *traumatic stressor* is one that occurs outside the range of normal human experience, i.e., the stressor is of such a magnitude that it would be experienced as traumatic by almost any person. This type of stress occurs in situations in which a person feels that his or her own, or a loved one's, physical integrity is under serious threat or that there is actual or threatened death or serious injury. Examples include natural catastrophes (earthquakes, floods), violent physical or sexual assault, fatal or near-fatal car accidents, terrorist attacks, torture, and military combat. Bereavement is a special case of traumatic stress that will be discussed later.

Nature and severity of patient's reaction

Some patients are of a durable disposition and seem to weather stressful or traumatic life events with minimal symptoms, whereas others seem more susceptible to the development of a diagnosable disorder. Depending on the severity of the stressor and their underlying vulnerability, patients may develop (1) an adjustment reaction; (2) an acute stress reaction or posttraumatic stress disorder; (3) a dissociative disorder; or (4) another major mental illness like a depressive, an anxiety, or a psychotic disorder.

Adjustment reaction

This reaction encompasses a wide, nonspecific range of emotional or behavioral symptoms that occur *in response* to a psychosocial stressor (significant life change or life event) to which a patient has had to adapt to or adjust. Examples include moving to a new area, changing schools or occupation, becoming a parent, or being promoted. An adjustment reaction may also occur after a traumatic stressor in an individual who is resilient enough not to develop a posttraumatic stress reaction (see later). The manifestations of an adjustment reaction include mild symptoms of depression and/or anxiety and feelings of being unable to cope. In some rarer cases, there may be disturbances of conduct (e.g., reckless driving, aggressive behavior, truancy). Although it is assumed that the reaction would not have arisen without the original stressor, an individual's personality and vulnerability to stress play an important contributing role.

A diagnosis of *adjustment disorder* is made when a patient has an adjustment reaction that occurs within 3 months of the stressful event or life change and the duration of symptoms does not usually *exceed 6 months*. Note that adjustment disorder is diagnosed by exclusion. The diagnosis is made when a patient develops symptoms, after any kind of stressor, that do not meet the criteria for any other, more specific, disorder.

You should diagnose an adjustment disorder only when patients do not meet the criteria for a more specific diagnosis such as a mood, psychotic, or anxiety disorder (including PTSD), or a normal bereavement reaction.

Stress reaction

For a diagnosis of posttraumatic stress disorder (PTSD) or acute stress disorder to be made, (1) the *stressor* must be classified as *traumatic* (see traumatic stressor above) and (2) the person's response must involve fear, helplessness, or horror. These conditions can occur in individuals with no prior history of mental illness.

The symptoms of an *acute stress disorder* (combat fatigue, psychic shock) develop within 4 weeks of the traumatic event. The reaction lasts

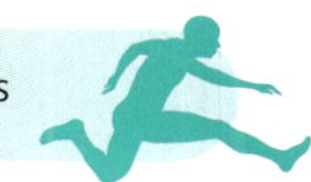

for a minimum of 2 days and a maximum of 4 weeks. Typically, patients will experience an initial "dazed" state followed by a narrowing of attention with an inability to process external stimuli and disorientation. This may be followed either by a period of diminished responsiveness to the extreme of a dissociative stupor or psychomotor agitation and overactivity (see Fig. 6.1 for dissociative disorders). Patients may also have amnesia for the episode – see dissociative amnesia later.

When assessing a patient with suspected PTSD, remember that head injuries and a seizure disorder are important differential diagnoses as they may present with similar symptoms and both may have been incurred at the time of the initial trauma. Alcohol and psychoactive substance intoxication or withdrawal may present similarly; this is also an important diagnostic consideration because patients with PTSD have high rates of comorbid substance use.

The symptoms of *posttraumatic stress disorder* usually develop within 6 months of a traumatic stressor. Symptoms include all of the following:

- Repetitive *re-experiencing* of the traumatic event in the form of:
  a. Flashbacks (a sense of reliving the original experience)
  b. Nightmares and illusions
  c. Recurrent images or thoughts
  d. Distress caused by internal or external cues that resemble the stressor.

  Note that, at times, patients may dissociate (see later) and experience the original event as though it were happening at that moment.
- *Avoidance* of stimuli associated with the stressor, amnesia for aspects of the trauma as well as emotional numbness and social withdrawal.
- Increased *arousal* (insomnia, anger outbursts, hypervigilance, poor concentration, exaggerated startle response).

Dissociation

In clinical psychiatry, *dissociation* describes the event where a disruption occurs in the usually integrated functions of consciousness, memory, identity, perception, and movement. In this rare phenomenon, memories of the past, awareness of identity, thoughts or emotions, movement and sensation, and control of behavior become separated from the rest of an individual's personality such that they function independently or are not open to voluntary control. Hypnosis is probably the most common example of a dissociative state in a normal person. Figure 6.1

Dissociative disorders	
Dissociative amnesia	Partial or complete memory loss for recent events of a traumatic or stressful nature not due to normal forgetfulness, organic brain disorders, or intoxication (e.g., alcoholic "blackouts")
Dissociative fugue	Sudden unexpected travel beyond the individual's usual range during which self-care and normal social interaction are maintained. There are features of dissociative amnesia for personal details and in some cases a new identity may be assumed
Depersonalization disorder	Persistent or recurrent episodes of detachment or estrangement from oneself. Patients will feel like automatons or as if they are living in a movie
Dissociative identity disorder	Apparent existence of two or more personalities within the same individual. This a rare and highly controversial diagnosis

Fig. 6.1 Dissociative disorders.

describes the most common *dissociative disorders*. Note that this diagnosis cannot be made if there is any evidence of a physical or psychiatric disorder that might explain the symptoms. Studies have shown that a noteworthy number of patients initially diagnosed with a dissociative disorder are eventually re-diagnosed with conditions such as epilepsy, depression, schizophrenia, and malingering. The psychoanalytic terms hysteria and conversion, which are often used synonymously with dissociation, are best avoided because of their varied and vague meanings.

Depersonalization and derealization are variants of dissociation that are not necessarily pathologic. *Depersonalization* is the term used to describe the experience when oneself or one's body feels somehow strange or unreal. *Derealization* is the term used to describe the experience when external reality seems strange or unreal. Depersonalization and derealization may be caused by psychiatric illness (e.g., depression, anxiety, schizophrenia), physical illness (e.g., epilepsy), psychosocial stress, and substance abuse.

Before accepting the diagnosis of a dissociative disorder, a central or peripheral nervous system affliction or other psychiatric illness should be aggressively sought for and ruled out.

Precipitation or exacerbation of an existing mental illness

The influence of a patient's environment on the development and course of mental illness cannot be overemphasized. Considerable research has indicated that almost all forms of mental illness (e.g., depression, suicidal behavior, psychotic illness, anxiety) can be precipitated or exacerbated by psychosocial ("life events") or traumatic stressors. However, unlike the above reactions in this group, there need not be a direct etiologic link with the stressor involved.

Bereavement

Note that bereavement is a unique kind of traumatic stress that is experienced by most people at some stage of their life and is therefore within the range of normal human experience. A bereavement reaction usually occurs after the loss of a loved person but can also result from other losses, like the loss of health (mental or physical), status, a national figure, or a dear pet. C. M. Parkes described the normal course of grief after bereavement as occurring in five phases (Fig. 6.2). Note that these phases of grief should not be regarded as a rigid sequence that is passed through only once. The bereaved person may pass back and forth between pining and depression repeatedly before coming to the final phase of reorganization.

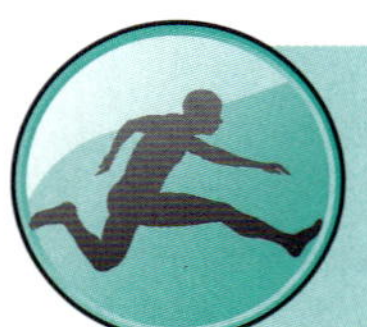

The length of a normal bereavement reaction is highly variable and tends to be longer if the death was sudden and unexpected. The DSM-IV-TR suggests that a bereavement reaction extending beyond 2 months should be coded as major depressive disorder.

Although most people will meet the criteria for a depressive episode at some stage during the grieving process, normal bereavement reactions are not pathologic and so no psychiatric diagnosis is made in these cases. However, patients who have been bereaved are at higher risk for developing a genuine depressive episode that will require treatment. The DSM-IV-TR notes the following symptoms that are not characteristic of a normal bereavement reaction and suggest the development of a major depressive episode:

1. Guilt about things *other than* actions taken or not taken by the patient at the time of the loved one's death
2. Thoughts of death *other than* that the patient would be better off dead or should have died with the deceased
3. Morbid preoccupation with worthlessness
4. Marked psychomotor retardation
5. Prolonged and marked functional impairment
6. Hallucinatory experiences *other than* patients thinking that they transiently see or hear the deceased.

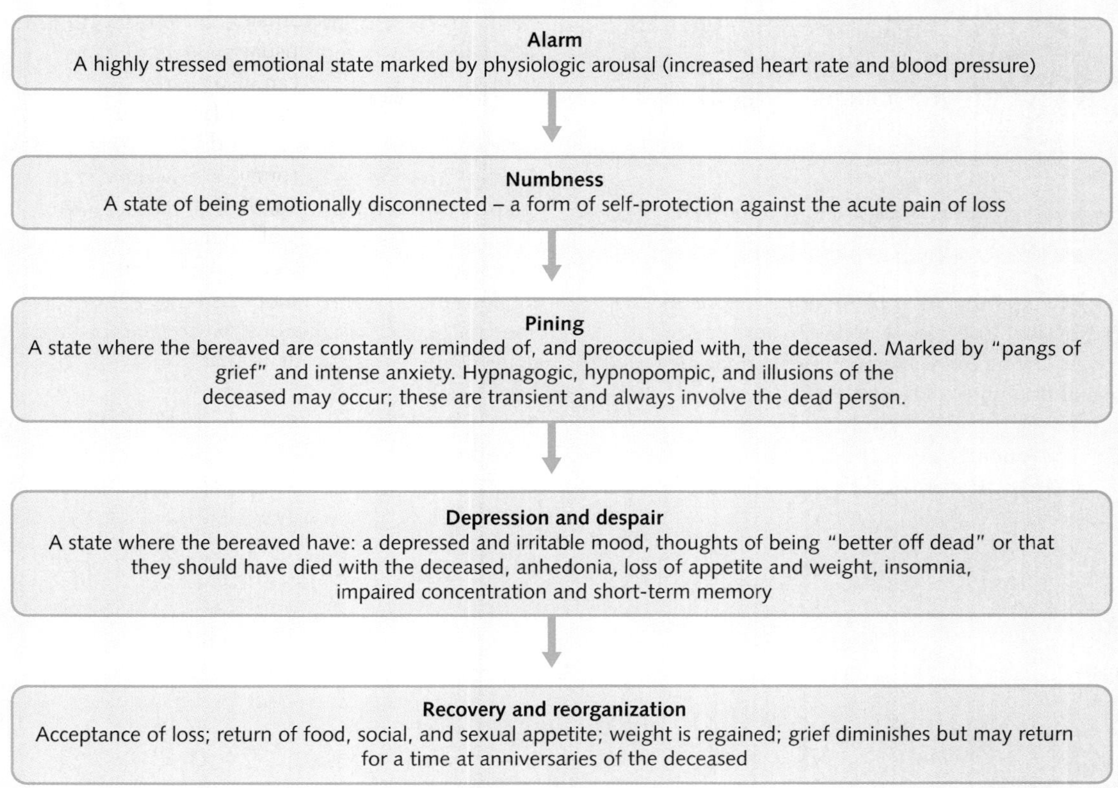

Fig. 6.2 Parkes' stages of normal bereavement.

Note that if a bereavement reaction, which is complicated by either a prolonged duration, or an abnormal quality of symptoms, does not meet the criteria for a depressive episode then a diagnosis of adjustment disorder is made.

Differential diagnosis

The diagnosis is usually clear if you have clearly elicited the nature and severity of the life event and the nature and severity of the patient's reaction. Remember that if the symptoms developed in response to a traumatic or psychosocial stressor meet the criteria for another major psychiatric diagnosis (mood disorder, psychotic disorder) then this diagnosis should be given instead of (or in clear cases of PTSD, in addition to) a diagnosis of adjustment, acute stress, or posttraumatic stress disorder. See Figure 6.3.

Differential diagnosis for patients presenting with a reaction to stress or trauma

Adjustment disorder
Acute stress disorder
Posttraumatic stress disorder
Normal bereavement reaction
Dissociative disorder
Exacerbation or precipitation of other psychiatric illness:

- Mood disorders
- Anxiety disorders
- Psychotic disorders (especially acute and transient psychotic disorders)

Malingering (see Ch. 8)

Fig. 6.3 Differential diagnosis for patients presenting with a reaction to stress or trauma.

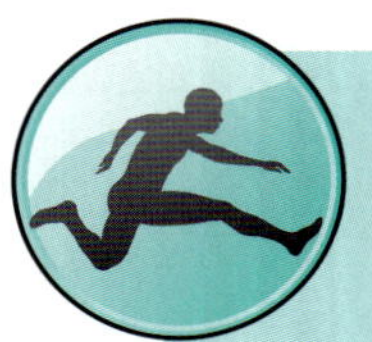

The risk of developing depression increases sixfold in the 6 months that follow a stressful event.

Discussion of case study

Mrs PT experienced a *traumatic* stressor in that her physical integrity was under immediate threat. The event was outside the range of normal human experience and thus would have been experienced as traumatic by most people. She subsequently developed *avoidance* of stimuli associated with the trauma (avoided talking or thinking about it, avoided public transportation and television), amnesia for aspects of the trauma, and social withdrawal. Later she showed signs of *increased arousal* (increased startle response, quick-tempered, "jumpy"). Finally, Mrs PT repetitively *re-experienced* the trauma through nightmares, flashbacks, and dissociation (reliving and behaving as though the trauma were occurring at that moment through mental imagery and hallucinations). All of the above suggest a diagnosis of *posttraumatic stress disorder*.

Now go to Chapter 15 to read about the anxiety disorders and their management.

7. The Patient with Obsessions and Compulsions

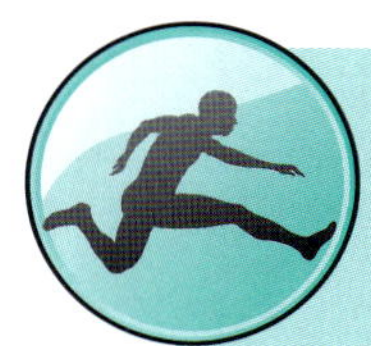

Mr OC is a 22-year-old medical student and has recently moved into his own flat. He describes a 5-month history of recurrent thoughts that he has behaved in a sexually inappropriate way toward his mother. He says that, even though on one level he knows that this is near impossible, he is unable to push these thoughts away despite trying "rigorous mental gymnastics." The only way he is able to relieve the distress he experiences is to actually contact his mother for reassurance that his fears are not true. On most days, he physically has to go and see his mother and will spend up to 2 hours analyzing his behavior with her until he feels reassured. Whenever he tries to stop himself from seeking reassurance, he feels a rapid escalation in anxiety, thinking that not contacting his mother is evidence that his thoughts "might be true." He shudders in horror when asked whether he has ever had any sexual feelings for his mother but admits that these distressing thoughts are "obviously" his own. He is heterosexual and has recently become engaged. He is extremely embarrassed and was eventually persuaded to see his family doctor by his mother and fiancée when he struggled to keep up with his studies. He says that the whole thing is starting to depress him and that he has lost weight.

(For a discussion of the case study see the end of the chapter)

Obsessions or compulsions are terms that are often used in everyday language, e.g., "she has an obsession with shoes" or "he is a compulsive liar." Psychiatrists, however, use these terms in a very specific way, and it is important to elicit, recognize, and understand obsessive-compulsive psychopathology.

Definitions and clinical features

Obsessions and compulsions

Obsessions are involuntary *thoughts*, *images*, or *impulses*, which have the following important characteristics:

- They are recurrent and intrusive and are experienced by patients as unpleasant or distressing.
- They enter the mind against conscious resistance. Patients try to resist but are unable to do so.
- Patients recognize obsessions as the product of their own mind (not from without, as in *thought insertion* [see Ch. 4]), even though they are involuntary and often repugnant.

Obsessions are not merely excessive concerns about normal life problems, and patients generally retain insight into the fact that their thoughts are irrational. In fact, patients often see their obsessions as foreign to, or against, their "essence" (*ego-dystonic*).

Compulsions are repetitive *mental operations* (counting, praying, or repeating a mantra silently) or *physical acts* (checking, seeking reassurance, handwashing, strict rituals) that have the following unique characteristics:

- Patients feel compelled to perform them in response to their own obsessions (see case study) or irrationally defined "rules" (e.g., "I must count to 10,000 four times before falling asleep").

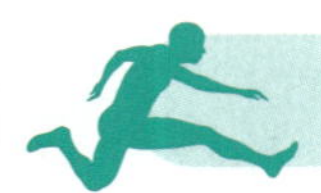

Examples of the most commonly occurring obsessions and their associated compulsions in descending order	
Obsession	**Compulsion**
Fear of contamination (feared object is usually impossible to avoid, e.g., feces, urine, germs)	Excessive washing and cleaning Avoidance of contaminated object
Pathological doubt ("Have I turned the stove off?" "Did I lock the door?")	Exhaustive checking of the possible omission
Reprehensible violent, blasphemous, or sexual thoughts, images, or impulses (e.g., impulse to stab husband, having thoughts that one might be a pedophile)*	Act of "redemption" (e.g., repeating "Forgive me, I have sinned" 15 times) or seeking reassurance (see case study)
Need for symmetry or precision	Repeatedly arranging objects to obtain perfect symmetry

** Patients often have these isolated obsessions without associated compulsions*

Fig. 7.1 Examples of the most commonly occurring obsessions and their associated compulsions in descending order.

- They are performed to reduce anxiety through the belief that they will prevent a "dreaded event" from occurring, even though they are not realistically connected to the event (e.g., compulsive counting each night to prevent "family catastrophe") or are ridiculously excessive (e.g., spending hours hand-washing in response to an obsessive fear of contamination).

Compulsions are experienced as unpleasant and serve no realistically useful purpose despite their tension-relieving properties. Similarly to obsessions, patients resist carrying out compulsions. Resisting compulsions, however, causes increased anxiety.

Obsessions and compulsions are often inextricably linked, as the desire to resist or neutralize an obsession produces a compulsive act (see Fig. 7.1 for examples of the most commonly occurring obsessions and compulsions). It can be difficult inquiring about obsessions and compulsions, especially when patients do not offer them as a presenting complaint. Figure 7.2 suggests some useful questions in eliciting these symptoms.

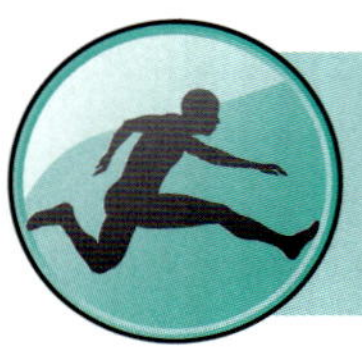

Make sure that you are able to explain what obsessions and compulsions are!

Questions used to elicit obsessions and compulsions

Do you worry about contamination with dirt even when you have already washed?
Do you have awful thoughts entering your mind despite trying hard to keep them out?
Do you repeatedly have to check things that you have already done (stoves, lights, faucets, etc.)?
Do you find that you have to arrange, touch, or count things many times over?

Fig. 7.2 Questions used to elicit obsessions and compulsions.

Differential diagnosis

Obsessions and compulsions may occur as a primary illness, as in *obsessive-compulsive disorder* (OCD), or may be clinical features of other psychiatric conditions. If patients have genuine obsessions or compulsions without other psychiatric symptoms then the diagnosis is invariably obsessive-compulsive disorder. For a definite diagnosis the DSM-IV-TR has proposed certain guidelines, as presented in Figure 7.3.

Many other psychiatric conditions may also present with repetitive or intrusive thoughts, impulses, images, or behaviors. However, it is usually possible to differentiate them from OCD by applying the strict definition of obsessions and compulsions as described earlier. Also, when repetitive thoughts occur in the context of other

Obsessive-compulsive disorder

A. Either obsessions or compulsions:

Obsessions as defined by (1), (2), (3), and (4):

(1) recurrent and persistent thoughts, impulses, or images that are experienced, at some time during the disturbance, as intrusive and inappropriate and that cause marked anxiety or distress
(2) the thoughts, impulses, or images are not simply excessive worries about real-life problems
(3) the person attempts to ignore or suppress such thoughts, impulses, or images, or to neutralize them with some other thought or action
(4) the person recognizes that the obsessional thoughts, impulses, or images are a product of his or her own mind (not imposed from without as in thought insertion)

Compulsions as defined by (1) and (2):

(1) repetitive behaviors (e.g., hand-washing, ordering, checking) or mental acts (e.g., praying, counting, repeating words silently) that the person feels driven to perform in response to an obsession, or according to rules that must be applied rigidly
(2) the behaviors or mental acts are aimed at preventing or reducing distress or preventing some dreaded event or situation; however, these behaviors or mental acts either are not connected in a realistic way with what they are designed to neutralize or prevent or are clearly excessive

B. At some point during the course of the disorder, the person has recognized that the obsessions or compulsions are excessive or unreasonable.

Note: This does not apply to children.

C. The obsessions or compulsions cause marked distress, are time-consuming (take more than 1 hour a day), or significantly interfere with the person's normal routine, occupational (or academic) functioning, or usual social activities or relationships.

D. If another Axis I disorder is present, the content of the obsessions or compulsions is not restricted to it (e.g., preoccupation with food in the presence of an Eating Disorder; hair pulling in the presence of Trichotillomania; concern with appearance in the presence of Body Dysmorphic Disorder; preoccupation with drugs in the presence of a Substance Use Disorder; preoccupation with having a serious illness in the presence of Hypochondriasis; preoccupation with sexual urges or fantasies in the presence of a Paraphilia; or guilty ruminations in the presence of Major Depressive Disorder).

E. The disturbance is not due to the direct physiologic effects of a substance (e.g., a drug of abuse, a medication) or a general medical condition.

Specify if:

With Poor Insight: if, for most of the time during the current episode, the person does not recognize that the obsessions and compulsions are excessive or unreasonable

Fig. 7.3 DSM-IV-TR diagnostic guidelines for obsessive-compulsive disorder.

mental disorders, the contents of these thoughts are limited exclusively to the type of disorder concerned (e.g., morbid fear of fatness in *anorexia nervosa*, ruminatory thoughts of worthlessness in *depression*, fear of dreaded objects in *phobias*). In these cases, obsessive-compulsive disorder is only diagnosed when the content of the obsessions or compulsions is unrelated to the other disorder. Figure 7.4 lists the differential diagnosis and key distinguishing features of patients presenting with obsessive-compulsive symptomatology. Figure 7.5 suggests a diagnosis algorithm that may be useful in differentiating OCD from other psychiatric conditions.

Discussion of case study

Mr OC has genuine obsessions (recurrent, intrusive thoughts that are distressing, resisted, and recognized as being from his own mind) and compulsions (repetitive reassurance seeking in response to obsessions to relieve anxiety, ridiculously excessive). He also describes symptoms of depression (depressed mood and weight loss).

His most likely diagnosis is obsessive-compulsive disorder (OCD); however, it is

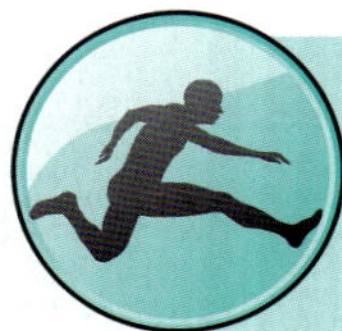

You should always consider depression in patients with obsessions or compulsions because:

- Over 20% of depressed patients can have obsessive-compulsive symptoms, which occur simultaneously at or after the onset of depression. They invariably resolve with treatment of the depression.
- Over two-thirds of patients with OCD experience a depressive episode in their lifetime. Obsessions and compulsions are present before and persist after the treatment of depression.
- OCD is a disabling illness, and patients often have chronic mild depressive symptoms that do not fully meet the criteria for a depressive episode. These symptoms usually resolve when the OCD is treated and the patient's quality of life improves.

Differential diagnosis for patients presenting with obsessions or compulsions

Diagnosis	**Diagnostic features**
Obsessive-compulsive disorder	Genuine obsessions and compulsions that cause marked distress, are time-consuming (>1 h/day), or significantly interfere with the person's normal routine or functioning (see Fig. 7.3)
Depressive disorder (see Ch. 1)	Obsessive-compulsive symptoms occur simultaneously with, or after the onset of, depression and resolve with treatment Obsessions are mood congruent e.g., ruminatory thoughts of worthlessness (i.e., ego-syntonic as opposed to ego-dystonic in OCD)
Other anxiety disorders (see Ch. 5)	Phobias: provoking stimulus comes from external object or situation rather than patient's own mind Generalized anxiety disorder: excessive concerns about real-life circumstances Absence of genuine obsessions or compulsions
Eating disorders (see Ch. 12)	Morbid fear of fatness (overvalued idea) Thoughts and actions are not recognized by patient as excessive or unreasonable and are not resisted (ego-syntonic) Thoughts do not necessarily provoke, or actions reduce, distress *Note: There is a higher incidence of true OCD in patients with anorexia nervosa*
Schizophrenia (see Ch. 4)	Thought insertion: patients believe that thoughts are not from their own mind Presence of other schizophrenic symptoms Lack of insight
Habit and impulse-control disorders: pathological gambling, kleptomania, trichotillomania (see Ch. 11)	Repetitious impulses and behavior (gambling, stealing, pulling out hair) with no other unrelated obsessions/compulsions Concordant with the patient's own wishes (therefore ego-syntonic)
Obsessive-compulsive personality disorder (see Ch. 11)	Enduring behaviour pattern of rigidity, doubt, perfectionism, and pedantry Ego-syntonic No true obsessions or compulsions
Hypochondriasis (see Ch. 8)	Obsessions only related to the fear of having a serious disease or bodily disfigurement
Gilles de la Tourette's syndrome (see Ch. 23)	Motor and vocal tics, echolalia, coprolalia *Note: 35–50% of patients with Gilles de la Tourette's syndrome meet the diagnostic criteria for OCD, whereas only 5–7% of patients with OCD have Tourette's syndrome*

Fig. 7.4 Differential diagnosis for patients presenting with obsessions or compulsions.

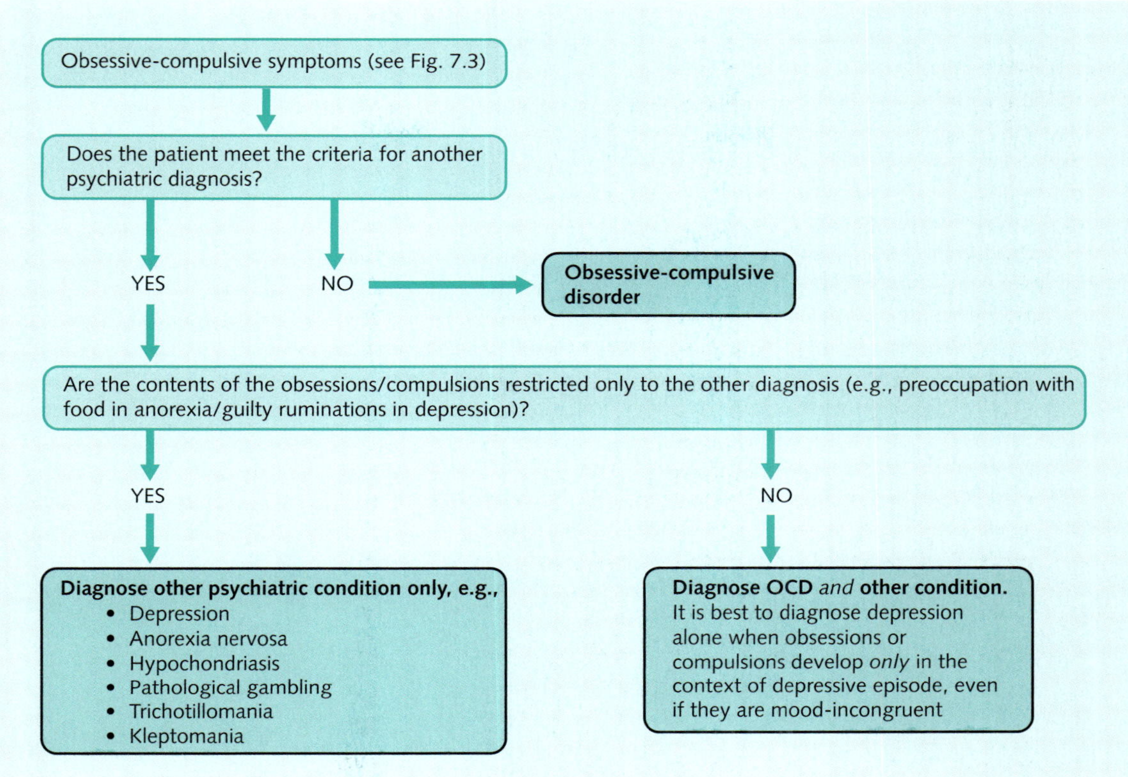

Fig. 7.5 Algorithm for the diagnosis of obsessions and compulsions.

important to consider depression. In this case the depressed mood developed after the obsessive-compulsive symptoms. If Mr OC now met the criteria for a depressive episode then OCD and depression would be diagnosed. He most probably has mild "reactive" depression, which will resolve when the OCD is treated (see Fig. 7.4).

Now go to Chapter 15 to read about obsessive-compulsive disorder and its management.

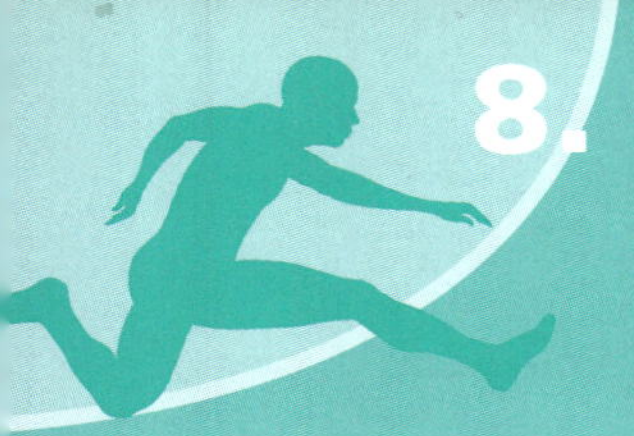

8. The Patient with Medically Unexplained Symptoms

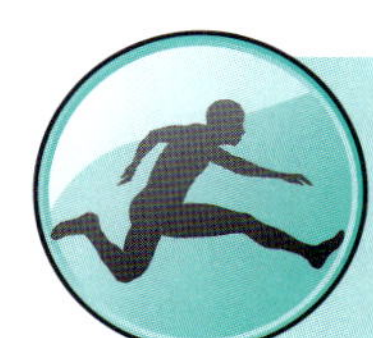

Mrs SD, a 32-year-old mother of three, had consulted her family doctor at least once every 2 weeks for the past year. Mrs SD's doctor had known her for just over a year since she had moved some distance after a prolonged divorce. Her medical history, part of which was obtained from her previous family doctor, was considerable for someone her age and had resulted in her being unemployed. At menarche, she was diagnosed with dysfunctional uterine bleeding and dysmenorrhea. Later, extensive investigations, which included three exploratory laparoscopies, revealed no cause for a persistent problem of upper abdominal pain with alternating diarrhea and constipation. Three years ago Mrs SD presented with urinary frequency and dysuria. Exhaustive investigations, including cystoscopy, bladder urodynamic studies, and radiography, were all normal. She had also been referred to various specialists, including a rheumatologist, for a problem of chronic neck pain that she had described as "the pain that has ruined mine and my kids' life!" Again, physical examination and investigations revealed no abnormalities. Mrs SD was taking up to 30 codeine tablets daily and could not sleep without two different types of sleeping tablets. Despite a difficult childhood, which featured a violent, alcohol-abusing father, and two abusive marriages that had ended in divorce, Mrs SD refused to contemplate her doctor's suggestion that there might be a psychological cause for her symptoms. However, she eventually agreed to one appointment with a psychiatrist when she developed hearing loss after her 13-year-old daughter became pregnant.

(For a discussion of the case study see the end of the chapter)

Although humans have historically been recognized as consisting of the two distinct components, body (soma) and mind (or soul), most insightful doctors will testify that there is an interrelated and perhaps indivisible relationship between them. Patients with numerous physical complaints are often referred to psychiatry as a last resort because no medical cause can be found for their symptoms. Having some understanding of the mental disorders that may mimic physical illness can provide an invaluable perspective for all health practitioners.

Definitions and clinical features

A so-called physical cause should always be sought in response to reported "physical symptoms." However, in certain cases, the reported symptoms:

- Do not correspond to, or are clearly not typical of, any known physical condition
- Are associated with an absence of any physical signs or structural abnormalities
- Are associated with an absence of any abnormalities in comprehensive laboratory, imaging, and invasive special investigations.

In these cases, a psychiatric illness should be considered, especially when unexplained physical symptoms bear a close relationship with stressful life events or psychological difficulties. In this regard you need to be able to distinguish between the *somatoform disorders* and *factitious disorder* and *malingering*.

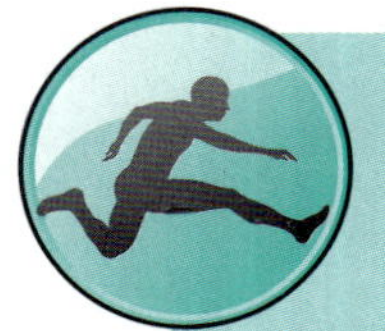

The term "psychosomatic" can also be used to describe physical symptoms that are presumed to be caused by psychological factors, but remember that the experience and expression of most physical symptoms are influenced by psychological factors.

Somatoform disorders

Soma means body, and so the somatoform disorders are a class of mental disorders which feature symptoms that are suggestive of, or take the *form* of, a physical disorder. However, there are no detectable organic or neurophysiologic abnormalities to explain these symptoms, leading to the presumption that they are caused by psychological factors. Note that these physical symptoms are not under voluntary control, i.e., they occur unintentionally, as opposed to the intentional feigning or production of symptoms in factitious disorder and malingering. *Somatization disorder* and *hypochondriasis* are the most common of the somatoform disorders, but you should also be aware of *somatoform autonomic dysfunction* and *persistent somatoform pain disorder*.

Somatization disorder (Briquet's syndrome)

According to the DSM-IV-TR, the essential feature of somatization disorder is multiple, recurrent, frequently changing physical symptoms which begin before age 30. These include:

- *Four pain symptoms:* head, abdomen, joints, extremities, chest, rectum, during menstruation, during sexual intercourse, during urination
- *Two gastrointestinal symptoms:* nausea, vomiting, diarrhea, food intolerance, belching, regurgitation, abdominal pain, constipation
- *One sexual symptom:* loss of libido, ejaculatory or erectile dysfunction, irregular menses, menorrhagia, dysmenorrhea
- *One pseudoneurologic symptom:* impaired coordination or balance, paralysis, localized weakness, difficulty swallowing, aphonia, urinary retention, hallucinations, loss of touch, double vision, blindness, deafness, seizures, loss of consciousness.

In addition, after appropriate investigation, each of these symptoms cannot be fully explained by a known general medical condition or the direct effects of a substance. When there is a related general medical condition, the physical complaints or resulting social or occupational impairment are in excess of what would be expected from the history, physical examination or lab findings.

Unlike factitious disorder or malingering, the patient is not intentionally producing or feigning these symptoms.

Most patients with somatization disorder will have had a long history of contact with the medical services during which numerous special investigations and operations will have been carried out – often leading to iatrogenic disease with explainable symptoms (e.g., abdominal adhesions from frequent exploratory surgery). Due to frequent courses of medication, they are very often dependent upon or abuse analgesics and sedatives.

The "somatic syndrome" refers to the biologic symptoms of depression (see Ch. 1) and has nothing to do with somatization disorder, which is one of the somatoform disorders.

Hypochondriasis

In somatization disorder, patients express concern about numerous physical symptoms, whereas in *hypochondriasis*, patients misinterpret normal bodily sensations, which lead them to believe that they have a *serious and progressive physical disease*. So patients with hypochondriasis will ask for investigations to definitively diagnose or confirm their underlying disease, whereas patients with somatization disorder will ask for treatment to remove their symptoms. However, despite these repeated examinations and investigations, which reveal no abnormalities, hypochondriacal patients refuse to accept the reassurance of numerous doctors that they do not suffer from a serious physical illness.

Body dysmorphic disorder

Body dysmorphic disorder (BDD) is a variant of hypochondriasis that features patients being preoccupied with an imagined defect in their appearance, or, if there is a slight physical anomaly, their preoccupation is markedly excessive. This imagined defect or deformity may concern any part of the body (e.g. a "crooked nose" or "ugly hands"). The preoccupation causes significant distress or impairment in functioning. Note that the psychopathology of hypochondriasis (and body dysmorphic disorder) takes the form of an *overvalued idea* (see Ch. 4), i.e., the belief that one has a serious disease or physical defect is *overvalued*. The belief is not delusional because patients are usually open to some form of explanation and their fears are allayed, at least for a short while, after yet another special investigation has been performed.

Conversion disorder

Patients with this disorder have one or more symptoms or deficits affecting a voluntary motor or sensory function that suggests a neurologic or general medical condition. However, the symptom(s), after appropriate investigation, cannot be fully explained by a general medical condition or substance. The symptoms are preceded by significant psychological conflict or stress. The patient is in significant distress and is not intentionally feigning the symptoms.

The patient often presents with *la belle indifference*: an inappropriately cavalier attitude toward apparently serious symptoms. The symptoms are often inconsistent with the physical examination.

Of note, one third of patients with conversion disorder have concurrent neurologic illness. More than one-half of patients with pseudoseizures may have a neurologic illness. Therefore, it is important to take a complete history and perform a thorough physical exam.

Pain disorder

The essential feature of this disorder is a complaint of severe and persistent pain at one or more anatomic sites that cannot be fully explained by any physical illness. The pain usually occurs in association with emotional difficulties or psychosocial stressors. It causes significant distress or impairment in social, occupational, or other areas of functioning. Patients are often disabled, and there is an increased use of health-care services and an increased use (or abuse) of medications as well as family problems.

The pain is not intentionally produced and is not due to a mood, anxiety, or psychotic disorder. Pain disorder can be associated with both psychological factors and/or a general medical condition.

Factitious disorder and malingering

In both factitious disorder and malingering, physical or psychological symptoms are *produced intentionally* or *feigned*. Patients may give convincing histories that fool even experienced clinicians and often manufacture signs (e.g., warfarin may be ingested to simulate bleeding disorders, insulin may be injected to produce hypoglycemia, and patients may contaminate their urine with blood or feces). Certain patients feign psychological symptoms such as hallucinations, delusions, depression, or dissociation. Because there are no definitive special investigations to diagnose psychiatric disorders, these patients often go undetected and may receive large doses of psychotropic medication and electroconvulsive therapy.

The patient's motivation differentiates between factitious disorder and malingering. In factitious disorder (Münchausen's syndrome), patients are focused on the *primary internal gain* of assuming the sick role, i.e., their only aim is to be treated like a patient and to be hospitalized. In malingering, patients are focused on a *secondary external gain*; they seek the secondary consequence of being diagnosed with an illness (e.g., avoidance of military service, evading criminal prosecution, obtaining illicit drugs, or obtaining financial or housing benefits).

Differential diagnosis

The differential diagnosis for patients presenting with medically unexplained symptoms is shown in Figure 8.1.

An underlying medical condition should be ruled out when patients present with unexplained physical symptoms. Somatization disorder can resemble insidious multisystemic diseases such as systemic lupus erythematosus, multiple sclerosis, acquired immune deficiency syndrome (AIDS),

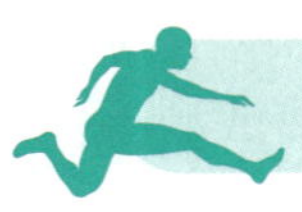

Differential diagnosis for patients presenting with medically unexplained symptoms

Somatoform disorders
- Hypochondriasis
- Conversion disorder
- Pain disorder
- Body dysmorphic disorder

Factitious disorder

Malingering

Other psychiatric conditions
- Anxiety disorders
- Mood disorders
- Psychotic disorders
- Dissociative disorders

General medical conditions
- Multiple sclerosis
- Myasthenia gravis
- Seizure disorder
- Dystonia
- Systemic lupus erythematosus (SLE)
- AIDS
- Acute intermittent porphyria
- Hyperparathyroidism
- Hypo- or hyperthyroidism
- Hemachromatosis
- Malignancy
- Lyme disease

Fig. 8.1 Differential diagnosis for patients presenting with medically unexplained symptoms.

acute intermittent porphyria, hyperparathyroidism, hyperthyroidism, myasthenia gravis, hemochromatosis, occult malignancy, and chronic infections.

Also remember that physical complaints often occur in the context of other psychiatric conditions. Patients with *schizophrenia* may have somatic delusions or visceral somatic hallucinations. However, the explanation of these symptoms is usually quite odd and there are usually other psychotic symptoms accompanying the physical complaints. Individuals with *depressed mood* often present with numerous somatic complaints; these tend to be episodic and resolve with the treatment of the depression. Distinguishing between the *anxiety disorders* and somatization disorder can be difficult. Patients with *panic disorder* have multiple somatic symptoms while having panic attacks, but these resolve when the panic subsides. Patients with *generalized anxiety disorder* may also have multiple somatic preoccupations, but their anxiety is not limited to physical symptoms.

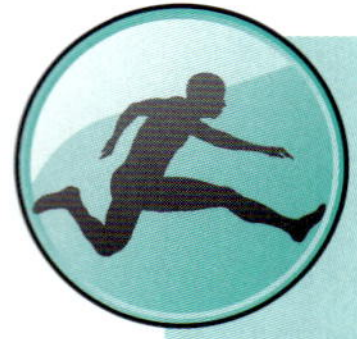

Somatization disorder usually has its onset in early adult life. The onset of multiple physical symptoms late in life is almost always due to a physical illness.

Assessment

Clinical

The following questions may be helpful in screening for somatoform disorders on mental state examination:

- Do you often worry about your health?
- Are you bothered by many different symptoms?
- Are you concerned that you might have a serious illness?
- Are you concerned about your facial or bodily appearance?
- Do you find it hard to believe doctors when they tell you that there is nothing wrong with you?

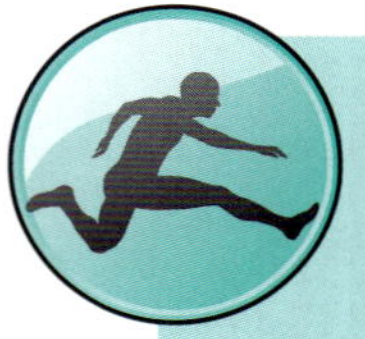

A thorough physical examination with special focus on the presenting problem is imperative when dealing with somatoform complaints.

Special investigations

Clinicians dealing with patients with a somatoform disorder need to investigate physical complaints judiciously. It is important to take all symptoms seriously, yet excessive and needless investigations to placate an anxious patient can result in a vicious circle with a worsening of symptoms. See Figure 15.4 in Chapter 15 for guidance on how to manage these patients.

Discussion of case study

Mrs SD has a long history of multiple, recurrent, frequently changing physical symptoms for which no physical causes have been found despite extensive investigation. She is resistant to the idea that there might be a psychological reason for her symptoms despite the association of her symptoms with psychosocial stress. Her functioning has been impaired and has probably affected her children's lives. Because she is focused on symptoms, not the idea that she has a serious and progressive illness, Mrs SD has *somatization disorder* as opposed to *hypochondriasis*. As is typical, Mrs SD has a secondary substance misuse problem (codeine and sleeping pills). It would be important to exclude other mental illness, such as depression and anxiety, as causative factors. If there was evidence that Mrs SD intentionally produced or feigned her symptoms, then *factitious disorder* or *malingering* should be considered.

Now go to Chapter 15 to read about the somatoform disorders and their management.

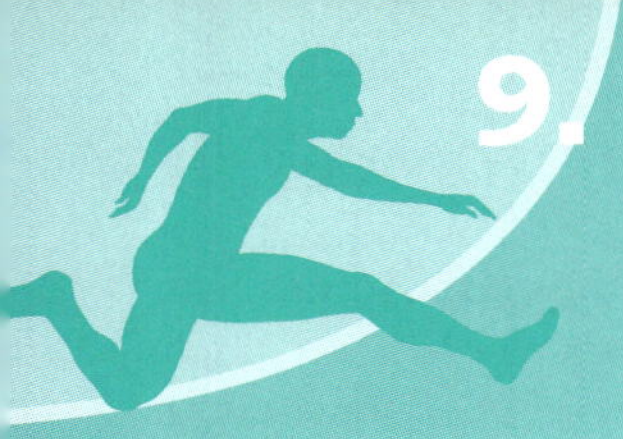

9. The Patient with Impairment of Consciousness, Memory, or Cognition

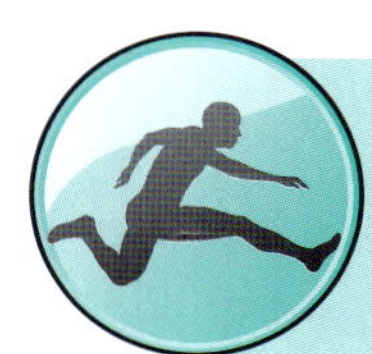

Mr DD, aged 78, had recently been admitted to a nursing home with a diagnosis of end-stage Alzheimer's disease. His family doctor had referred him to a psychiatrist 6 years ago after he started experiencing difficulty remembering things. At first he would forget things like the social arrangements he had made. Later he started forgetting activities he had engaged in only the day before. His wife had noticed a gradual change in his personality in that he became increasingly withdrawn and sullen and, at times, verbally abusive. His language deteriorated to the point where he would ramble incoherently, even when there was no one else in the room. Despite having smoked for many years, Mr DD seemed unable to recognize his pipe and would stare at it quizzically for hours. He lost the ability to dress himself or complete simple multistep tasks like making a cup of coffee. His wife discussed hospitalization with his psychiatrist when Mr DD no longer recognized her and refused to allow her to feed him. At the time of admission he was not orientated to place and time but displayed a normal consciousness level.

Two days after admission Mr DD's mental state changed dramatically. Nurses were concerned because his consciousness level was fluctuating from hour to hour. He slept through most of the day but would wander around the ward at night looking very agitated and appeared to have visual hallucinations. The senior nurse pointed out that he had developed a productive cough.

(For a discussion of the case study see the end of the chapter)

The human cognitive faculty is the most highly developed of all species. Apart from enabling us to ponder intangible abstract concepts, our cognitive faculty is the cornerstone of basic survival. There are many temporary and progressive conditions that cause an impairment of cognitive functioning and thus result in the most debilitating deterioration in functioning. The ability to assess and evaluate cognition should therefore be a fundamental skill for all health practitioners, not just psychiatrists.

Cognition: basic concepts and psychopathology

The term *cognition* is used in two ways by psychiatrists and psychologists. This chapter concerns cognition in its broadest sense as meaning: all the mental activities that allow us to perceive, integrate and conceptualize the world around us. These include: attention and concentration, memory, orientation, reading, writing, calculation, comprehension, learning, language, judgment, reasoning, and visuospatial ability. A narrower use of the term is found in cognitive psychology and cognitive therapy, where individual thoughts or ideas are also to be referred to as "cognitions."

This section will discuss the basic concepts of impaired consciousness and memory and then define the three syndromes that are characterized by impaired cognitive functioning, namely *dementia*, *delirium*, and the *amnesic syndrome*.

Consciousness

To be conscious is to be aware, both of objects that are perceivable and of oneself as a subjective being. Consciousness is said to be normal, heightened, or lowered.

Heightened consciousness involves an enhanced sense of awareness or arousal: colors are brighter and more vivid, sounds seem louder and crisper, and there is a greater sense of alertness. Heightened consciousness may be induced by psychoactive stimulants (amphetamines) or hallucinogens (LSD) and may also be found in early mania (see Ch. 2). Heightened awareness can be on the continuum of normal experience (e.g., being in love, religious experiences).

Unfortunately, the many terms describing *lowered consciousness* are muddled and confusing. Lowered consciousness needs to be distinguished from reduced wakefulness or sleep. There is a qualitative difference between the pathway from clear consciousness to sleep and the pathway from clear consciousness to coma. The difference is that the individual who is asleep can always be aroused to a state of clear consciousness with stimulation, unlike the patient with lowered or clouded consciousness. Consciousness can be seen as existing on a continuum of decreasing alertness, from clear consciousness to coma, with *clouding of consciousness* as an intermediate level in between. Figure 9.1 describes the pathway from clear consciousness to coma.

Abnormalities of consciousness often involve both a quantitative lowering of consciousness and a qualitative alteration of consciousness (the nature of awareness is altered). Most of the psychopathology described in this book concerns a qualitative alteration of awareness (e.g., hallucinations, illusions, delusions, mood changes, and anxiety) and these symptoms often accompany states of quantitatively impaired consciousness, as in delirium. Two further qualitative alterations in consciousness should be clarified: *confusion* and *stupor.*

Confusion

Patients are described as being confused when their thinking lacks its normal clarity and coherence. Confusion can occur in a state of normal or impaired consciousness. It may be a subjective complaint by the patient or be objectively inferred from the patient's speech and behavior. The cause of confusion is nonspecific. It may be caused by a lowering of consciousness, as in delirium; by a global impairment of cognitive functioning, as in dementia; by the deranged thinking or perceptual abnormalities of a psychotic patient; or simply when strong emotions or anxiety interfere with logical thinking.

Stupor

This term is best used to mean a clinical presentation of *akinesis* (lack of voluntary movement), *mutism*, and *extreme unresponsiveness* in an otherwise alert patient (there may be slight clouding of consciousness). Although apparently alert, the stuporous patient will initiate no spontaneous movement or speech, stare blankly

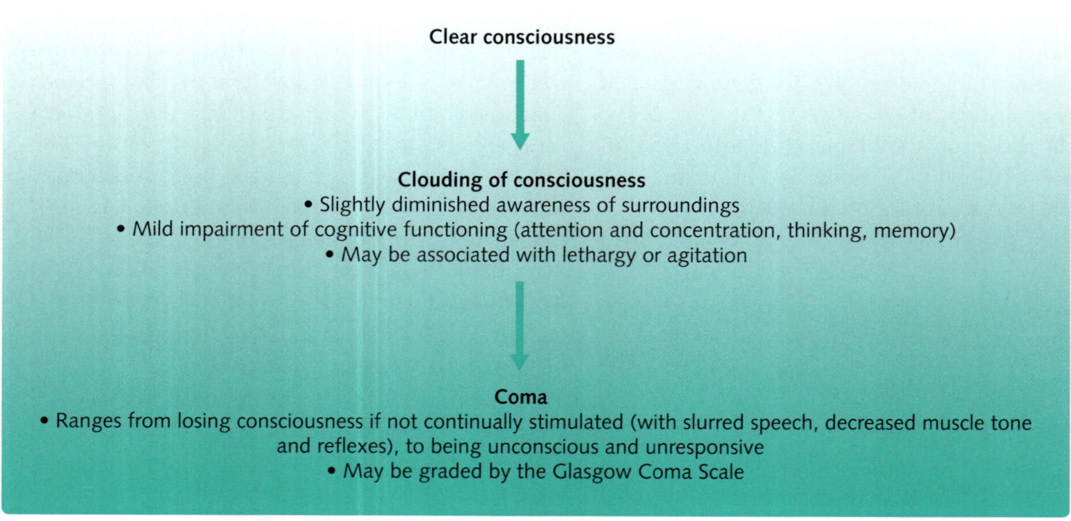

Fig. 9.1 The pathway from clear consciousness to coma.

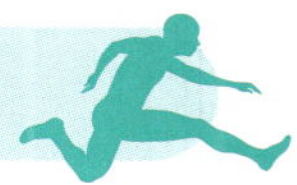

and seemingly take nothing in. Psychiatric causes of stupor include schizophrenia (catatonic stupor), depression, mania, and dissociative states. Organic causes of stupor include dementia, delirium, cerebral tumors or cysts, neurosyphilis, encephalitis, and postictal states.

> The vast number of confusing terms used to describe consciousness underscores the importance of documenting a patient's state of awareness in as much detail as possible, instead of describing a complex quantitative and qualitative presentation with one word.

Memory

The quantity of contemporary literature on memory is daunting and some of the terms used to define the types of memory have varied meanings. This section will describe the most commonly used definitions and provide a framework that has clinical applicability.

The process of retaining data is termed *storage*. Memory storage can be sensory, short-term, and long-term.

Immediate memory (also called sensory memory)

Immediate sensory information is held for less than a second, unprocessed, in the form that it was perceived by the sense organ. This allows the brain time to process the vast amount of visual (iconic memory), auditory (echoic memory), and touch (haptic memory) input it receives every second. This type of memory has limited clinical relevance.

Short-term memory (also called primary or working memory)

Once immediate memory has been attended to, it may be transferred to a temporary memory store, which has a limited capacity for 7 ± 2 items at a time (e.g., a telephone number). This will be forgotten in 15–30 seconds if it is not rehearsed or converted into long-term memory. Short-term memory is tested clinically with the digit span test (Fig. 9.2).

Long-term memory (also called secondary memory)

All data that have been processed and understood may be added to an existing memory store. This long-term memory store is probably limitless in terms of capacity and features a duration of storage from minutes to decades:

- *Recent memory* refers to memories stored minutes, hours, days, weeks, or months ago

Memory function tests	
Short-term memory	**Digit span test:** Ask the patient to repeat after you. Start with 2 different digits and deliver them in an even tone at a rate of one per second. If the patient repeats correctly, increase the number of digits by one each time (using different digits) until the patient's limit or digit span is reached. A normal digit span is 7 ± 2
Long-term memory	**Ability to store new memories (anterograde memory):** Ask patients to commit to memory three unrelated objects (e.g., apple, table, and penny.) Test recall 3–5 minutes later after interposition of other cognitive tests **Remote memory:** Ask patients about important events (personal or general knowledge) that occurred in childhood or decades ago. Correlate with collateral information **Recent memory:** Ask patients about events over the past few days (e.g., what they had for breakfast, what they did the day before, etc.)

Fig. 9.2 Memory function tests.

- *Remote memory* refers to memories stored many years or decades ago.

Note that committing a telephone number to memory for 1 hour and remembering childhood events from decades ago are both examples of long-term memory – recent and remote, respectively.

Long-term memory stores may be *explicit* or *implicit*. Explicit memory (sometimes called *declarative memory*) includes all stored material of which the individual is consciously aware and which the individual can thus "declare" to others. Implicit memory (sometimes called *procedural memory*) includes all material that is stored without the individual's conscious awareness (e.g., the ability to speak a language or ride a bicycle).

Some clinicians use the term "short-term memory" to mean recent memory (as defined in the text) and the term "immediate memory span" to mean short-term or primary memory (as defined in the text). For this reason many authors designate the type of memory to which they are referring with the qualification: *as measured by the digit span test* (see Fig. 9.2).

Amnesia refers to the loss of the ability to *store* new memories or *retrieve* memories that have previously been stored. Amnesia may be caused by a physical brain affliction (e.g., head injury, dementia) or it may be secondary to some form of emotional stress (e.g., dissociative amnesia – see Ch. 6).

Anterograde amnesia occurs after an amnesia-causing event and results in the patient being unable to store new memories from the event onward (impaired learning of new material), although the ability to retrieve memories stored before the event may remain unimpaired. Anterograde amnesia usually results from damage to the medial temporal lobes, especially the hippocampal formation.

Retrograde amnesia occurs after an amnesia-causing event and results in the patient being unable to retrieve memories stored before the event, although the ability to store new memories from the event onwards may remain unaffected. Retrograde amnesia usually results from damage to the frontal or temporal cortex.

Figure 9.2 describes how to clinically test the different types of memory.

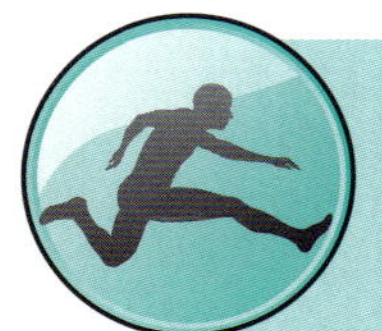

Implicit memory (procedural memory) is typically preserved despite severe disruptions to explicit (declarative) memory, probably because of its independent neural location. Implicit memory is associated with the striatum and neocortex. Explicit memory is associated with the hippocampal and diencephalic structures.

The cognitive disorders

It is useful to describe patients presenting with an impairment of cognition in terms of one of three commonly occurring syndromes: *dementia*, *delirium*, and the *amnesic syndrome*.

A delirium is characterized by an acute impairment of consciousness with cognitive deficits. A dementia is characterized by multiple cognitive deficits, including memory, *without an impairment of consciousness*. An amnesic syndrome is characterized by memory impairment in the absence of other significant cognitive deficits.

Remember that identification of one of these syndromes does not mean that a final diagnosis has been made. Instead, it serves as an intermediate guide, which is then used to prompt further investigation until a definitive diagnosis is reached. For example, the definitive cause of a delirium might be a subdural hematoma or hepatic encephalopathy.

Dementia

Dementia is an acquired syndrome characterized by a global impairment of cognitive function and personality without an impairment of consciousness. It is irreversible and chronic in course with a progressive deterioration in social and occupational functioning. Symptoms should be present for 6 months before a diagnosis is made.

The following text describes the general categories of impairment in dementia:

Memory impairment

Impairment of memory is a common feature of dementia. Recent memory is first affected (e.g., forgetting where objects are placed, conversations, and events of the previous day). With disease progression, all aspects of memory are affected, although highly personal information (e.g., name, previous occupation) is usually retained until late in the disease. Note that memory is essential for orientation to person, place, and time, and this will also be gradually affected (e.g., patients may lose their way in their own house).

Loss of language ability (aphasia)

Both receptive and expressive dysphasias may occur manifested by difficulty understanding commands or by vague, circumstantial speech with a reduced ability to read or write. Ultimately, patients may exhibit echolalia (repeating what is heard) or palilalia (repeating their own words over and over), or become mute.

Apraxia

Patients may lose the ability to carry out skilled motor movements despite an intact motor and sensory function (e.g., putting a letter in an envelope).

Agnosia

Patients may lose the ability to recognize or identify previously familiar objects or people despite intact sensory function.

Impairment of executive functioning

Patients may have difficulty in planning and sequencing complex activities.

Personality and behavior changes

Close family members are first to notice this. Patients may become introverted and socially withdrawn or hostile, irritable, and socially disinhibited. Pre-existing personality traits may become unpleasantly accentuated.

Psychiatric symptoms

Hallucinations in all sensory modalities (visual more common) may occur in up to 30% of patients. Delusions, especially persecutory, may occur in up to 40% of patients. Depression and anxiety may occur in up to half of all demented patients. Patients with dementia are more susceptible to the development of a delirium.

Neurologic symptoms

In addition to aphasia, apraxia, and agnosia, 10–20% of patients will experience seizures. Primitive reflexes (e.g., grasp, snout, suck) may also be evident, as well as myoclonic jerks.

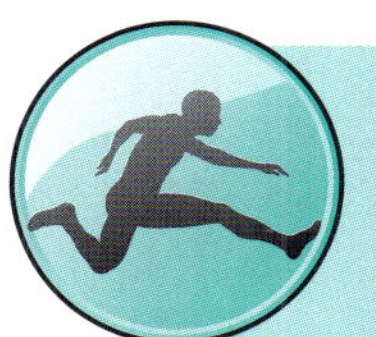

The diagnosis of dementia cannot be made on the basis of memory impairment alone. It is a syndrome that includes numerous cognitive deficits, including the inability to learn new complex material or adapt to novel situations, personality changes, and impaired executive functioning.

Distinguishing the type of dementia

The term senile or late-onset dementia is used if the onset of dementia is after age 65 and presenile or early-onset dementia if at or before age 65. Figure 9.3 lists the many disease processes that can cause dementia. The most common type of dementia is Alzheimer's disease which accounts for up to 60% of dementia cases. Vascular dementia is the second most common type and accounts for 15–30% of cases. Another form is called dementia with Lewy Body (DLB) which is characterized by problems with gait and balance, frequent falls, prominent visual hallucinations or delusions, fluctuations in alertness, and periods of unresponsiveness. Another type of dementia is frontotemporal (e.g., Pick's disease) which is characterized by personality changes, poor judgment, inappropriate behaviors, and lack of planning and goal setting. Finally, other diseases such as HIV/AIDS, Parkinson's disease, Huntingdon's disease and rare infectious diseases (e.g., Creutzfeldt-Jacob) can all cause dementia. All of these dementias result from a *primary neurodegenerative process*.

It is important to establish the underlying type of dementia because:

- A secondary dementia-causing process (e.g., brain tumor) may be detected and possibly halted

Diseases that may cause dementia

Neurodegenerative
- Alzheimer's disease
- Vascular dementia
- Frontotemporal dementia (includes Pick's disease)
- Dementia with Lewy bodies (DLB)
- Parkinson's disease
- Huntington's disease
- Progressive supranuclear palsy
- Normal pressure hydrocephalus

Space-occupying lesions
- Cysts, abscesses, hematomas
- Primary versus metastatic carcinoma, paraneoplastic syndrome

Trauma
- Head injury
- Punch-drunk syndrome (dementia pugilistica)

Infection
- Creutzfeldt–Jakob disease (including "new variant CJD")
- HIV-related dementia
- Neurosyphilis
- Viral encephalitis
- Progressive multifocal leukoencephalopathy (PMLE)
- Tuberculosis
- Sarcoidosis
- Whipple's disease

Metabolic and endocrine
- Chronic uremia
- Liver failure
- Wilson's disease
- Hyper- and hypothyroidism
- Hypo- and hyperparathyroidism
- Cushing's syndrome and Addison's disease
- Inherited enzyme deficits

Nutritional
- Thiamin deficiency (Wernicke's encephalopathy)
- Vitamin B_{12} or folic acid deficiency
- Niacin deficiency (pellagra)

Anoxia

Inflammatory disorders
- Multiple sclerosis
- Systemic lupus erythematosus and other collagen vascular diseases

Fig. 9.3 Diseases that may cause dementia.

- The progress of certain types of dementia may be slowed with specific medication (e.g. acetylcholinesterase inhibitors in Alzheimer's disease)
- Certain drugs may be contraindicated in some dementias (e.g., antipsychotics can cause a catastrophic parkinsonian reaction in patients with dementia with Lewy bodies)
- The prognoses of the various dementias differ; this may have practical implications for patients and their families as regards final arrangements (e.g., wills)
- The patient's relatives may inquire about genetic counseling (e.g., Huntington's disease, early-onset Alzheimer's disease).

In a minority of cases the distinction will be obvious, based on other symptoms produced by the disease process (e.g., jerky movements of the face and body [chorea]) and a positive family history will be indicative of Huntington's disease. In the majority of cases, the different dementias may be distinguished to some degree based on a detailed history from the patient and an informant, physical examination, relevant special investigations, and follow-up over time. However, the definitive diagnosis of dementia can only be established with absolute certainty on detailed microscopic examination of the brain at autopsy – and not always then. Figure 9.4 describes the distinguishing clinical features of the various types of dementia, which account for up to 95% of all cases.

To aid the clinical distinction of dementia, some authors differentiate *cortical*, *subcortical*, and *mixed* dementias based on the predominance of cortical or subcortical dysfunction – or a mixture of the two (see Fig. 9.5 for the features of cortical and subcortical dementias). Unfortunately, in advanced dementia, of whatever type, there is often a considerable overlap.

At this point you might find it helpful to read up on the etiology and neuropathology of the various neurodegenerative dementias in Chapter 16.

Delirium

The essential feature of a delirium is an impairment of consciousness with a reduced ability to focus or maintain attention. The delirious state tends to develop over a short period of time and is transient. The following text describes the prominent symptoms of delirium.

Impaired consciousness

Patients may have a reduced awareness of the environment from clouding of consciousness to

Distinguishing clinical features of the commonest types of dementia	
Alzheimer's disease	Gradual onset with progressive cognitive decline Diagnosis by exclusion of other causes of dementia
Vascular dementia (multi-infarct dementia)	Focal neurological signs and symptoms Evidence of cerebrovascular disease or stroke Uneven or stepwise deterioration in cognitive function
Dementia with Lewy bodies (DLB)	Day to day (or shorter) fluctuations in cognitive performance Recurrent visual hallucinations Spontaneous motor signs of parkinsonism (rigidity, bradykinesia, tremor) Recurrent falls and syncope Transient disturbances of consciousness Extreme sensitivity to antipsychotics (induces parkinsonism)
Frontotemporal dementia (including Pick's disease)	Early decline in social and personal conduct (disinhibition, tactlessness) Early emotional blunting Attenuated speech output, echolalia, perseveration, mutism Early loss of insight Relative sparing of other cognitive functions

Fig. 9.4 Distinguishing clinical features of the commonest types of dementia.

Features of cortical and subcortical dementias

Characteristic	Cortical dementia	Subcortical dementia
Language	Aphasia early	Normal
Speech	Normal until late	Dysarthric
Praxis	Apraxia	Normal
Agnosia	Present	Usually absent
Calculation	Early impairment	Normal until late
Motor system	Usually normal posture/tone	Stooped or extended posture, increased tone
Extra movements	None (may have myoclonus in Alzheimer's disease)	Tremor, chorea, tics

Cortical: Alzheimer's disease and the frontotemporal dementias (including Pick's disease)
Subcortical: Parkinson's disease, dementia with Lewy bodies, Huntington's disease, progressive supranuclear palsy, Wilson's disease, normal pressure hydrocephalus, multiple sclerosis, HIV-related dementia
Mixed: Vascular dementias, infection-induced dementias (Creutzfeldt–Jakob disease, neurosyphilis, and chronic meningitis)

Fig. 9.5 Features of cortical and subcortical dementias.

coma. Their ability to sustain attention is reduced and they are easily distractible.

Impaired cognitive function

Short-term memory (primary memory) and recent memory are impaired, with relative preservation of remote memory. Delirious patients are almost always disorientated to time and often to place. Orientation to self is seldom lost. Language abnormalities such as rambling, incoherent speech and an impaired ability to understand are common.

Perceptual and thought disturbance

Patients may have perceptual disturbances ranging from misinterpretations (e.g., a door slamming is mistaken for an explosion) to illusions (e.g., a crack in the wall is perceived as a snake) to hallucinations (especially visual and, to

Causes of delirium

CNS pathology

Neurodegenerative
Dementia with Lewy bodies (DLB)
Other dementias complicated by infection, anoxia, etc.

Space-occupying lesions
Tumors, cysts, abscesses, hematomas

Head injury (especially concussion)

Infection
Meningitis
Encephalitis
Syphilis

Normal pressure hydrocephalus

Cerebrovascular disorders
Transient ischemic attack
Cerebral thrombosis or embolism
Intracerebral or subarachnoid hemorrhage
Hypertensive encephalopathy
Vasculitis (e.g., from systemic lupus erythematosus)

Systemic causes

Drugs (ingestion or withdrawal)
Alcohol (Wernicke's encephalopathy, delirium tremens)
Anticholinergics
Anticonvulsants
Antidepressants
Antihypertensive drugs
Antiparkinsonian drugs
Antipsychotics
Cannabis
Cimetidine
Disulfiram

Drugs (ingestion or withdrawal) (cont'd)
Digoxin
Insulin
Opiates
Phencyclidine
Salicylates
Steroids
Sedatives (benzodiazepines)

Poisons
Heavy metals (lead, mercury, manganese)
Carbon monoxide

Metabolic and endocrine
Electrolyte disturbances
Uremia
Hepatic encephalopathy
Porphyria
Hypoglycemia
Hyper- and hypothyroidism
Hyper- and hypoadrenocorticism (Cushing's syndrome, Addison's disease)
Hypopituitarism

Nutritional
Thiamine (Wernicke's encephalopathy), vitamin B_{12}, folic acid, or niacin deficiency

Infections and sepsis

Hypoxia
Respiratory failure
Heart failure
Anemia
Hypotension

Fig. 9.6 Causes of delirium.

a lesser extent, auditory). Transient persecutory delusions and delusions of misidentification may occur.

Psychomotor abnormalities

Patients may be hyper-or hypoactive or fluctuate from one to the other and may also have an enhanced startle reaction.

Sleep–wake cycle disturbance

Sleep is characteristically disturbed and can range from daytime drowsiness and night-time hyperactivity to a complete reversal of the normal cycle. The nightmares of delirious patients may continue as hallucinations after awakening.

Mood disturbance

Emotional disturbances such as depression, euphoria, anxiety, anger, fear, and apathy are common.

Note that a delirium is a medical emergency, and the cause should be found and treated (see Ch. 16). Figure 9.6 lists the causes of delirium.

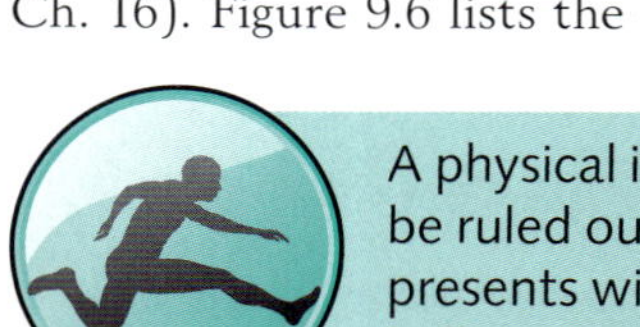

A physical illness should always be ruled out whenever a patient presents with prominent visual hallucinations because patients with schizophrenia and other functional psychotic disorders usually experience auditory hallucinations.

Distinguishing between delirium and dementia

Although the syndromes of delirium and dementia both consist of memory and cognitive impairment, they differ dramatically in cause, management, and prognosis. It is imperative that you understand how

Factors diferentiating delirium from dementia		
Feature	**Delirium**	**Dementia**
Onset	Acute	Gradual
Duration	Hours to weeks	Months to years
Course	Fluctuating	Progressive deterioration
Consciousness	Impaired	Normal
Perceptual disturbance	Common	Occurs in late stages
Sleep–wake cycle	Disrupted	Usually normal

Fig. 9.7 Factors differentiating delirium from dementia.

Causes of amnesic syndrome	
Diencephalic damage	**Hippocampal damage**
Vitamin B_1 (thiamine) deficiency (Korsakoff's syndrome) Chronic alcohol abuse Gastric carcinoma Severe malnutrition Hyperemesis gravidarum Bilateral thalamic infarction Multiple sclerosis Post subarachnoid hemorrhage Third ventricle tumors/cysts	Bilateral posterior cerebral artery occlusion Carbon monoxide poisoning Closed head injury Herpes simplex virus encephalitis

Fig. 9.8 Causes of amnesic syndrome.

to differentiate between the two. Figure 9.7 summarizes the factors differentiating delirium from dementia. Learn it well.

Amnesic syndrome

While dementia is the most common cause of chronic memory dysfunction, certain brain diseases can cause a severe disruption of memory with minimal or no deterioration in global cognitive functioning (i.e., aphasia, apraxia, agnosia, or disturbance of executive functioning). This clinical scenario is termed the *amnesic syndrome* and usually results from damage to the hypothalamic–diencephalic system or the hippocampal region.

Note that dementia with Lewy bodies is the only dementia that features transient episodes of impaired consciousness as a typical feature. All other dementias do not feature an impairment of consciousness unless complicated by a delirium (i.e., as result of infection, anoxia, etc.).

Figure 9.8 summarizes the causes of amnesic syndrome.

The amnesic syndrome is characterized by all of the following:

- Anterograde and retrograde amnesia. The impairment of memory for past events is in reverse order of their occurrence; i.e. recent memories are the most affected.
- There is no impairment of attention or consciousness or global intellectual functioning. There is also no defect of short-term (primary or working) memory as tested by digit span.
- There is strong evidence of a brain disease known to cause the amnesic syndrome (Fig. 9.8).

Although there is no impairment of global cognitive functioning, patients with the amnesic syndrome are usually *disorientated in time* because of their inability to learn new material (anterograde amnesia). *Confabulation* (filling of gaps in memory with fictitious details), *lack of insight*, and *apathy* are also associated features.

Note that when the lesions in the hypothalamus and diencephalon are due to a thiamine deficiency, the term *Korsakoff's syndrome* may be used. The most common cause of amnesic syndrome due to thiamine deficiency, or Korsakoff's syndrome, is chronic alcohol abuse. *Wernicke's encephalopathy* is the acute neuropsychiatric consequence of a severe thiamine deficiency and characterized by an acute onset of (1) ophthalmoplegia (nystagmus and abducens and conjugate gaze palsies); (2) an ataxic gait; and (3) confusion. Wernicke's encephalopathy and Korsakoff's syndrome ultimately result from the same pathologic process, the former being the acute reaction and the latter the residual defect – hence the term: *Wernicke–Korsakoff encephalopathy*. An untreated Wernicke's encephalopathy will result in a Korsakoff's amnesic syndrome in about 85% of cases. See also Chapters 10 and 16.

> Because of their unimpaired intellectual functioning, tendency to confabulate, and lack of insight, patients with an amnesic syndrome can appear deceptively "normal." This highlights the importance of obtaining collateral information as well as doing memory tests on mental state examination.

Differential diagnosis

Figure 9.9 shows the differential diagnosis for the patient presenting with cognitive impairment.

When patients present with a significant impairment of cognitive function, it is important to firstly establish their level of consciousness and then do a comprehensive psychiatric history and mental state examination that includes a global assessment of the various domains of cognitive functioning (see MMSE, p. 71). The differentiation between and the causes of dementia, delirium, and the amnesic syndrome have already been discussed. Remember that it is possible, and common, to have a delirium complicating a dementia (e.g., a patient with Alzheimer's disease develops delirium secondary to a urinary tract infection).

Psychoactive substance intoxication and withdrawal, most commonly alcohol, can cause multiple cognitive deficits and a lowered level of consciousness. Remember, however, that when a psychoactive substance causes symptoms which are in excess of that which is usually associated with its intoxication or withdrawal syndrome, then substance intoxication or withdrawal *delirium* should be diagnosed. For example, the cessation of drinking in an alcohol-dependent patient can precipitate an alcohol withdrawal syndrome or, in a smaller number of cases, precipitate a life-threatening delirium. Chapter 10 discusses this in more detail.

Patients with *learning disability* characteristically have below-average intellectual functioning with an impaired ability to adapt to their social environment. Unlike dementia, learning disability manifests in the developmental period (before age 18), and the level of cognitive functioning tends to be stable over time, not progressively deteriorating.

Patients with *chronic schizophrenia* may have multiple cognitive deficits, but unlike dementia, the age of onset is earlier and psychotic symptoms are present from the start. Also, the cognitive impairment in schizophrenia tends to be milder than in dementia. The disturbed behavior, vivid hallucinations, distractibility, and thought disorder of *acutely psychotic* patients may resemble a delirium. However, careful examination will reveal that the consciousness level is not lowered.

Depressive pseudodementia is the term used when patients present with clinical features resembling a dementia that results from an underlying depression (also called *depression-related cognitive dysfunction*). There is some debate as to whether this syndrome reflects true cognitive impairment (in which case pseudodementia is a misnomer) or whether the depression-associated psychomotor retardation, social withdrawal, difficulty thinking, and poor concentration give a misleading impression of

Differential diagnosis of cognitive impairment
Dementia
Delirium
Amnesic syndrome
Psychoactive substance intoxication or withdrawal
Mental retardation (learning disability)
Psychotic disorders
Mood disorders
Dissociative disorders
Age-related cognitive decline
Factitious disorder and malingering

Fig. 9.9 Differential diagnosis of cognitive impairment.

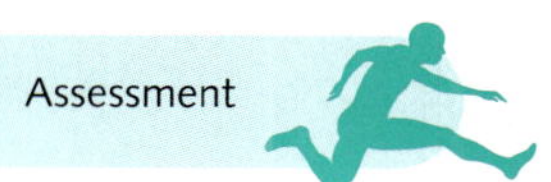

dementia in the presence of an intact cognitive faculty. In either case, the situation usually responds to antidepressant treatment. Depressive pseudodementia is differentiated from dementia by the abrupt onset of cognitive impairment with relatively normal premorbid functioning.

Memory loss, confusion, and stupor can occur in the *dissociative disorders* (see Ch. 6), such as dissociative amnesia, fugue, and stupor. They are distinguished from dementia and the amnesic syndrome by the lack of evidence of a physical cause and because they are usually precipitated by a psychosocial stressor.

Dementia and the amnesic syndrome must be differentiated from the normal decline in cognitive function that occurs with aging. This is usually of minor severity and does not interfere with the individual's social and occupational functioning.

Assessment

Clinical

When doing a mental state examination, a cognitive assessment should always be done. Figure 9.2 demonstrates how to test specifically for memory function. Now that you are aware of the many aspects comprising cognition, you might find the *Mini-Mental State Examination* (MMSE) a useful tool for doing a global test of cognitive functioning (see Fig. 9.10 for a description of the MMSE). This is a standardized set of questions that test the

Mini Mental State Examination

Cognitive ability tested	Questions	Maximum score
1. Orientation	What is the (year) (season) (month) (day of month) (day of week)? Where are we: (country) (county) (city/town) (building) (floor level)?	5 5
2. Registration	Name three common objects (e.g. "apple," "ball," "table"). Now ask the patient to repeat all three. Give one point for each correct answer. Repeat them until patient learns all three. Record the number of trials needed	3 Number of trials:
3. Attention and calculation	*Serial 7s*: Ask the patient to subtract 7 from 100 and then again up to five times (93→86→79→72→65) *OR* Ask the patient to spell WORLD backwards (D→L→R→O→W)	5
4. Recall	Ask the patient to name the three objects mentioned in "registration"	3
5. Naming	Ask the patient to name two objects (show a pencil) (show a watch)	2
6. Repeating	Ask the patient to repeat: "NO IFS, ANDS OR BUTS"	1
7. Three stage command	Ask the patient to: "Take this paper in your right hand, fold it in half, and put it on the floor"	3
8. Reading	Ask the patient to read and obey the following: **CLOSE YOUR EYES**	1
9. Writing	Ask the patient to write a short sentence	1
10. Construction	Ask the patient to copy the following drawing (overlapping pentagons):	1 TOTAL: /30

Fig. 9.10 Mini-Mental State Examination. (Adapted from Folstein MF et al 1995 Mini-Mental State: a practical method for grading the cognitive state of patients for the clinician. Journal of Psychiatric Research 12:189–198.)

most important aspects of cognition such as orientation, registration, attention, calculation, language, executive functioning, and visuospatial skills. It is often used to screen for or monitor the progress of dementia but is very useful as a general test for assessing global cognitive ability. A score below 25/30 suggests dementia. Note that the MMSE score naturally declines with age, so that the mean score at 90 years is 23/30.

The main aim of the *physical examination* is to identify treatable underlying causes of dementia, such as hypothyroidism or a space-occupying lesion. In addition, consideration should be given to complications of dementia, such as malnutrition or falls. Cardiovascular and neurologic examinations are particularly important. Evidence of hypertension or circulatory disease has obvious implications for the likelihood of vascular dementia, and neurologic examination may identify focal signs necessitating further investigation.

Special investigations

Apart from HIV-testing for AIDS-associated dementia and genetic tests for Huntington's disease, there are no specific tests that are diagnostic for the neurodegenerative forms of dementia in living individuals. A number of tests are usually performed soon after the diagnosis of dementia to screen for the general medical causes of dementia or to differentiate between the different types of dementia (see Fig. 9.3).

The EEG in Alzheimer's disease reveals diffuse slowing in the early stages followed by reduced alpha and beta activity and increased theta and delta activity. The EEG is of limited use diagnostically and is rarely used unless the clinical picture is atypical. The characteristic EEG in Creutzfeldt–Jakob disease is a slow background rhythm with paroxysmal sharp waves.

Individual units vary in their use of neuroimaging techniques to help diagnose dementia. Computed tomography (CT) and magnetic resonance imaging (MRI) are most often used to exclude other causes of cognitive impairment (e.g. tumors, hematomas). They may also be supportive but not essential in the diagnosis of Alzheimer's disease. MRI is particularly good at identifying small cerebral infarcts, especially in the white brain matter. Figure 9.11 summarizes the CT-scan features of the main forms of dementia.

Where available, functional imaging, especially single photon emission computed tomography

Typical CT appearances for the main forms of dementia

Condition	CT appearance
Normal aging	Progressive cortical atrophy and increasing ventricular size
Alzheimer's disease	Generalized cerebral atrophy Widened sulci Dilated ventricles Thinning of the width of the medial temporal lobe (in temporal-lobe-oriented CT scans)
Vascular dementia	Single/multiple areas of infarction Cerebral atrophy Dilated ventricles
Frontotemporal dementia (including Pick's disease)	Greater relative atrophy of frontal and temporal lobes Knife-blade atrophy (appearance of atrophied gyri)
Huntington's disease	Dilated ventricles Atrophy of caudate nuclei (loss of shouldering)
Creutzfeldt–Jakob disease (CJD)	Usually appears normal Note that nvCJD does have a characteristic MRI picture: a bilaterally evident high signal in the pulvinar (postthalamic) region

nv – new variant

Fig. 9.11 Typical CT appearances for the main forms of dementia.

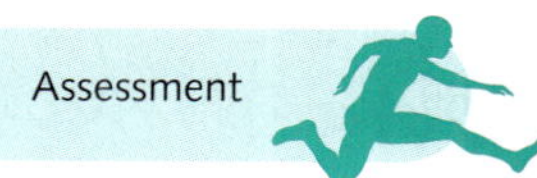

(SPECT), can be very helpful in differentiating the various forms of dementia.

Genetic testing is not recommended for late-onset Alzheimer's disease. Three genes may be tested for in the extremely rare families that have autosomal dominant early-onset familial Alzheimer's disease. These are amyloid precursor protein, presenilin-1, and presenilin-2. However, these three genes may only account for 30–50% of all autosomal dominant early-onset cases. See Chapter 16 for a full discussion of the genetics of Alzheimer's disease.

Psychological investigations are used to diagnose cognitive impairment (e.g., MMSE, clock drawing test) and when investigating atypical (e.g., predominantly frontal lobe signs) or presenile presentations. Specific tests of frontal lobe functioning include the Wisconsin Card Sorting Test. Intelligence scales (e.g., Wechsler Adult Intelligence Scale) may be useful in distinguishing cases of pseudodementia. A comprehensive cognitive assessment is usually performed by a specialist clinical psychologist.

Figure 9.12 summarizes a typical dementia work-up.

Similar principles apply to the investigation of delirium, particularly since there is invariably an identifiable organic cause. Additional investigations to consider include C-reactive protein (marker of inflammation), arterial blood gases, blood and urine cultures, virology, and urine drug screen. The EEG shows diffuse slowing and may be useful if encephalitis is suspected.

Work-up of dementia

Psychiatric and medical history including review of medications and alcohol/drug use

Mental state examination

Complete physical examination with special focus on neurologic examination
Physical investigations
- Urine
  - Culture (exclude urinary tract infection)
  - Drug and heavy metal screen
- Bloods
  - Complete blood count
  - Urea and electrolytes, magnesium, calcium, glucose
  - Liver function tests
  - Thyroid function tests
  - B_{12} and folate
  - Erythrocyte sedimentation rate (ESR)
  - Syphilis serology
  - HIV test if indicated
  - Other screening tests if indicated (e.g. antinuclear antibodies)
- Chest X-ray
- ECG
- EEG – if indicated by history or psychiatric/physical examination, e.g., suspicion of CJD
- CT or MRI scan of the head – if indicated by history or psychiatric/physical examination
- SPECT scan – if indicated by history or psychiatric/physical examination

Psychologic
- Mini-Mental State Examination (MMSE) – useful screening and monitoring tool
- Neuropsychologic tests may be useful when dealing with an atypical dementia (e.g., Wisconsin Card Sorting Test for frontal lobe function) or when the diagnosis of dementia is in question (e.g. Wechsler Adult Intelligence Scale in cases of depressive pseudodementia). The Alzheimer's Disease Assessment Scale (ADAS-cog) is a comprehensive assessment scale used in research settings

Social
- Collateral information from family doctor, community mental health team, family
- Consider home visit to assess self-care, current driving status, risks to self

Fig. 9.12 Work-up of dementia.

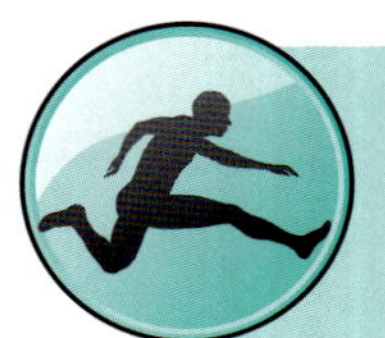

In addition to doing the MMSE on patients you might want to add the specific memory tests that you have already learned (see Fig. 9.2) to make your cognitive assessment more comprehensive.

Discussion of case study

Mr DD first presented with memory loss for recent events. His personality gradually changed (withdrawn, prone to verbal abuse), and he also developed numerous other cognitive deficits: aphasia (rambling incoherently), agnosia (unable to recognize pipe and, later, wife), apraxia (unable to dress himself), and impaired executive functioning (unable to make a cup of coffee). This 6-year deterioration in cognitive functioning associated with a normal level of consciousness confirms the diagnosis of dementia. It is important that the type of dementia is determined; Alzheimer's disease, the commonest form of dementia, is diagnosed when other types of dementia have been excluded.

Two days after admission, Mr DD developed delirium, as evidenced by the rapid onset of a fluctuating consciousness level, disturbed sleep–wake cycle, psychomotor agitation, and apparent perceptual disturbances (visual hallucinations). It is crucial that the cause of the delirium is diagnosed and treated. In this case, it could be pneumonia, as Mr DD had developed a productive cough.

Now go to Chapter 16 to read about delirium and dementia and their management.

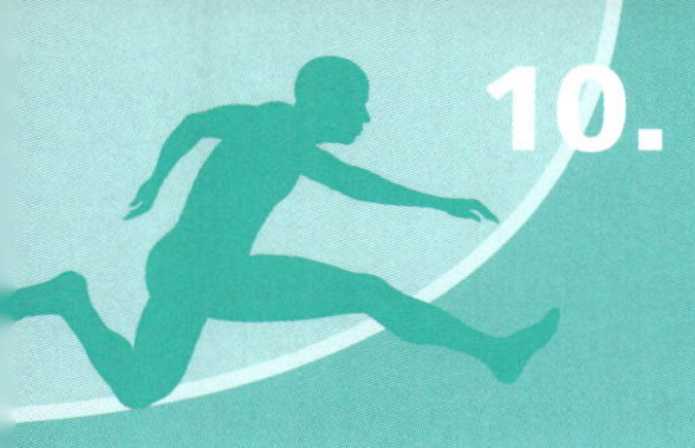

10. The Patient with Alcohol or Substance Use Problems

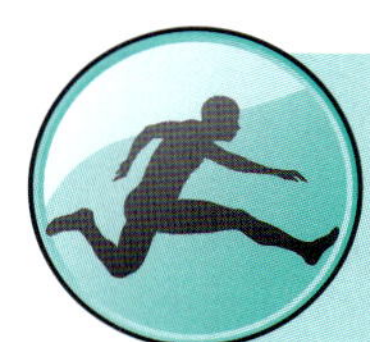

Mr AD, aged 42, presented to his family doctor smelling of alcohol and complaining of depression, anxiety, marital problems, and impotence. On further questioning, it transpired that he was drinking heavily, up to 10 cans of strong beer and half a bottle of whisky per day. He had been using increasing amounts over the past 2 years because alcohol no longer gave him the same feeling of well-being. Now, for the first time, he noticed that he *had* to drink in order to avoid shaking, sweating, vomiting, and feeling "on edge." These symptoms were worse in the morning, resulting in his having two shots of whisky before breakfast. Mr AD admitted that he had neglected his family and work because keeping up his drinking habit was taking all of his time. Whereas in the past he would vary what and when he drank, he now tended to drink exactly the same thing at the same time each day, regardless of his mood or the occasion. Mr AD maintained that he continued to drink although he knew it was harming his liver. He was also concerned about his mental health because, on more than one occasion, he thought he saw a man-size parrot walking around the room, which he knew "wasn't really there." Mr AD had no previous psychiatric history or family history of psychiatric illness and was not on any medication.

(For a discussion of the case study see the end of the chapter)

Psychoactive substances have been used for centuries, and the use of these drugs, especially alcohol, is seen in some segments of society as socially and culturally acceptable. However, it is important to keep in mind that psychoactive substances either activate or inhibit specific parts of the brain, which can lead to a range of subjective feelings or behavioral changes. Brain-altering substances can cause psychiatric symptoms that are indistinguishable from common psychiatric disorders such as schizophrenia and depression.

Definitions and clinical features

The term *psychoactive substance* refers to any substance that has an effect on the central nervous system. This includes drugs of abuse or recreational drugs (including alcohol and nicotine), prescribed or over-the-counter medication, and poisons or toxins.

There are a large number of different types of psychoactive substances in existence. However, whenever an external chemical or drug is added to the central nervous system, the brain has a finite number of nonspecific ways that reveal that the delicate homeostasis has been "upset." Therefore, in psychiatry, it is possible to describe a limited number of typical disorders or psychopathologic states that may be caused by any number of different drugs.

It is useful to divide psychoactive substance related disorders into the *substance use disorders*, which describe *pathologic patterns of substance use*, and the *substance-induced disorders*, which describe *pathologic states directly induced by substances*. Figure 10.1 provides an overview of the substance-related disorders.

Each of the substance-induced disorders that mimic other primary psychiatric illnesses (e.g., dementia, psychotic, mood, and anxiety disorders) is discussed in the differential diagnosis section in

Framework of the psychoactive substance related disorders

Substance use disorders
- Substance abuse or harmful use
- Substance dependence (dependence syndrome)

Substance-induced disorders
- Substance intoxication
- Substance withdrawal
- Substance intoxication delirium
- Substance withdrawal delirium (delirium tremens)
- Substance-induced dementia syndrome
- Substance-induced amnesic syndrome
- Substance-induced psychotic disorder
- Substance-induced mood disorder
- Substance-induced anxiety disorder
- Other substance-induced disorders (sexual dysfunction/sleep disorder)

Fig. 10.1 Framework of the psychoactive substance related disorders.

the chapters on those specific disorders. This is done so that psychoactive substances are always thought of as a potential cause of the psychiatric illness in question.

This section will introduce four new concepts specifically in relation to psychoactive substance use: substance abuse, substance dependence, substance intoxication, and substance withdrawal.

Substance abuse (misuse)

Substance abuse describes a maladaptive pattern of substance use that results in a failure to fulfill work, home, or school obligations; physically hazardous behavior (e.g., driving a vehicle); legal problems (e.g., arrest for disorderly conduct), and recurrent interpersonal problems (e.g., arguments/fights with spouse). *Harmful use* describes a pattern of substance use that is harmful to physical or mental health.

Substance dependence

Substance dependence describes a syndrome that incorporates physiologic, psychological, and behavioral elements (i.e., physiologic and psychological dependence). If patients exhibit either tolerance or withdrawal (see below), they may be specified as having physiologic dependence. However, it is important to note that dependence does not only imply physiologic dependence, and patients can meet the criteria for the dependence syndrome without having developed tolerance or withdrawal. The dependence syndrome (DSM-IV-TR criteria) is diagnosed if *three or more* of the following have been present together at some time during the previous 12 months:

1. Physiologic withdrawal state when substance use has reduced or ceased; or continued use of the substance to relieve or avoid withdrawal symptoms
2. Signs of tolerance: increased quantities of substance are required to produce the same effect originally produced by lower doses – or simply diminished effect with the same amount of the substance
3. The substance is often taken in larger amounts or over a longer period than was intended
4. There is a persistent desire or unsuccessful efforts to cut down or control substance use
5. A great deal of time is spent acquiring, taking, and recovering from the substance
6. Important social, occupational, or recreational activities are given up or reduced because of substance abuse
7. Persistence with substance use despite clear awareness of harmful consequences (physical or mental).

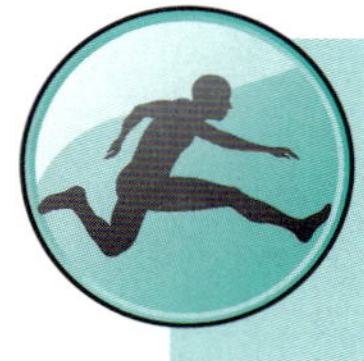

Patients are physiologically dependent on a psychoactive substance when they exhibit signs of tolerance or withdrawal.

Substance intoxication

Substance intoxication describes a transient, substance-specific condition that occurs following the use of a psychoactive substance and features disturbances of consciousness, perception, mood, behavior, and physiologic functions, and is closely related to dose levels.

Substance withdrawal

Substance withdrawal describes a substance-specific syndrome that occurs on reduction or cessation of a psychoactive substance that has usually been used repeatedly, in high doses, for a prolonged period. It is also one of the criteria of the dependence syndrome.

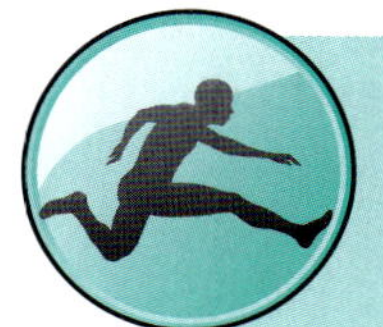

The confusion regarding use of the term "addiction" led the World Health Organization (1964) to recommend that the term be abandoned in scientific literature in favor of the term "dependence."

Alcohol-related disorders

Alcohol use disorders

Any individual who uses alcohol can be classified into one of three categories: the social drinker, the problem drinker, and the alcohol-dependent drinker:

Social drinker

This category includes the majority of drinkers, whose drinking remains within healthy limits and does not cause any harmful effects to themselves or those around them. Some argue that a daily safe alcohol consumption level is one beer or glass of wine or shot for women and two beers, glasses of wine, or shots for men. However, this is controversial as it does not take into account an individual's unique circumstances (e.g., history of substance dependence or family history of alcoholism that could increase the risk of dependence for that individual.)

Problem drinker (includes substance abuse and harmful use)

This category is used when drinking causes secondary physical, psychological, or social harm to the patient. The majority of problem drinkers will not necessarily be dependent on alcohol. Figure 10.2 lists the adverse physical, psychological, and social consequences of drinking.

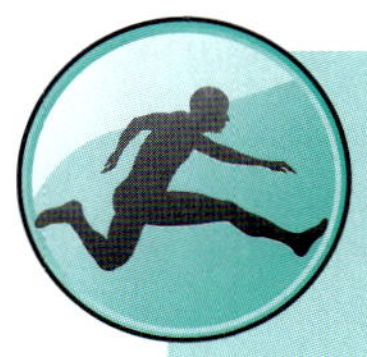

Although many drinkers may not be suffering from alcohol dependence, they could, in fact, be problem drinkers who might benefit from an alcohol treatment program.

Complications of excessive alcohol use

Psychological
- See substance-induced disorders – Fig. 10.1

Social
- Absenteeism from, or poor performance at, work or school
- Legal problems (increased risk of violent crime, drunk driving, alcohol-related disorderly conduct)
- Interpersonal problems (arguments with family due to alcohol)
- Financial problems (expense of drinking, unemployment)
- Vagrancy and homelessness

Physical
- *Nervous system*
  Intoxication or withdrawal delirium (delirium tremens)
  Withdrawal seizures
  Cerebellar degeneration
  Hemorrhagic stroke
  Peripheral and optic neuropathy
  Wernicke's encephalopathy/Korsakoff's syndrome
  Alcohol "dementia"
- *Gastroenterologic system*
  Alcoholic liver disease (fatty liver, alcoholic hepatitis, alcoholic cirrhosis)
  Acute and chronic pancreatitis
  Peptic ulceration and gastritis
  Cancers: oropharynx, larynx, esophagus, liver
- *Cardiovascular system*
  Hypertension
  Arrhythmias
  Ischemic heart disease (in heavy drinkers)
  Alcoholic cardiomyopathy
- *Immune system*
  Increased risk of infections (especially meningitis and pneumonia)
- *Metabolic and endocrine system*
  Hypoglycemia
  Hyperlipidemia
  Hyperuricemia
  Hypomagnesemia, hypophosphatemia, hyponatremia
  Alcohol-induced pseudo-Cushing's syndrome
- *Hematologic system*
  Red cell macrocytosis
  Anemia
  Neutropenia
  Thrombocytopenia
- *Musculoskeletal system*
  Acute and chronic myopathy
  Osteoporosis
- *Reproductive system*
  Intrauterine growth retardation
  Fetal alcohol syndrome
- *Increased incidence of trauma*

Fig. 10.2 Complications of excessive alcohol use.

Alcohol dependence

There are many reasons why individuals start, and continue, drinking in a problematic way. However, after a significant time of heavy, regular drinking, they may develop the *added* problem of alcohol dependence. This means that, in addition to the original reasons that initiated their drinking, they now have an extra problem that further perpetuates it. In 1976, Edwards and Gross formulated a detailed description of *alcohol dependence syndrome* – a repeated cluster of symptoms and signs that occur in heavy drinkers (Fig. 10.3). It is important to note that alcohol dependence does not just mean physical dependence (although that is an important part of it) but describes a heterogeneous collection of symptoms, signs, and behaviors that are determined by biologic, psychological, and sociocultural factors. Also note that the dependence syndrome is not simply said to be present or not, but is described as *degrees of dependence*. There is a difference between the dependent drinker who experiences an irksome tremor while at work and the dependent drinker who shakes so much after waking that he is unable to drink a cup of coffee in the morning without spilling it.

Alcohol-induced disorders

Acute intoxication (including delirium)

Ingestion of significant quantities of alcohol results in transient psychological, behavioral, and neurologic changes, the severity of which are roughly correlated to the alcohol concentration in the brain. Low blood alcohol concentrations may produce an enhanced sense of well-being, greater confidence, and relief of anxiety, which may lead to individuals becoming disinhibited, talkative, and flirtatious. As blood levels increase, some drinkers may exhibit inappropriate sexual or aggressive behavior, whereas others may become sullen and withdrawn. Lability of mood is common, and certain patients become maudlin and overdramatic and may engage in parasuicidal behavior. Incoordination, slurred speech, ataxia, amnesia (see later), and impaired reaction times ensue, followed by lowered level of consciousness, respiratory depression, coma, and death.

An *alcohol intoxication delirium* (see Ch. 9) is diagnosed when there is lowered consciousness or ability to sustain attention, and global cognitive impairment that is in excess of that usually associated with alcohol intoxication.

Alcohol dependence syndrome (Adapted from Edwards and Gross 1976)

1. **Narrowing of repertoire**: The range of cues, internal and external, that affect drinking in a normal person influence the pattern of drinking in a dependent person less and less, i.e., drinking becomes increasingly stereotyped. The dependent person will drink the same type of alcohol at the same time each day in the same place.
2. **Increased salience of drinking**: Maintaining the stereotyped pattern of drinking is given priority over other aspects of the patient's life such as home and family life, career, and previously enjoyed recreational activities.
3. **Increased tolerance to alcohol**: Increased quantities of alcohol are required to produce the same effect. Patients are able to tolerate blood alcohol levels that would incapacitate nontolerant drinkers. Note that tolerance to alcohol can sometimes decrease considerably in patients who have been drinking heavily for many years.
4. **Withdrawal symptoms**: A fall in blood alcohol level results in withdrawal symptoms. This will occur when drinkers reduce or stop their alcohol intake. Heavier degrees of dependence may result in early morning withdrawal symptoms after a night's sleep. Withdrawal symptoms include tremors (shakes), nausea and vomiting, sweating, and mood disturbances (anxiety, depression, agitation).
5. **Relief or avoidance of withdrawal symptoms by further drinking**: Dependent drinkers may need to nip off to the local bar at midday or, worse, have a stiff drink in the morning or, worse still, have a drink in the middle of the night to fend off incipient withdrawal.
6. **Subjective awareness of the compulsion to drink**: Patients sometimes describe this highly subjective symptom as a "compulsive craving" that is extremely difficult to resist.
7. **Rapid reinstatement after abstinence**: Although the dependence syndrome may take many years of heavy drinking to develop, many drinkers may rapidly redevelop dependence when they start drinking again after a significant period of abstinence. For example, within 3 days a drinker might develop severe withdrawal symptoms and be able to tolerate vast quantities of alcohol despite 2 previous years of abstinence.

Fig. 10.3 Alcohol dependence syndrome. (Adapted from Edwards G, Gross MM 1976 Alcohol dependence: provisional description of a clinical syndrome. British Medical Journal 1:1058–1061.)

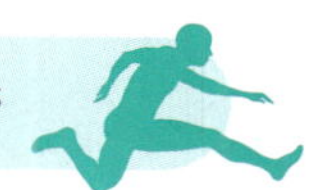

The term *pathologic intoxication* describes the sudden onset of aggressive, often violent behavior, not typical of the individual when sober, occurring soon after drinking small amounts of alcohol that would not produce intoxication in most people. Many authors question whether such a pathologic entity truly exists.

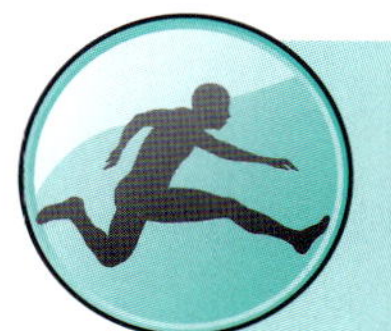

Alcohol intoxication is a potentially life-threatening condition because of the risk of respiratory depression, aspiration of vomitus, hypoglycemia, hypothermia, and trauma (e.g., subdural hematomas, fractures).

Alcohol withdrawal (including delirium)

The development of withdrawal symptoms is one of the criteria of the dependence syndrome. The severity of alcohol withdrawal can be seen as existing on a continuum from uncomplicated withdrawal to life-threatening withdrawal delirium (delirium tremens). Figure 10.4 summarizes the continuum of clinical features of alcohol withdrawal, from uncomplicated withdrawal to delirium. Remember, however, that uncomplicated does not mean: not serious. All withdrawal states are potentially life-threatening, as they are associated with autonomic hyperactivity and can include perceptual disturbances and seizures – and might herald the onset of a delirium.

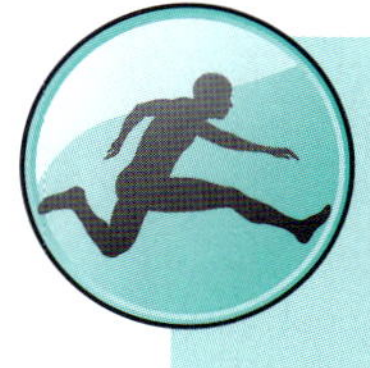

Although withdrawal seizures commonly precede an alcohol withdrawal delirium, the delirium can also appear without forewarning.

Alcohol-induced dementia syndrome

Chronic, heavy alcohol use can lead to mild to moderate impairment of memory, learning, visuospatial skills, and impulse control associated with cortical atrophy and ventricular enlargement. In addition to the toxic effects of alcohol, the brain is also damaged by years of malnutrition, alcohol-associated trauma (head injury), and the effects of multiorgan dysfunction (alcohol-induced liver and pancreatic disease). Subsequent abstinence from alcohol does lead to some improvement in cognitive functioning. See Chapter 9 for more on dementia.

Alcohol-induced amnesia

Alcohol-induced amnesic syndrome, or *Korsakoff's syndrome*, occurs because of a thiamine (vitamin B_1) deficiency and is a common sequela to Wernicke's encephalopathy. Whereas Wernicke's encephalopathy (and progression to Korsakoff's syndrome) is treatable with prompt doses of parenteral thiamine, only about 20% of patients with developed Korsakoff's syndrome recover. See also Chapters 9 and 16.

Episodes of anterograde amnesia or *alcoholic blackouts* can occur during acute alcohol intoxication. Memory loss may be patchy for a discrete block of time during which nothing can be remembered. Blackouts are common and have been experienced by two-thirds of dependent drinkers and one-third of young men in the general population.

Alcohol-induced psychotic disorder

Both hallucinations and delusions can occur in the context of heavy alcohol consumption. A number of syndromes have been described, ranging from fleeting perceptual disturbances with retained insight (*transient hallucinatory experience*) to more persistent, vivid, auditory (predominantly) or visual hallucinations with lack of insight (*alcoholic hallucinosis*) to a syndrome characterized by persecutory or grandiose delusions. These syndromes are distinguished from an intoxication or withdrawal delirium by the absence of clouding of consciousness. They do not appear to be related to schizophrenia and should clear with abstinence from alcohol.

Alcohol-induced mood disorder

The relationship between alcohol and depression is complex. Heavy alcohol consumption may cause patients to become maudlin and dramatic, which may make distinguishing true depressive illness difficult. This problem is compounded by the damage alcohol does to patients' personal lives, giving them ample reason to bemoan their

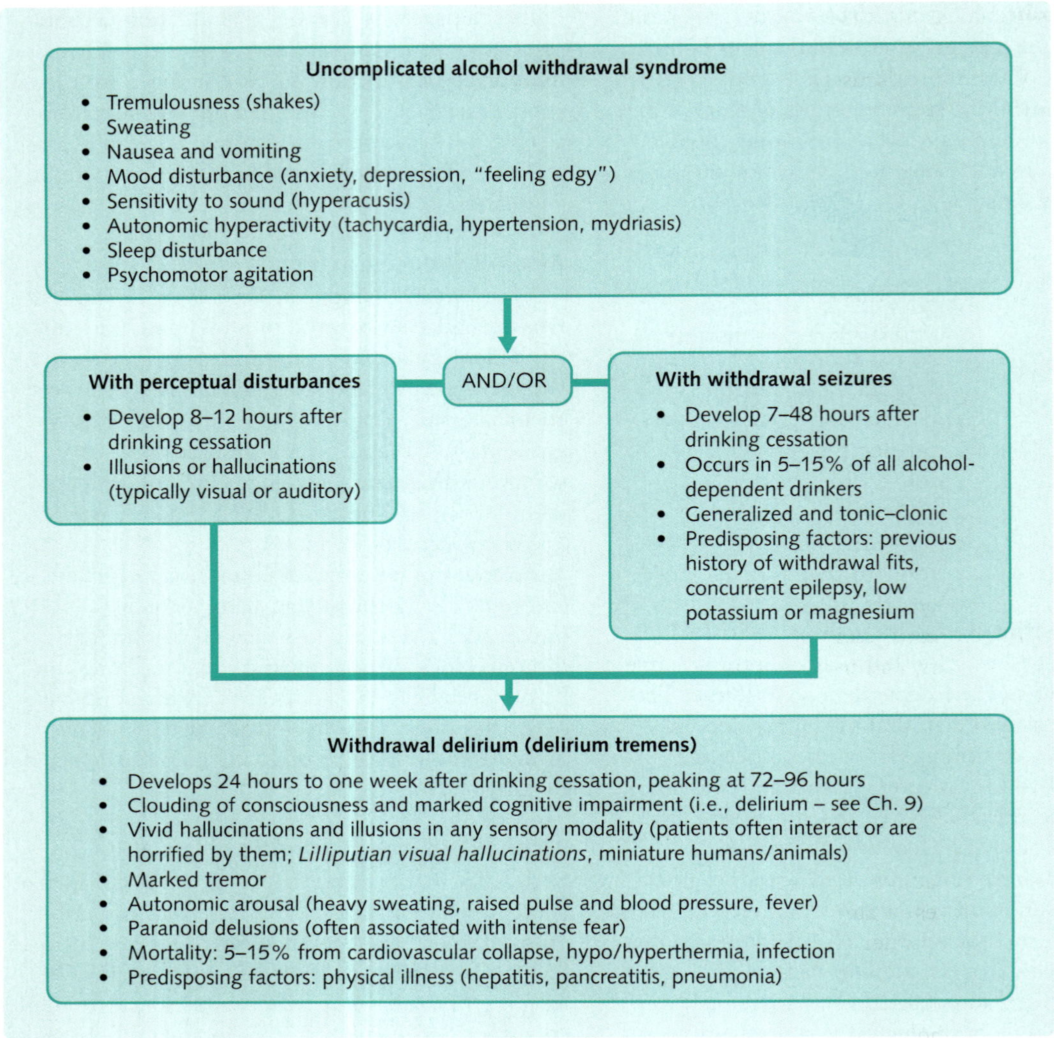

Uncomplicated alcohol withdrawal syndrome

- Tremulousness (shakes)
- Sweating
- Nausea and vomiting
- Mood disturbance (anxiety, depression, "feeling edgy")
- Sensitivity to sound (hyperacusis)
- Autonomic hyperactivity (tachycardia, hypertension, mydriasis)
- Sleep disturbance
- Psychomotor agitation

↓ AND/OR

With perceptual disturbances

- Develop 8–12 hours after drinking cessation
- Illusions or hallucinations (typically visual or auditory)

With withdrawal seizures

- Develop 7–48 hours after drinking cessation
- Occurs in 5–15% of all alcohol-dependent drinkers
- Generalized and tonic–clonic
- Predisposing factors: previous history of withdrawal fits, concurrent epilepsy, low potassium or magnesium

↓

Withdrawal delirium (delirium tremens)

- Develops 24 hours to one week after drinking cessation, peaking at 72–96 hours
- Clouding of consciousness and marked cognitive impairment (i.e., delirium – see Ch. 9)
- Vivid hallucinations and illusions in any sensory modality (patients often interact or are horrified by them; *Lilliputian visual hallucinations*, miniature humans/animals)
- Marked tremor
- Autonomic arousal (heavy sweating, raised pulse and blood pressure, fever)
- Paranoid delusions (often associated with intense fear)
- Mortality: 5–15% from cardiovascular collapse, hypo/hyperthermia, infection
- Predisposing factors: physical illness (hepatitis, pancreatitis, pneumonia)

Fig. 10.4 Clinical features of alcohol withdrawal.

existence. Many patients, however, do develop genuine depressive illness, which will require treatment in addition to abstinence from alcohol. The difficulty in these cases is deciding whether alcohol caused, or is merely associated with, the depression. Note that the lifetime risk of suicide in problem drinkers is 3–4%, which is 60–120 times greater than the normal population.

Problematic drinking is more often a consequence of mania (as a form of self-medication) than a persistently elevated mood state induced by alcohol.

Alcohol-induced anxiety disorder

Up to one-third of drinkers have significant anxiety symptoms. As in depression, establishing alcohol as a causal factor in anxiety disorders is difficult. The anxiolytic properties of alcohol often result in attempts at self-medication in patients with agoraphobia and social phobia, and alcohol withdrawal symptoms can mimic anxiety and panic symptoms. Nevertheless, alcohol use should always be considered as a direct causal factor for patients presenting with an anxiety disorder.

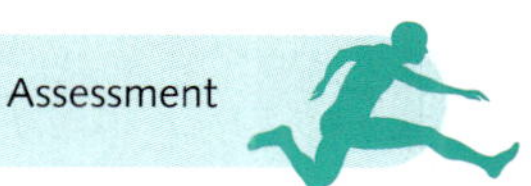

Other alcohol-induced disorders

Alcohol can cause sleep disorders and sexual dysfunction, which are discussed in Chapters 21 and 22.

Other substance-related disorders

It is beyond the scope of this book to describe the individual psychiatric consequences of each of the illicit drugs in detail, as has been done with alcohol. However, like alcohol, other substance-related disorders are classified as substance use disorders (harmful use or dependence syndrome) or substance-induced disorders (e.g., acute intoxication, psychotic disorder) – see Figure 10.1. Try to think of the many drugs of abuse in principal groups according to their characteristics and effects, namely, *opiates*, *stimulants*, *hallucinogens*, *depressants*, *cannabinoids*, *dissociative anesthetics*, and *inhalants*, as described in Figure 10.5.

Differential diagnosis of patients using alcohol or other drugs

Patients using psychoactive substances can present with the exact features of almost any known primary psychiatric disorder (psychotic disorders, mood disorders, dementia, delirium, amnesic disorders, anxiety disorders). Therefore, patients presenting with psychological symptoms and concurrent psychoactive drug use are a diagnostic challenge. There are three diagnostic possibilities:

1. There is a primary psychiatric disorder such as depression or schizophrenia and the patient is coincidentally using drugs or alcohol (remember that patients suffering from mental illness often use psychoactive substances to obtain relief from their symptoms, which is also described as self-medication).
2. The symptoms are entirely due to the direct effect of the drug and no primary psychiatric diagnosis exists.
3. Or, as is often the case, psychiatric symptoms may be due to a combination of the above, as occurs when psychoactive drugs act on patients with a *predisposing vulnerability* to the development of mental illness.

The following features suggest a drug-induced psychiatric disorder:

- The psychological symptoms are known to be associated with the specific drug in question (e.g., psychotic features with amphetamine use).
- There is a temporal relationship (hours or days) between the use of the suspected drug and the development of psychological symptoms.
- There is a complete recovery from all psychological symptoms after termination of the suspected drug use.
- There is an absence of evidence to suggest an alternative explanation for psychological symptoms (e.g., previous history of primary psychiatric illness or family history of psychiatric illness).

Assessment

Clinical

The **CAGE** questionnaire is a simple tool to screen for alcohol dependence. If patients answer affirmatively to two or more questions, regard the screen as positive and check whether they meet the definitive criteria for the alcohol dependence syndrome.

1. Have you ever felt you ought to **C**ut down on your drinking?
2. Have people ever **A**nnoyed you by criticizing your drinking?
3. Have you ever felt **G**uilty about your drinking?
4. Have you ever needed a drink first thing in the morning to steady your nerves or get rid of a hangover ("**e**ye-opener")?

The Alcohol Use Disorders Identification Test (AUDIT), which was developed by the World Health Organization, is a 10-item screening questionnaire for problem drinking with three questions on the amount and frequency of drinking, four questions on harmful alcohol use and three questions on alcohol dependence. It takes 3 minutes to complete and score, and is being used increasingly in many segments of health care.

The *physical examination* requires an awareness of the acute and long-term effects of alcohol or substance use and should focus on:

- Evidence of acute use or intoxication (e.g., pupil constriction with opiate use; incoordination and slurred speech with alcohol use)

Effects of the drugs of abuse			
Drug group	**Common examples**	**Psychological effects**	**Physical effects**
Opiates and morphine derivatives	Morphine, heroin or diamorphine (*smack*), codeine, methadone, opium	Euphoria, drowsiness, apathy, personality change	Miosis, conjuctival injection, nausea, pruritus, constipation, bradycardia, respiratory depression, coma
Stimulants	Amphetamine (*speed*), cocaine, crack cocaine, methylenedioxy-methamphetamine (*MDMA*, *Ecstasy*, *E*), nicotine, methylphenidate	Alertness, hyperactivity, euphoria, irritability, aggression, paranoid ideas, hallucinations (e.g., formication – cocaine), psychosis	Mydriasis, tremor, hypertension, tachycardia, arrhythmias, perspiration, fever (esp. *Ecstasy*), convulsions, perforated nasal septum (cocaine)
Hallucinogens	Lysergic acid diethylamine (*LSD*, *acid*), mescaline, psilocybin (*magic mushrooms*)	Marked perceptual disturbances including chronic flashbacks, paranoid ideas, suicidal and homicidal ideas, psychosis	Mydriasis, conjunctival injection, hypertension, tachycardia, perspiration, fever, loss of appetite, weakness, tremors
Central nervous system depressants	Benzodiazepines, barbiturates	Drowsiness, disinhibition, confusion, poor concentration, reduced anxiety, feeling of well-being	Miosis, hypotension, seizures, impaired coordination, respiratory depression
Cannabinoids	Cannabis (*dope*, *weed*, *grass*), hashish, hash oil	Euphoria, relaxation, altered time perception, psychosis	Impaired coordination and reaction time, conjunctival injection, nystagmus, dry mouth
Dissociative anesthetics	Ketamine, phencyclidine (*PCP*, *angel dust*)	Hallucinations, paranoid ideas, thought disorganization, aggression	Mydriasis, tachycardia, hypertension
Inhalants	Aerosols, paint, glue, lighter fluid, benzene, gases	Disinhibition, stimulation, euphoria, clouded consciousness, hallucinations, psychosis	Headache, nausea, slurred speech, loss of motor coordination, muscle weakness, damage to brain/ bone marrow/liver/ kidneys/myocardium, sudden death

Fig. 10.5 Effects of the drugs of abuse.

- Signs of withdrawal (e.g., tremulousness, sweating, nausea and vomiting, tachycardia, and pupil dilatation with alcohol withdrawal)
- Immediate and short-term medical complications of substance use (e.g., head injury following alcohol intoxication, local and systemic infection caused by intravenous drug use)
- Long-term medical complications (e.g., alcohol-related liver disease, hepatitis B or C, or HIV infection with intravenous drug use).

Special investigations

Nonspecific investigations are useful to exclude longer-term complications of alcohol (see Fig. 10.2) and substance misuse, and include a complete blood count, BUN and electrolytes, liver function tests, ECG, chest X-ray, hepatitis serology, and an HIV test. If the patient is suffering from a withdrawal delirium, specific investigations may be necessary to exclude an additional complication (e.g., infection, head injury, brain abscess). A urine

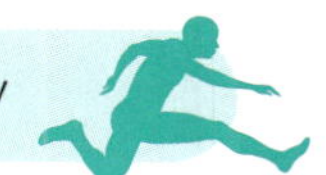

drug-screening test is essential whenever the use of psychoactive substances is suspected.

There is no 100% sensitive and 100% specific test for heavy drinking. Therefore, the following screening tests are of use only in a population with a high prevalence of excess alcohol consumption (to limit the false positives) and when used in combination (to improve the sensitivity and specificity):

- The *mean corpuscular volume* (MCV) measures the size of red blood cells. However, an increased MCV only has a sensitivity of 20–50% and a specificity of 55–100% for heavy drinking. Remember that, because of the long life of red blood cells (120 days), the MCV may remain elevated for some time after drinking cessation.
- The raised liver enzymes, *gamma glutamyl transpeptidase (GGT)*, *aspartate aminotransferase (AST)*, and *alanine aminotransferase (ALT)*, all indicate alcohol-related liver damage. The most useful of these, GGT, only has a sensitivity of 20–90% and a specificity of 55–100%, making its reliability questionable. The GGT will fall more rapidly after drinking cessation than the MCV.
- *Blood alcohol concentration (BAC)*, or breath alcohol (via a breathalyzer) as an indirect measure, only detects recent alcohol use. However, the finding of a high alcohol concentration (more than 100 mg/100 mL) in the absence of signs of intoxication suggests some degree of tolerance, which is likely to be indicative of chronic heavy drinking.
- Elevated *triglycerides*, *cholesterol*, and *uric acid* can all be increased secondary to alcohol use but are very nonspecific and of limited clinical use.

All patients, especially young psychotic patients who are suspected of having a substance-induced psychiatric disorder, should have a urine drug-screening test. It is important to collect the urine as soon as possible because the half-lives of some drugs are short.

The sensitivity and specificity of the blood investigations as screening tests for heavy drinking may be improved when they are used in combination. For example, a measurement of MCV and GGT in combination is far more useful than any of these in isolation.

Discussion of case study

Mr AD is a problem drinker (alcohol causing physical, psychological, and social harm). He also has the added problem of alcohol dependence, as evidenced by the tolerance, withdrawal symptoms, relief of withdrawal by drinking, salience of drinking, narrowing of repertoire (Edwards and Gross criteria), and also continued drinking despite awareness of harmful consequences (DSM-IV-TR criteria). He has physical (sexual, possibly other systems), social (marital discord, neglect of family and work), and psychological (depression, anxiety, hallucinations) complications of his alcohol use. In relation to the depression, anxiety, and hallucinations, it is important to rule out a mental illness, which will require extraclinical attention, apart from treating the alcohol dependence. The absence of family or personal history for psychiatric illness suggests that the depression, anxiety, and hallucinations will resolve with abstinence. The visual hallucinations may be symptomatic of a withdrawal syndrome or be one of the perceptual disturbances sometimes caused by heavy alcohol use – in this case, *transient hallucinatory experience*, as Mr AD has retained insight.

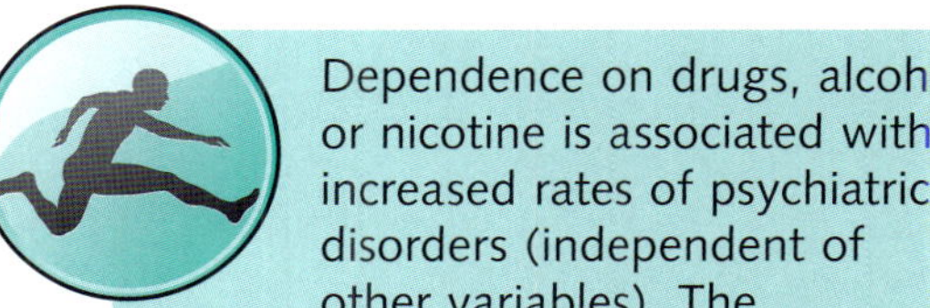

Dependence on drugs, alcohol, or nicotine is associated with increased rates of psychiatric disorders (independent of other variables). The importance of this is that clinicians should screen for other psychiatric disorders when assessing individuals with dependence.

Now go to Chapter 17 to read about the alcohol and substance disorders and their management.

11. The Patient with Personality and Impulse-Control Problems

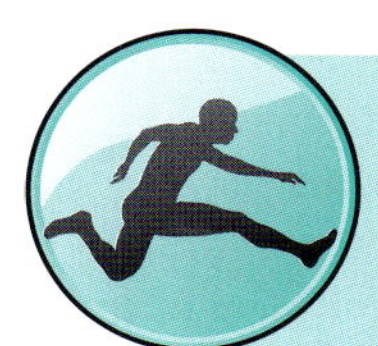

The on-call psychiatrist was asked to assess Ms BP, a 27-year-old woman who had been known to the mental health services since the age of 17 with a condition that had changed little in 10 years. She lived with her mother, who had contacted the PCP because Ms BP was threatening to throw herself in front of a bus. From her notes, the PCP noted that Ms BP had a long history of deliberate self-harm that included self-inflicted cuts to her arms, thighs, and torso and repeated overdoses. Ms BP had been sexually abused as a child by her father, who was serving a prison sentence. She had a "love–hate" relationship with her mother, who was inclined to challenge Ms BP's promiscuous behavior and binge drinking, which led to many heated arguments. Despite maintaining that all she ever wanted was love, Ms BP was unable to form any lasting relationships. She had a pattern of either idealizing or devaluing the virtues of those close to her and alternated between the extremes of helpless submissiveness and aggressive dominance. After the psychiatrist arrived, Ms BP told him that she was feeling "more depressed than ever" because her mother had suggested that she move into her own house. With gentle questioning it transpired that she was afraid that her mother would stop caring for her if she moved out. The psychiatrist, who had known Ms BP for years, recognized that this behavior was not unusual for her and was able to comfort her by helping her to see another perspective to her mother's suggestion. Ms BP's mood lifted and her suicidal ideation resolved.

(For a discussion of the case study see the end of the chapter)

People use the term "personality" in varying contexts to mean any number of things. In fact, the term has over 100 different definitions in the psychological literature. Amid the lack of consensus on what defines personality, there is little doubt that certain people seem to experience and interact with the world in a way that is relatively different to similar individuals in their culture, and some of these people may come to the attention of health workers. The description and management of what has been arbitrarily designated "personality disorder" is one of the most controversial subjects in psychiatry. Not only are personality disorders associated with significant distress to the sufferer, but they also place a substantial burden on health-care, social, and criminal justice agencies.

Definitions and clinical features

The DSM-IV-TR defines *personality traits* as enduring patterns of perceiving, thinking about, and relating to the environment and oneself that are exhibited in a wide range of social and personal contexts. It is only when an individual has traits that are persistently inflexible and maladaptive but stable over time and that cause significant personal distress or functional impairment that a *personality disorder* is said to exist.

Patients with a personality disorder do not regard their patterns of behavior and coping style as inherently abnormal and therefore will not present with that as their primary complaint. Instead, they usually present to the health-care services with a wide range of problems related or

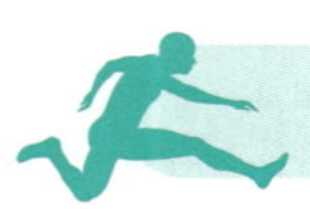

consequent to their abnormal personality traits (e.g., deliberate self-harm, feelings of depression or anxiety, violence or disorderly conduct, posttraumatic stress disorder, eating disorders, dissociative disorders, somatoform disorders, factitious disorders). Also note that having a significant major psychiatric illness such as schizophrenia does not preclude patients from also having a personality disorder (30–60% of patients with a psychotic disorder also have a personality disorder).

The DSM-IV-TR separates axis II conditions (personality disorders and mental retardation) from axis I conditions (major mental illnesses, e.g., psychotic and mood disorders) so that both are considered when diagnosing a patient with florid mental illness.

Classification

The personality disorders can be classified into two groups according to their etiology. The first group includes "acquired" personality disorders in which the disordered personality clearly develops after, and is directly related to, a recognizable "insult." *Organic personality disorder* results when this "insult" is some form of brain damage or disease (e.g., a brain tumor or stroke). It is characterized by social disinhibition (e.g., stealing, sexual inappropriateness) and abnormalities of emotional expression (e.g., shallow cheerfulness, aggression, apathy) and is typically seen in frontal lobe lesions. Patients can also exhibit an enduring personality change after *experiencing a catastrophic event* (e.g., concentration camp or hostage situation) or after the *development of a severe psychiatric illness*.

The second group include what is known in the ICD-10 as the *specific personality disorders* (note that this group is far more prevalent and is, therefore, simply referred to as the "personality disorders" – as will be done for the rest of the chapter). In personality disorders, it is difficult to find a direct causal relationship with any one specific thing, although genetic and environmental factors have been implicated (see Ch. 18). The specific personality disorders usually have their onset in adolescence or early adulthood and remain relatively stable over time.

Personality disorders can also be classified according to which particular maladaptive personality traits individuals display, i.e., based on clinical presentation. In this regard there are two approaches: the dimensional and categorical classification. The *dimensional approach* hypothesizes that the personality traits of patients with a personality disorder differ from the normal population only in terms of degree. Maladaptive personality traits can therefore be seen as existing on a continuum that merges into normality. The dimensional approach is used predominantly in the research of personality disorders and is measured by personality inventories (e.g., Minnesota Multiphasic Personality Inventory [MMPI]). The DSM-IV-TR primarily use the *categorical approach*, which assumes the existence of distinct types of personality disorder and therefore classifies patients into discrete categories as summarized in Figure 11.1. Despite the widespread use of the categorical approach in clinical practice, it seldom conforms to reality as there is a considerable overlap of traits and most individuals do not fit perfectly into these described categories.

In an attempt to simplify the classification of personality disorders even further, the DSM-IV-TR has designated three personality clusters based on general similarities. *Cluster A*, which includes paranoid, schizoid, and schizotypal personality disorders, describes individuals who appear odd or eccentric. *Cluster B*, which includes borderline, antisocial (dyssocial), histrionic, and narcissistic personality disorders, describes individuals who appear dramatic, emotional, or erratic. *Cluster C*, which includes avoidant, dependent, and obsessive-compulsive (anankastic) personality disorders, describes individuals who appear anxious or fearful.

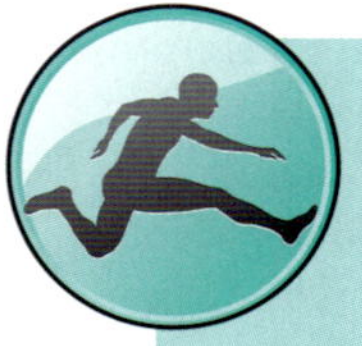

Despite the name, the majority of patients with obsessive-compulsive disorder do not meet the criteria for obsessive-compulsive personality disorder.

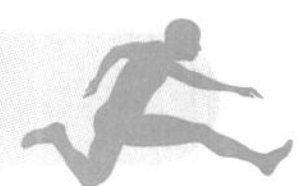

Categorical classification of the personality disorders	
Cluster A: "odd or eccentric"	
Paranoid personality disorder	Suspects others are exploiting, harming, or deceiving them; doubts about spouse's fidelity; bears grudges; tenacious sense of personal rights; litigious
Schizoid personality disorder	Emotional coldness; neither enjoys nor desires close or sexual relationships; prefers solitary activities; takes pleasure in few activities; indifferent to praise or criticism
Schizotypal personality disorder	Eccentric behavior; odd beliefs or magical thinking; unusual perceptual experiences (e.g., "sensing" another's presence); ideas of reference; suspicious or paranoid ideas; vague or circumstantial thinking; social withdrawal
Cluster B: "dramatic, emotional, erratic"	
Borderline personality disorder	Unstable, intense relationships (fluctuating between extremes of idealization and devaluation); unstable self-image; impulsivity (sex, binge eating, substance abuse, spending money); repetitive suicidal or self-harm behavior fluctuations in mood, frantic efforts to avoid abandonment (real or imagined), transient paranoid ideation or dissociation
Antisocial personality disorder	Repeated unlawful or aggressive behavior; deceitfulness; lying; reckless irresponsibility; lack of remorse or incapacity to experience guilt; often have *conduct disorder* in childhood – see p. 166
Histrionic personality disorder	Dramatic, exaggerated expressions of emotion; attention seeking; seductive behavior; labile, shallow emotions
Narcissistic personality disorder	Grandiose sense of self-importance, need for admiration
Cluster C: "anxious or fearful"	
Dependent personality disorder	Excessive need to be cared for; submissive, clinging behavior; needs others to assume responsibility for major life areas; fear of separation
Avoidant personality disorder	Hypersensitivity to critical remarks or rejection; inhibited in social situations; fears of inadequacy
Obsessive-compulsive personality disorder	Preoccupation with orderliness, perfectionism, and control; devoted to work at expense of leisure; pedantic, rigid, and stubborn; overly cautious

Fig. 11.1 Categorical classification of the personality disorders.

Habit and impulse-control disorders

There are many psychiatric conditions that feature poor impulse control (e.g., substance-related disorders, personality disorders, psychotic disorders, mood disorders). This category of behavioral disorders includes those conditions that are not classified in other categories. They are characterized by a repeated failure to resist an impulse or temptation to perform an act that is harmful to the patient's own or others' interests. The individual may experience tension or arousal prior to the act, followed by pleasure, gratification, or relief at the time of carrying out the act.

Examples include pathologic gambling, pathologic fire setting (pyromania), pathologic stealing (kleptomania), and trichotillomania (pulling out one's hair).

> The term "borderline personality disorder" is derived from the early 20th century psychoanalysts, who described a group of patients who stood "on the borderline" between the neuroses and the psychoses.

Assessment

Clinical

As with all other mental illnesses, giving a patient a label of personality disorder gives those involved with their care only a limited amount of information. In fact, the clinical classification of personality disorders is often unreliable and, although psychiatrists usually agree that a patient has a personality disorder, there are often differing points of view as regards the subtype of the disorder.

A practical approach includes making a comprehensive assessment of:

- Sources of distress (thoughts, emotions, behavior, and relationships) to self and others
- Other comorbid mental illness
- Specific impairments of functioning at work or home or in social circumstances.

It is usually possible to establish some idea of a patient's personality by taking a detailed history of their life focusing on the areas of education, work, forensic, relationship, and sexual history. When patients are not able to describe aspects of their personality it may be useful to ask them how those close to them might describe them. It is also useful to obtain collateral information from the patient's family, teachers (including school records), employer, and family doctor, all of whom might be able to distinguish between transient and enduring patterns of behavior.

Self-rating instruments

In these self-report questionnaires, patients respond to numerous questions describing various personality traits. Examples include the Minnesota Multiphasic Personality Inventory (MMPI) and Millon Clinical Multiaxial Inventory (MCMI).

Structured interviews

In this assessment, data are obtained from a semistructured interview with preset questions; for example, the Structured Clinical Interview for DSM-IV Personality Disorders (SCID-II).

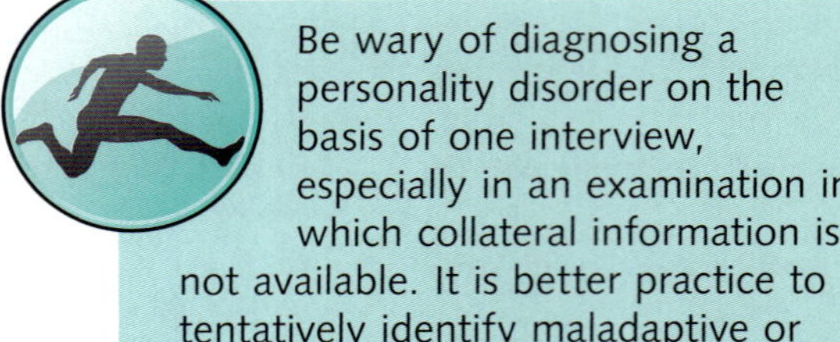

Be wary of diagnosing a personality disorder on the basis of one interview, especially in an examination in which collateral information is not available. It is better practice to tentatively identify maladaptive or inflexible personality traits that would require further assessment.

Differential diagnosis

Almost all the mental illnesses described in this book can feature some of the behaviors that characterize the personality disorders. For example, social withdrawal, suspiciousness, and eccentric ideas in schizophrenia; self-harm, low mood, and poor self-image in depression; and aggression, irresponsibility, and impulsivity in substance abuse or mania. The diagnostic task is also complicated by the observation that many patients with a major mental illness also have a concurrent personality disorder. Therefore, you should always consider the possibility of an underlying major mental illness (DSM-IV: Axis I) before diagnosing a personality disorder (DSM-IV: Axis II), although both can be diagnosed together. A personality disorder should only be diagnosed when the clinical features begin in adolescence or early adulthood, are stable over time and do not only occur during an episode of a major mental illness (e.g. depressive, manic, psychotic episode).

When an individual develops a dramatic personality change after a period of normal personality functioning consider an *organic personality disorder* or a personality disorder that occurs secondary to experiencing a catastrophic event or developing a severe psychiatric illness.

Remember that the cluster A personality disorders may present with features similar to the psychotic disorders (e.g., suspiciousness, social withdrawal, and eccentric beliefs) but are differentiated by the absence of true delusions or hallucinations.

Discussion of case study

Ms BP has a chronic condition that first presented in adolescence and has remained stable over time. She has a number of maladaptive and inflexible personality traits that have manifested as repeated self-mutilation and suicidal behavior; intense unstable relationships; relationships characterized by alternating idealization and devaluation; unstable self-image (alternating between submission and dominance); impulsivity (promiscuity, binge drinking); fluctuations in mood; and a desperate fear of abandonment by her mother. These characteristics are consistent with a diagnosis of borderline personality disorder. It would be important to exclude another mental illness that may coexist with the personality disorder, such as depression or alcohol abuse/dependence. Note that there is an association between borderline personality disorder and childhood sexual abuse.

Now go to Chapter 18 to read about the personality disorders and their management.

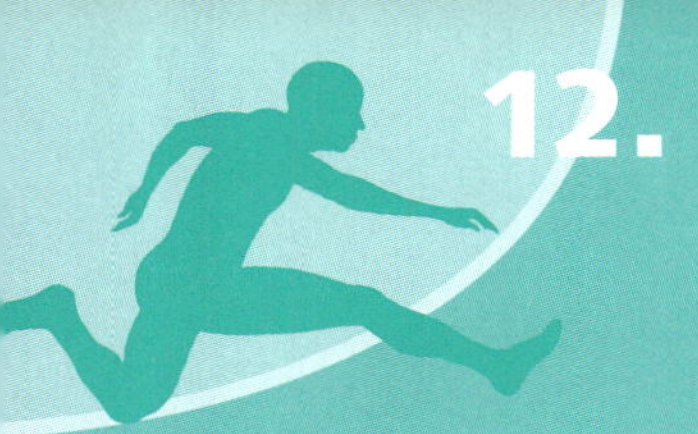

12. The Patient with Eating or Weight Problems

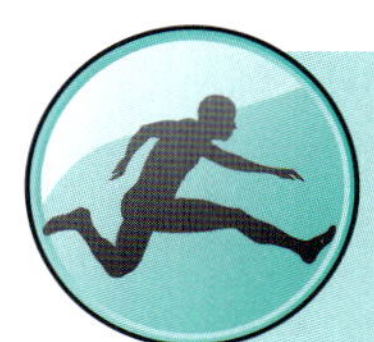

Ms ED, an 18-year-old undergraduate, eventually agreed to see a psychiatrist after much persuasion from her mother and family doctor. Her weight had fallen from 143 lb to 90 lb over the previous 6 months and she appeared emaciated. Her family doctor had measured her height at 5 ft 4¾ in and had calculated her body mass index (BMI) to be 15. The psychiatrist saw Ms ED alone and spent some time putting her at ease and reassuring her that the interview would remain confidential. After an initial reluctance, she admitted that she was repelled by the thought of being fat and felt that she was still overweight and needed to lose "just a few more pounds." She had stopped menstruating 4 months ago and had also noted that she was feeling tired and cold all the time and was finding it difficult to concentrate. The psychiatrist elicited that she only ate one small meal a day and was exercising to the point of collapse. She denied binge eating or self-induced vomiting but did admit to using 20 senna tablets daily. She reported symptoms of depression but no suicidal ideation. Physical examination revealed a pulse rate of 50 beats per minute and fine downy hair covering her torso.

(For a discussion of the case study see the end of the chapter)

Many people are concerned about what and how much they eat. However, certain individuals become so morbidly concerned with their body image that their life revolves around the relentless pursuit of thinness. This life-threatening form of psychopathology needs to be distinguished from other causes of appetite and weight loss.

Definitions and clinical features

Weight loss can be deliberately intended or occur as a secondary consequence to a medical condition, psychiatric illness, or use of a substance. There are two syndromes characterized by conscious and deliberate attempts to reduce body weight: anorexia nervosa and bulimia nervosa.

Anorexia nervosa and bulimia nervosa

A desire to be fashionably thin and shapely should be distinguished from the specific psychopathology that occurs in both anorexia and bulimia nervosa. This takes the form of an overvalued idea (see Ch. 4), which is characterized by a dread of fatness, resulting in patients imposing a low target weight on themselves. This desired weight may be achieved by poor caloric intake, self-induced vomiting, excessive exercise, or the use of drugs (e.g., appetite suppressants, laxatives, thyroid preparations, diuretics).

In anorexia nervosa, body weight is maintained at least 15% below that expected. A body mass index (Fig. 12.1) less than 17.5 is consistent with anorexia nervosa. There is also a generalized endocrine disturbance, as evidenced by amenorrhea in postmenarchal women, loss of sexual interest and potency in men, raised growth hormone and cortisol levels, and reduced T_3. In prepubertal anorectics, expected weight gain during the growth period is impaired and pubertal events (menarche, breast development) may be delayed or arrested.

In bulimia nervosa, patients usually have a normal body weight (may even be increased). The characteristic feature is a preoccupation with

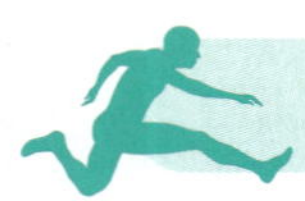

The body mass index

The body mass index (BMI) relates height to weight and is used as a crude test to assess nutritional status in patients age 16 and over.

$$\text{BMI} = \frac{\text{weight in pounds}}{(\text{height in inches}) \times (\text{height in inches})} \times 703$$

Consistent with anorexia nervosa	<17.5
Below normal	<18.5
Normal	18.5–24.9
Overweight	25–29.9
Obese	30–39

Fig. 12.1 The body mass index (BMI).

eating and an irresistible craving for food that results in binge eating, which is associated with a sense of lack of control and is invariably followed by feelings of shame and disgust. To counteract this caloric load, patients engage in purging (self-induced vomiting, laxative and diuretic use), fasting, or excessive exercise, but may employ any number of ingenious, even dangerous, strategies (e.g., diabetic patients refusing to administer insulin).

Figure 12.2 summarizes the DSM-IV-TR criteria for anorexia and bulimia nervosa.

Some patients with anorexia may also engage in binge eating and purging behavior, which is characteristic of bulimia. This does not preclude the diagnosis of anorexia; the DSM-IV terms this "anorexia nervosa, binge eating/purging type." The key diagnostic difference between anorexia and bulimia is that patients with anorexia are significantly underweight and have amenorrhea.

Women who use oral contraception may still experience menstrual bleeding, despite having a low body weight with widespread endocrine abnormalities.

Assessment

Clinical

It is important to define the extent of the eating disorder, yet at the same time not alienate a patient who might be ambivalent about treatment. The following are some questions that might be useful on mental state examination:

Anorexic symptoms

- Body weight and shape can be very important to some people. Do you find that you are quite concerned about your weight?
- A common way of losing weight is to eat less or to exercise a lot. Are these things that you do?
- Sometimes when women lose weight, their periods can become irregular or stop. Has this happened to you?

Bulimic symptoms

- Are there times when you feel that your eating seems excessive or out of control?
- During these times, do you ever try to make yourself sick so that you feel better?
- Sometimes people might use pharmaceutical or street drugs to help control their weight. Have you ever had to do this?

Hypokalemia is a potentially life-threatening complication of vomiting, as well as laxative and diuretic abuse, that usually develops insidiously. Gradual correction is safer than rapid correction so advise patients to eat high-potassium foods (e.g., bananas) or to use potassium supplements. Severe hypokalemia is an indication for hospitalization.

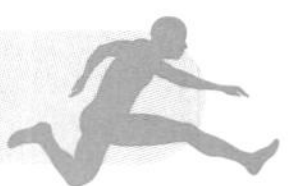

Anorexia nervosa

A. Refusal to maintain body weight at or above a minimally normal weight for age and height (e.g., weight loss leading to maintenance of body weight less than 85% of that expected; or failure to make expected weight gain during period of growth, leading to body weight less than 85% of that expected).
B. Intense fear of gaining weight or becoming fat, even though underweight.
C. Disturbance in the way in which one's body weight or shape is experienced, undue influence of body weight or shape on self-evaluation, or denial of the seriousness of the current low body weight.
D. In postmenarcheal females, amenorrhea, i.e., the absence of at least three consecutive menstrual cycles. (A woman is considered to have amenorrhea if her periods occur only following hormone, e.g., estrogen, administration.)

Specify type:
Restricting Type: during the current episode of Anorexia Nervosa, the person has not regularly engaged in binge-eating or purging behavior (i.e., self-induced vomiting or the misuse of laxatives, diuretics, or enemas)
Binge-Eating/Purging Type: during the current episode of Anorexia Nervosa, the person has regularly engaged in binge-eating or purging behavior (i.e., self-induced vomiting or the misuse of laxatives, diuretics, or enemas)

Bulimia nervosa

A. Recurrent episodes of binge eating. An episode of binge eating is characterized by both of the following:
  (1) eating, in a discrete period of time (e.g., within any 2-hour period), an amount of food that is definitely larger than most people would eat during a similar period of time and under similar circumstances.
  (2) a sense of lack of control over eating during the episode (e.g., a feeling that one cannot stop eating or control what or how much one is eating).
B. Recurrent inappropriate compensatory behavior in order to prevent weight gain, such as self-induced vomiting; misuse of laxatives, diuretics, enemas, or other medications; fasting; or excessive exercise.
C. The binge eating and inappropriate compensatory behaviors both occur, on average, at least twice a week for 3 months.
D. Self-evaluation is unduly influenced by body shape and weight.
E. The disturbance does not occur exclusively during episodes of Anorexia Nervosa.

Specify type:
Purging Type: during the current episode of Bulimia Nervosa, the person has regularly engaged in self-induced vomiting or the misuse of laxatives, diuretics, or enemas
Nonpurging Type: during the current episode of Bulimia Nervosa, the person has used other inappropriate compensatory behaviors, such as fasting or excessive exercise, but has not regularly engaged in self-induced vomiting or the misuse of laxatives, diuretics, or enemas

Fig. 12.2 DSM-IV-TR criteria for anorexia nervosa and bulimia nervosa.

Physical and special investigations

There is no diagnostic special investigation for anorexia or bulimia. However, numerous physical and metabolic changes are associated with being underweight and engaging in excessive purging, as summarized in Figure 12.3. It is important to know and search for these complications because they may be associated with long-term complications or result in sudden death. Special investigations should therefore include: BUN and electrolytes, complete blood count, liver function tests, thyroid function tests, glucose, amylase, cholesterol level, dexamethasone-suppression test and electrocardiogram (ECG). Because of the risk of osteoporosis, a DEXA bone density scan is indicated for those patients with a 2-year history of anorexia.

Differential diagnosis of patients with low weight

Patients with *anorexia nervosa* or *bulimia nervosa* may deny or be secretive about their symptoms, as they are often reluctant to seek treatment. Therefore, it is often difficult establishing: (1) the body image distortion associated with the overvalued idea of dread of fatness; (2) the various

Medical complications of eating disorders	
Related to starvation	**Related to vomiting**
Emaciation Amenorrhea; infertility; reproductive system atrophy Constipation; abdominal pain Cold intolerance; lethargy Bradycardia; hypotension; cardiac arrythmias; heart failure Lanugo: fine, downy hair on trunk; loss of head hair Peripheral edema Proximal myopathy; muscle wasting Osteoporosis; fractures Seizures; mild cognitive impairment; depression *Laboratory tests:* Abnormal liver functions Raised BUN (dehydration) Raised cortisol Raised growth hormone Reduced T_3 Reduced FSH and LH Hypercholesterolemia Hypoglycemia Hypercarotenemia (yellowing of skin) Normocytic anemia Leukopenia	Permanent erosion of dental enamel; dental cavities Enlargement of salivary glands (especially parotid) Calluses on the back of hands from repeated teeth trauma (Russell's sign) Esophageal tears; gastric rupture Serious cardiac and skeletal cardiomyopathies from regular use of ipecac syrup *Laboratory tests*: Hypokalemic, hypochloremic alkalosis Hyponatremia Hypomagnesemia Raised serum amylase

Fig. 12.3 Medical complications of eating disorders.

Differential diagnosis for patient presenting with weight loss
Anorexia nervosa Bulimia nervosa Medical causes of low weight Depression Obsessive-compulsive disorder Psychotic disorders Alcohol or substance abuse Dementia

Fig. 12.4 Differential diagnosis for patient presenting with weight loss.

methods of weight loss; and (3) the presence of binge eating with associated feelings of shame and disgust. Figure 12.4 lists the other causes of significant weight loss that should be considered, especially when the onset of illness is later than adolescence or early adulthood.

Medical causes of low weight include malignancies, gastrointestinal disease, endocrine diseases (e.g., diabetes mellitus, hyperthyroidism), chronic infections, chronic inflammatory conditions, and the acquired immunodeficiency syndrome (AIDS). Note that rare neurologic syndromes associated with gross overeating include the Kleine–Levin, Klüver–Bucy, and Prader–Willi syndromes.

Severe weight loss may occur in *depression*, but this is usually associated with a marked loss of appetite and interest in food. Patients with anorexia maintain their appetite until late in the disease and remain interested in food-related subjects (e.g., low calorie recipes). Note that patients with anorexia and bulimia often have comorbid depression and that depressive symptoms may be secondary to the biologic consequences of starvation and thus resolve with subsequent weight gain.

Patients *with obsessive-compulsive disorder* may lose weight when time-consuming compulsions prevent an adequate diet. Also, obsessions of contamination of food might curtail their caloric intake. As with depression, the issue is clouded by the observation that patients with anorexia also have an increased incidence of obsessive-compulsive disorder (which should only be diagnosed when they exhibit obsessions or compulsions unrelated to food or body shape). Note that obsessive-compulsive behavior may be caused or exacerbated by significant malnutrition.

Psychotic patients may not eat because of delusions about food or hallucinations commanding them not to. The negative symptoms of schizophrenia (see Ch. 4) with self-neglect can also result in substantial weight loss.

Poor nutrition often occurs in patients with *alcohol or substance abuse* and *dementia*.

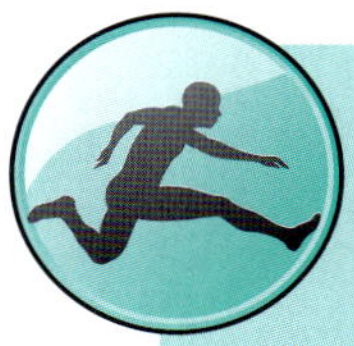

In the differential diagnosis of weight loss, only anorexia and bulimia nervosa are associated with the overvalued idea of dread of fatness.

Discussion of case study

Ms ED's body mass index is less than 85% of her expected weight. She admits to a dread of fatness and consequently pursues a target weight significantly below that which is normal or healthy. Thus, her body image distortion is an overvalued idea. Her weight loss methods include poor caloric intake, excessive exercise, and laxative abuse. Her extreme fear of fatness and low body weight coupled with an endocrine disturbance (amenorrhea) are characteristic of anorexia nervosa. The absence of binge eating precludes a diagnosis of bulimia nervosa, but Ms ED does engage in purging (use of laxatives). Medical complications include amenorrhea, lethargy, hypothermia, mild cognitive impairment (difficulty concentrating), bradycardia, and lanugo (fine downy hair on torso). The depressive symptoms may signify a comorbid disorder or be secondary to the biologic effects of malnutrition.

Now go to Chapter 19 to read about the eating disorders and their management.

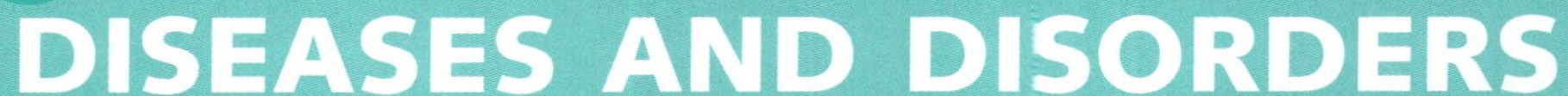

DISEASES AND DISORDERS

13. The Mood (Affective) Disorders

This chapter discusses the disorders associated with the presenting complaints in Chapters 1, 2, and 3, which you might find helpful to read first:

- Depressive disorders (Ch. 1)
- Bipolar affective disorder (Ch. 2)
- Cyclothymia and dysthymia (Ch. 1 and 2)
- Suicide and deliberate self-harm (Ch. 3).

Depressive disorders

Epidemiology

Figure 13.1 summarizes the epidemiology of the mood disorders.

Etiology

Biologic and genetic factors

The monoamine theory suggests that depression is due to a shortage of norepinephrine, serotonin, and possibly dopamine, and, thus, offers an explanation why antidepressants are effective in treating depression. Tricyclic antidepressants primarily prevent the reuptake of norepinephrine and serotonin, which increases their concentration in the synaptic cleft. Selective serotonin reuptake inhibitors (SSRIs) have a similar action, selectively on serotonin. Monoamine oxidase inhibitors (MAOIs) prevent norepinephrine, serotonin, and dopamine breakdown presynaptically, so that more is available for release. Each class of drug makes more monoamine molecules available in the synaptic cleft; these then act postsynaptically, stimulating second messenger systems. Over time this may correct intracellular abnormalities, leading to a remission of symptoms.

It is likely that the monoamine theory is an oversimplification and that other neurotransmitters such as gamma-aminobutyric acid (GABA) and various peptides (e.g., vasopressin) are also involved. It has been suggested that depression may be linked to abnormalities of corticosteroid regulation by the hypothalamic–pituitary–adrenal axis, or to disturbances in the lipid constituents of neuronal membranes.

Twin and family studies have shown that there is a genetic component to depression; thus, a history of depression in first-degree relatives is a significant risk factor.

Psychological and social factors

There is strong evidence that psychological factors may predispose to the development of depression. Families that show high expressed emotion (EE), especially in the form of critical remarks, have been shown to increase the risk of relapse in depressed patients. The risk of developing depression is increased in patients with certain personality disorders (e.g., borderline personality disorder, obsessive-compulsive personality disorder). The risk is also increased after significant adverse life events such as marital separation and job loss. Other vulnerability factors in women include:

- Having three or more children at home under the age of 14
- Not working outside the home
- Lacking a confiding relationship
- Loss of a mother before the age of 11.

Assessment, clinical features, investigations, and differential diagnosis

Discussed in Chapters 1, 2, and 3.

Management

A *biopsychosocial* approach is taken to the management of depression, which means that consideration should be given to treating biologic, psychological, and social aspects of the depression.

Treatment setting

Most patients with depression can be treated successfully in primary care, or in a psychiatric outpatient clinic. Day-hospital attendance may be helpful in patients with chronic or recurrent illness, especially if poor motivation or low self-esteem has led to a reluctance to go outside the home and make contact with others. Inpatient admission is advisable for assessment of patients with:

Epidemiology of the mood disorders			
	Lifetime risk	**Average age of onset**	**Sex ratio (female:male)**
Recurrent depressive disorder	10–25% (women) 5–12% (men)	Late 20s	2:1
Bipolar affective disorder	1%	20	Equal incidence
Cyclothymia	0.5–1%	Adolescence, early adulthood	Equal incidence
Dysthymia	3–6%	Childhood, adolescence, early adulthood	2–3:1

Fig. 13.1 Epidemiology of the mood disorders.

- Distressing hallucinations or delusions or other psychotic phenomena
- Active suicidal ideation or planning, especially if suicide has previously been attempted or risk factors for suicide are present (see Ch. 3)
- Lack of motivation leading to self-neglect (e.g., dehydration or starvation).

Involuntary commitment may be necessary for patients who need admission but are unwilling to accept inpatient treatment because of reduced insight.

Pharmacologic treatment

The antidepressants are equally effective if prescribed at the correct dose and taken for an adequate length of time (with the possible exception of venlafaxine – some studies have shown greater efficacy at dose of 150 mg or greater). Clinicians therefore tend to choose an antidepressant based upon its side-effect profile after discussion with the patient. The SSRIs (sertraline, paroxetine, citalopram, fluoxetine, and escitalopram) are usually used as first-line treatments for depression, although the newer antidepressants such as bupropion, venlafaxine, and mirtazapine can also be used. Some psychiatrists still use the older tricyclic antidepressants (amitriptyline, imipramine) despite their adverse side-effect profile and cardiotoxicity in overdose. Figure 13.2 summarizes some of the factors guiding the choice of an antidepressant.

Prescribed at an adequate dose for a sufficiently long period (usually 4–6 weeks), with appropriate patient education and encouragement, an antidepressant will produce a remission in 60–70% of cases (compared with 30% on placebo). When an antidepressant has brought remission of symptoms, it should be continued at full dose (i.e., at the dose that induced the remission) for at least 12 months to reduce the relapse rate. Patients with a history of recurrent depressive disorder may need to take antidepressants for a longer period, perhaps even lifelong in severe cases. The

Choosing an antidepressant

The antidepressants all have a similar efficacy for the treatment of depression. Therefore, the choice of which drug to prescribe depends on:

- Their side effects; SSRIs have a more favorable side-effect profile than TCAs. Also, side effects should be matched to a patient's lifestyle, e.g., the weight gain caused by mirtazapine may be preferable to the sexual dysfunction caused by the SSRIs; some patients benefit from the sedation caused by some antidepressants, e.g., amitriptyline, trazodone, mirtazapine (see Ch. 27).
- Previous good response to a specific drug: this is usually re-prescribed.
- Safety in overdose; SSRIs are safer in overdose than TCAs.
- For severe depression requiring hospitalization, antidepressants that affect both norepinephrine and serotonin may be preferable, i.e., TCAs and high-dose venlafaxine (SSRIs may be slightly less effective in hospitalized patients).
- Atypical depression (i.e., hypersomnia, overeating, and anxiety) may respond preferably to MAOIs.
- Associated psychiatric symptoms, e.g., patients with obsessions or compulsions, may respond preferably to the SSRIs or clomipramine.
- Concomitant physical illnesses, e.g., TCAs, are contraindicated in patients with a recent myocardial infarction, or arrhythmias.

SSRI, selective serotonin reuptake inhibitor; TCA, tricyclic antidepressant; MAOI, monoamine oxidase inhibitor

Fig. 13.2 Choosing an antidepressant.

prophylactic effect of antidepressants of reducing relapse has been demonstrated for up to 5 years (with imipramine).

Treatment often fails as a result of inadequate dose of drug, duration of treatment, or poor compliance; therefore, these factors should always be ruled out. However, when a patient has not responded to an antidepressant at the correct dose for the length of treatment the following strategies may be employed (often in this order):

- Increase the dose of the current antidepressant (e.g., increasing fluoxetine from 20 mg to 40 mg)
- Change to another antidepressant within the same class (e.g., from fluoxetine to sertraline)
- Change to another antidepressant from a different class (e.g., from sertraline [SSRI] to venlafaxine [SSNRI] or bupropion [NDRI])
- Consider augmenting the current antidepressant with bupropion or lithium (usually done by a psychiatrist). Tri-iodothyronine (T_3) has also been used as an augmenting agent in treatment-resistant depression
- Consider other treatment modalities such as psychotherapy and ECT.

A depressive episode with psychotic features usually requires the adjunctive use of antipsychotic medication.

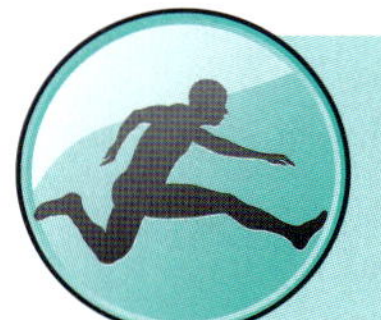

- Patients may respond idiosyncratically to different antidepressants of the same class (e.g., SSRIs), so it is worthwhile trying a different antidepressant from within the same class.
- Depressed patients who are treated with tricyclic antidepressants are often prescribed inadequate doses. A dose greater than 125 mg per day is required to treat depression.

Psychological treatment

Both drug treatments and psychotherapy are effective in the treatment of an acute depressive episode and in the prevention of relapse. Psychotherapeutic approaches (see Ch. 28) may be used as an alternative to medications or in combination with them. Options include:

- *Cognitive-behavioral therapy (CBT):* cognitive therapy identifies distorted or illogical thoughts (cognitions) and assumptions and then attempts to replace them with more "reality-based" thinking and behaviors. Behavior therapy involves behavioral experiments (testing irrational thoughts against reality), target setting, and activity scheduling. Requires between six and 20 sessions. See pp. 211–213.
- *Interpersonal therapy (IPT):* identifies interpersonal problems resulting from grief, role disputes, role transitions, or interpersonal deficits and attempts to modify these. See Chapter 28.
- *Psychodynamic therapy:* see Chapter 28.
- *Family and marital interventions* may be useful for family or marital discord.
- *Dialectical behavioral therapy:* therapy comprised of four skills: mindfulness, distress tolerance, emotion regulation, interpersonal skills. Has been shown to reduce suicidality in patients with borderline personality disorder.

Studies have shown that cognitive-behavioral therapy (CBT) can be as effective as antidepressants in treating moderate depressive episodes. Also, patients who receive CBT following standard antidepressant treatment have significantly lower rates of relapse 4 years later than patients receiving standard clinical treatment alone (35% versus 70%).

Electroconvulsive therapy (ECT)

Indications for ECT in depression include:

- Poor response to adequate trials of antidepressants
- Intolerance of antidepressants due to side effects
- Depression with severe suicidal ideation
- Depression with psychotic features, severe psychomotor retardation or stupor
- Depression with severe self-neglect (poor fluid and food intake)
- Previous good response to ECT.

Course and prognosis

Depression is self-limiting, and without treatment a first depressive episode will generally remit within 6 months to 1 year. However, the course of depression is often chronic and relapsing and at least 60% of patients may have a further depressive episode, with the risk of future episodes increasing with each relapse.

Depression is one of the most important risk factors for suicide; rates of suicide are over 20 times greater in patients with depression compared with those in the general population.

Bipolar affective disorder

Epidemiology

Figure 13.1 summarizes the epidemiology of the mood disorders.

Etiology

Biologic and genetic factors

The monoamine hypothesis is as applicable to elevated mood as it is to low mood, with manic episodes thought to be associated with increased central norepinephrine or serotonin.

Evidence from twin studies has shown a strong genetic component to the etiology of bipolar affective disorder (more pronounced than in depression) and many patients have a positive family history. Concordance rates in monozygotic twins range from 65 to 75%; rates for dizygotic twins are 14%.

Significant life events and severe stressors may provoke the onset of a first manic or hypomanic episode (e.g., there is an increased risk of manic episodes in the early postpartum period). However, there are no personality traits strongly associated with the development of bipolar affective disorder.

Assessment, clinical features, investigations, and differential diagnosis

Discussed in Chapters 1, 2, and 3.

Management

Management considerations include:

- Treatment of an acute manic or hypomanic episode
- Treatment of an acute depressive episode
- Maintenance treatment (prevention of relapse).

Treatment setting

The initial treatment setting depends on the presentation and severity of illness. A manic episode may necessitate a period of hospitalization in cases of:

- Reckless behavior endangering the patient or others around them
- Significant psychotic symptoms
- Impaired judgment (e.g., sexual indiscretions, overspending)
- Excessive psychomotor agitation with risk of self-injury, dehydration, and exhaustion
- Thoughts of harming self or others.

Involuntary commitment is often necessary in patients with reduced insight. Bipolar patients may also require hospital admission for depressive episodes.

Pharmacologic treatment

The mainstay of acute and maintenance treatment of bipolar illness are the mood stabilizers, which include lithium and the anticonvulsants (sodium valproate/valproic acid and carbamazepine as well as lamotrigine, oxcarbazepine, and topiramate). Although lithium and valproate (Depakote) are approved by the FDA for acute mania, they may not provide the immediate behavioral control needed in acutely manic patients. The initial treatment of acute mania often requires antipsychotic medication in the form of an atypical antipsychotic, such as olanzapine or risperidone, or typical antipsychotic, such as haloperidol. Benzodiazepines (e.g., lorazepam or clonazepam) are often given concurrently as they work synergistically to control agitation. These drugs are then tapered off as the initial phase of mania subsides and the mood stabilizers begin to take effect.

Lithium is approved by the FDA for the prophylaxis of bipolar affective disorder, although valproic acid and carbamazepine are often used off-label by psychiatrists for the same purpose. In general, maintenance treatment for the prophylaxis of bipolar affective disorder is indicated in patients who have had more than one episode.

Before commencing lithium, valproic acid, and/or carbamazepine, patients should be provided with information on its potential side effects and toxicity and the need for periodic blood tests (usually 3-monthly) to assess the plasma level (see Ch. 27).

Liver and hematologic functioning should be assessed before and soon after starting patients on valproate or carbamazepine. Research is emerging that atypical antipsychotics such as olanzapine and clozapine may also be effective in preventing relapse. However, if prescribed atypicals the patient must be monitored for weight gain, hyperlipidemia/hypercholesterolemia and glucose dysregulation.

Carbamazepine and valproic acid are particularly effective in patients with rapid cycling bipolar affective disorder, i.e., four or more mood episodes (depressive, manic, or mixed) per year.

In depressive episodes associated with bipolar affective disorder, antidepressants should be used with the utmost caution because of their tendency to push mood beyond normal and provoke hypomanic or manic episodes. In cases where their use is necessary it is prudent to make concurrent use of a mood stabilizer. Lithium, olanzapine, and the newer anticonvulsant lamotrigine also appear to have antidepressant properties in bipolar illness.

Approximately half of all bipolar patients who discontinue lithium will have a recurrence of mania within 5 months. In addition, in some patients, discontinuation of lithium leads to recurrent mood swings that cannot be controlled by the reintroduction of lithium. This emphasizes the need for patient education about compliance as well as the correct selection of patients for lithium treatment.

Psychological treatment

Psychotherapy is performed much less commonly in bipolar affective disorder than in unipolar depression; however, it plays a supportive role and helps to improve compliance.

Electroconvulsive therapy (ECT)

Although ECT may precipitate a manic episode in bipolar patients, it can be an effective antimanic agent, superior even to lithium, especially in severe mania and mixed states – 80% of patients can be expected to show a marked improvement.

Course and prognosis

The prognosis is generally poor as more than 90% of patients who have a single manic episode go on to have future episodes. The frequency of episodes varies considerably, but averages out to four mood episodes in 10 years. Between 5% and 15% of patients have four or more mood episodes (depressive, manic, or mixed) within a year, which is termed *rapid cycling* and is associated with a poor prognosis. Completed suicide occurs in 10–15% of patients.

Dysthymia and cyclothymia

Etiology

The extent to which the etiologies of dysthymia and cyclothymia resemble those of depression and bipolar affective disorder is unclear. There are biologic similarities between dysthymia and depression; for example, REM latency is decreased in both conditions. Genetic studies link cyclothymia and bipolar affective disorder, as up to a third of patients with the former have a positive family history of the latter.

Epidemiology and course

Figure 13.1 summarizes the epidemiology of the mood disorders. Both dysthymia and cyclothymia have an insidious onset and a chronic course, often beginning in childhood or adolescence. A significant number of patients with cyclothymia will go on to suffer more severe affective disorders, most notably bipolar affective disorder. Dysthymia may coexist with depressive episodes ("double depression"), anxiety disorders, and borderline personality disorder.

Assessment, clinical features, investigations, and differential diagnosis

Discussed in Chapters 1, 2, and 3.

Treatment

The two conditions may be treated pharmacologically with the same drugs used in depressive and bipolar affective disorder, depending on the patient's clinical presentation. However, antidepressants should be used with caution in both bipolar disorders and cyclothymia because of their tendency to induce a hypomanic/manic episode. Psychological therapy may be useful for both conditions.

- What are the epidemiologic differences between recurrent depressive disorder and bipolar affective disorder?
- How does the monoamine theory of depression relate to antidepressants?
- Name four vulnerability factors for depression.
- When would you consider hospitalization for a depressive or manic episode respectively?
- What is the role of psychological therapies in the treatment of depression?
- What strategies would you employ when a patient does not respond to 4 weeks of treatment with an SSRI?
- What medications may be used to augment antidepressants in treatment-resistant cases?
- What is the initial treatment of the acutely manic patient?
- What are the advantages and disadvantages of the use of ECT in bipolar affective disorder?
- How would you counsel patients regarding their prognosis after one manic episode?
- What is the relationship between cyclothymia and bipolar affective disorder?

Suggested further reading

Anderson I M, Edwards J G 2001 Guidelines for choice of selective serotonin reuptake inhibitor in depressive illness. Advances in Psychiatric Treatment 7: 170–180

Clark A 2001 Proposed treatment for adolescent psychosis. 2: Bipolar illness. Advances in Psychiatric Treatment 7: 143–149

Keck P 2002 Clinical management of bipolar disorder. Available on line at: http://www.medscape.com/viewprogram/135

MacHale S 2002 Managing depression in physical illness. Advances in Psychiatric Treatment 8: 297–306

Porter R, Linsley K, Ferrier N 2001 Treatment of severe depression – non-pharmacological aspects. Advances in Psychiatric Treatment 7: 117–124

14. The Psychotic Disorders: Schizophrenia

Among the psychotic disorders, the main ones that should be distinguished are schizophrenia, delusional disorder, schizoaffective disorder, and acute and transient psychoses. This chapter will concentrate on schizophrenia, the most prevalent and widely researched disorder in this group.

Schizophrenia

History

Ideas about the disorder we now term schizophrenia crystallized toward the end of the past century. The concept of this disorder has evolved during this century. Important landmarks in the definition of this disorder are:

- 1893: Emil Kraepelin separated affective psychoses (e.g., mania) from nonaffective psychoses; he gave the term "dementia praecox" to clinical conditions resembling the main forms of schizophrenia.
- 1911: Eugen Bleuler coined the term "schizophrenia" ("splitting of the mind"); his description placed more emphasis on thought disorder and negative symptoms than on positive symptoms.
- 1959: Kurt Schneider described 11 "first-rank" symptoms of schizophrenia, including hallucinations, delusions, thought withdrawal, and thought insertion.
- 1970 to the present: the main international classification systems, ICD-10 and DSM-IV-TR, have further clarified the diagnostic criteria. The main distinction between ICD-10 and DSM-IV-TR is that the DSM-IV-TR specifies a 6-month duration of symptoms and places great emphasis on social or occupational dysfunction.

Epidemiology

- The *incidence* ranges from 5 to 50/100,000 individuals per year.
- The *prevalence* varies geographically but is approximately 1%.
- The *lifetime risk* is approximately 1% (see also Fig. 14.1).
- The *age of onset* is between late teens and mid-30s. Women have a later age of onset. Men: 18–25 years; women: 25–35 years.
- Men have a slightly higher incidence than women, although comparisons are difficult because of the differing ages of onset between sexes.
- There is an increased prevalence in lower socioeconomic classes. The *social drift* (impairment of functioning caused by schizophrenia results in a "drift" down the social scale) and *social causation* (poor socioeconomic conditions contribute to the development of schizophrenia) theories attempt to explain this phenomenon.
- Similarly, there is an increased prevalence in urban (inner city) compared to rural areas. Social drift and social causation theories apply here too.

Etiology

The etiology of schizophrenia involves a complex interaction of biologic and environmental factors.

Genetic

There is a strong tendency for schizophrenia to run in families. Figure 14.1 shows the lifetime risk of developing schizophrenia if relatives have schizophrenia. Twin studies show a higher concordance rate for monozygotic twins (50%) than for dizygotic twins (10%). Evaluation of adoption studies provides further supporting evidence for a genetic factor: babies adopted away from schizophrenic parents to nonschizophrenic parents retain their increased risk, whereas the risk is not increased when babies are adopted to schizophrenic parents from nonschizophrenic biologic parents. The mechanism for this inheritance is unknown, although several candidate genes are emerging.

Developmental factors

Strong evidence is now emerging that schizophrenia is associated with complications during pregnancy and birth. In addition, the observation that more schizophrenics are born in late winter or spring has

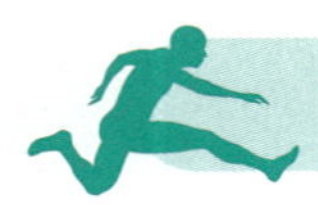

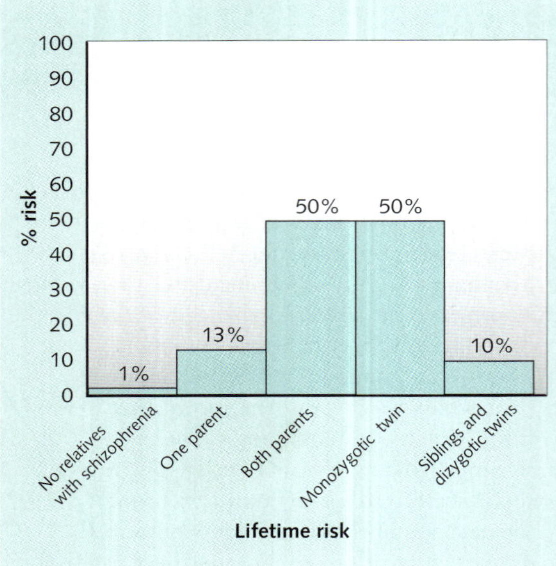

Fig. 14.1 Lifetime risk of developing schizophrenia if relatives have schizophrenia.

If schizophrenia were entirely a genetic disease, the concordance rate for monozygotic twins would be 100%. A concordance rate of 50% suggests that, although a significant genetic factor is involved, there must be an environmental factor contributing to its development as well.

led to the theory that schizophrenia is linked to second-trimester influenza infection.

Brain abnormalities

Increasingly sophisticated neuroimaging techniques are starting to consistently identify structural and functional abnormalities associated with schizophrenia; the findings may be secondary to the disorder itself or its treatment. They include:

- Ventricular enlargement (appears to be associated with negative symptoms)
- Reduced brain size (frontal and temporal lobes, hippocampus, amygdala, parahippocampal gyrus).

Furthermore, schizophrenics have been found to perform worse at specific tests of frontal lobe function and demonstrate "soft" neurologic signs (e.g., abnormalities of stereognosis or proprioception).

Neurotransmitter abnormalities

Based largely on the effects of the conventional antipsychotics, which block dopamine D_2 receptors, the dopamine hypothesis suggests that schizophrenia is secondary to overactivity of the mesolimbic dopamine pathway in the brain. Furthermore, drugs that potentiate this pathway (e.g., amphetamines, antiparkinsonian drugs) are known to cause psychotic symptoms. The recent identification of several dopamine receptor subtypes and successful use of clozapine, which has little affinity for the D_2 receptor but is a strong antagonist of D_1, D_4, and serotonin receptors, suggests a more complex mechanism than previously thought.

Life events

Stressful life events occur more frequently in the month before a first psychotic episode or relapse and may, therefore, precipitate the illness. It may also be that the early stages of the illness itself exacerbate the stressful events.

Expressed emotion

When family or carers become *overinvolved*, *overcritical*, or *hostile* toward a schizophrenic patient, he or she is more likely to relapse. This interaction has been termed "high expressed emotion" and exerts an influence if contact exceeds 35 hours a week.

Assessment, clinical features, investigations, and differential diagnosis

Discussed in Chapter 4.

Management

There is no known cure for schizophrenia. Management is aimed at improving symptoms and preventing relapse. Long-term medication is the mainstay of treatment, although psychosocial treatment is also very important.

Treatment setting

The initial treatment setting depends on the presentation and severity of illness. Hospitalization is often necessary in cases of first episode psychosis and when there is a significant risk that psychotic symptoms may lead to harm to self or others or self-neglect. Involuntary commitment is often necessary in patients with reduced insight.

When patients are stable, they are managed in the community with the help of a case manager and regular follow-up in a psychiatric outpatient clinic.

Pharmacologic treatment

Typical antipsychotics (e.g., haloperidol) have traditionally been the first-line treatment for schizophrenia. However, atypical antipsychotics (e.g., olanzapine, risperidone) are now recommended as first-line treatments for newly diagnosed patients and for patients on typical antipsychotics who experience either inadequate symptom control or unsatisfactory side effects.

Typical antipsychotics (first-generation or conventional) have been used since the 1950s. They are effective at treating positive symptoms (delusions, hallucinations, disorganized thinking) but may fail to treat, or even worsen, negative symptoms (apathy, poverty of thought and speech). They are also associated with extrapyramidal side effects (EPS), including parkinson-like symptoms, acute dystonia, and akathisia, as well as tardive dyskinesia (24% of patients), neuroleptic malignant syndrome, and hyperprolactinemia. Parkinsonism and acute dystonias (e.g., oculogyric crisis) should be promptly treated with anticholinergics (e.g., benztropine).

Atypical antipsychotics (second-generation or novel) have been used in the US since 1990. They are as effective as the typical antipsychotics in treating positive symptoms and may improve negative symptoms, mood symptoms, and perhaps cognition as well. They are less likely to cause EPS and tardive dyskinesia and thus lead to improved compliance. Clozapine and quetiapine are prolactin-sparing. Despite these major benefits, several side effects have emerged that may limit the utility of some of these medications, including:

- Agranulocytosis: clozapine
- Diabetes, weight gain, lipid abnormalities: clozapine, olanzapine, and quetiapine
- Increased prolactin levels (galactorrhea, sexual dysfunction, osteoporosis): risperidone.

With the exception of clozapine, which is indicated for treatment-resistant schizophrenia, no atypical has been consistently shown to be more effective than any other.

Treatment-resistant schizophrenia (TRS) is defined as a lack of satisfactory clinical improvement despite the sequential use of at least two antipsychotics for 6–8 weeks, one of which should be an atypical. In these instances, patients should be started on clozapine at the earliest opportunity. Clozapine is not used as a first-line medication because of its potential to cause life-threatening agranulocytosis in just less than 1% of patients. Thus, regular hematologic monitoring is obligatory, and patients are required to be registered with a monitoring service. Clozapine will benefit over 60% of treatment-resistant patients.

Compliance with medication is poor in schizophrenia, with up to 80% of patients failing to comply. This frequently leads to relapse. Compliance can be increased by the use of depot intramuscular medication (atypical preparations now available, such as risperidone), which is administered every 2–4 weeks, as well as increased social support and patient education.

The length of treatment requires careful consideration as single episodes cannot be predicted and most patients with schizophrenia relapse. After a first episode, treatment may be gradually stopped after 12 months, depending on each patient's particular presentation and situation. For most patients, antipsychotics are a long-term, perhaps lifelong, treatment.

Other medical treatments

Benzodiazepines can be of significant benefit in short-term relief of behavior disturbance, insomnia, aggression, and agitation, but they do not have any specific antipsychotic effect.

Antidepressants and lithium are sometimes used to augment antipsychotics in treatment-resistant cases, especially when there are significant affective symptoms, as is the case in schizoaffective disorders or post-schizophrenia depression.

ECT is now rarely used in schizophrenia. The usual indication is the rare case with severe catatonic symptoms.

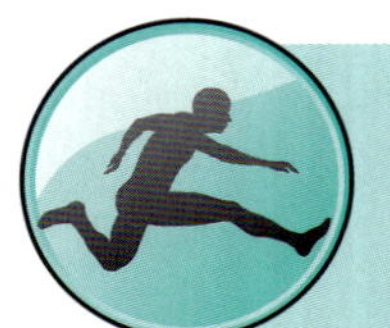

The duration of untreated illness prior to starting effective antipsychotic medication has been shown to be the most important predictor of relapse. In addition, the prognosis improves when patients are treated early with appropriate medication. This underscores the importance of early detection and treatment of schizophrenia.

Psychological treatments

Until recently, psychotic disorders were thought to be unresponsive to psychological interventions, but increasing evidence points toward their value in augmenting drug treatments:

- Cognitive-behavioral therapy has been shown to be effective in reducing symptoms in schizophrenia. It is also useful for helping patients with poor insight come to terms with their illness, thereby increasing compliance with medication.
- Family psychological interventions focus on alliance building, reduction of expressions of hostility and criticism (expressed emotion), setting of appropriate expectations and limits, and effecting change in relatives' behavior and belief systems. Family intervention has been shown to reduce relapse and admission rates.
- Schizophrenia can be a devastating condition and is associated with significant social morbidity. Therefore, the importance of support, advice, reassurance, and education to both patients and carers cannot be overemphasized.
- Social-skills training can improve social competence and help with adaptive functioning in the community.
- Psychodynamic psychotherapy is generally not used in schizophrenia.

Social treatments

Issues beyond drug and psychological treatment should be addressed to enable successful rehabilitation into the community; these include financial benefits, occupation, accommodation, daytime activities, social supports, and support for carers. A variety of agencies can provide these services, notably, health services, social services, local authorities, local support groups, and national support groups (NAMI).

All patients with schizophrenia should be assigned to a case manager and have close follow-up with their psychiatrist to achieve optimum coordination in the delivery of services.

After discharge from hospital and during exacerbation of symptoms, some patients benefit from attending a day hospital, which provides structure and social support during the day.

Assertive community treatment has been shown to reduce hospital admissions and time spent in hospital.

Acute behavior disturbance

Severe psychomotor agitation or aggressive behavior frequently occurs in acutely ill psychotic patients. Note that, in patients who are not well known, it is vital that the correct diagnosis is established. Many other conditions (e.g., mania, delirium, alcohol and substance withdrawal, and dementia) can present with acute aggression and agitation, all of which require special consideration. The algorithm in Figure 14.2 describes the principles of acute management.

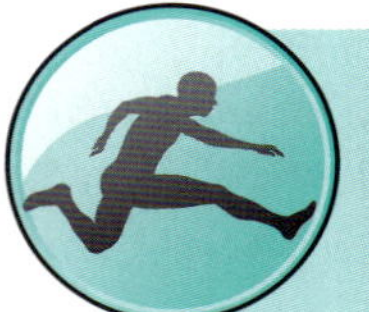

Lorazepam is the only benzodiazepine that has a reliable rate of absorption from muscle tissue and therefore should always be used, if at all possible, when benzodiazepines are given intramuscularly. Other advantages include its relatively short half-life (10–20 hours) and its lack of active metabolites during elimination (no accumulation).

Course and prognosis

The course of schizophrenia is highly variable and difficult to predict for individual patients. In general, the disorder is chronic, showing a relapsing and remitting pattern. About 20% have a single lifetime episode with no further relapses. However, more than 50% of patients have a poor outcome

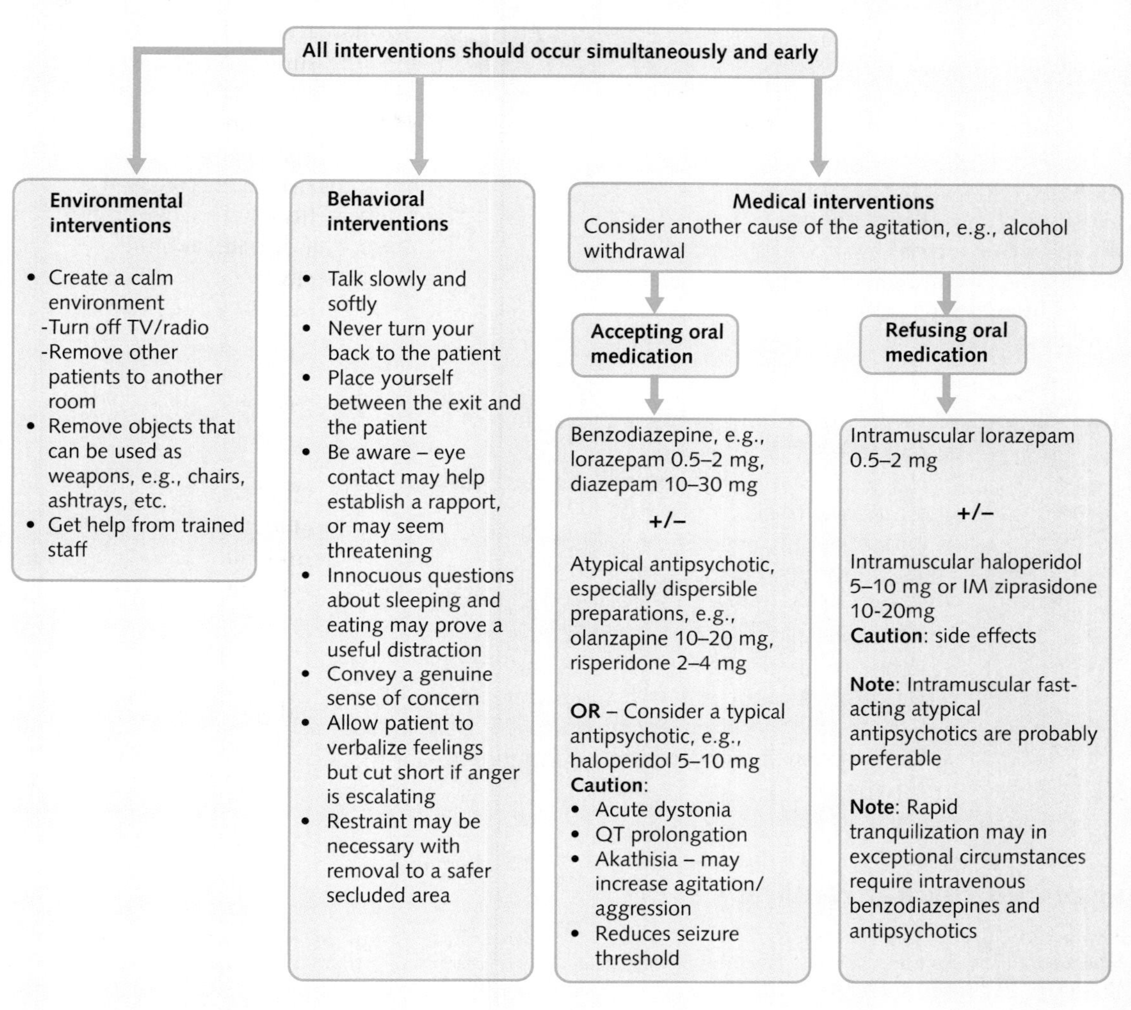

Fig. 14.2 Acute management of the agitated or aggressive patient.

characterized by repeated psychotic episodes with hospitalizations, depression, and suicide attempts.

About 10% of schizophrenic patients will successfully complete suicide. Those most at risk are young men who have attained a high level of education and who have some insight into their illness. The periods soon after the onset of illness and in the months following discharge from hospital are particularly vulnerable.

The lifespan for schizophrenic patients is on average 10 years shorter than for the general population. Causal factors include suicide, increased smoking, socioeconomic deprivation, neglect of diet, and accidents.

The overall prognosis for schizophrenia appears to be better in developing as opposed to developed countries; the reasons are unclear but may reflect better extended-family social support or greater social acceptance once recovered. The factors associated with a good prognosis are:

- Female sex
- Married
- Older age of onset

- Abrupt onset of illness (as opposed to insidious onset)
- Onset precipitated by life stress
- Short duration of illness prior to treatment
- Good response to medication
- Paranoid subtype, as opposed to disorganized subtype (see Ch. 4)
- Absence of negative symptoms
- Illness characterized by prominent mood symptoms or family history of mood disorders
- Good premorbid functioning.

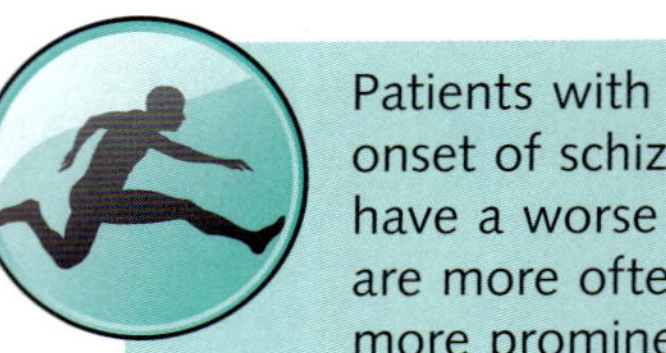

Patients with an early age of onset of schizophrenia tend to have a worse outcome. They are more often male, have more prominent negative symptoms, more evidence of cognitive impairment, and more evidence of structural brain abnormalities.

- Why is there an increased prevalence of schizophrenia in lower socioeconomic classes?
- What are the epidemiologic and prognostic differences between men and women with schizophrenia?
- What is your response to parents who ask you whether their other child will also develop schizophrenia?
- What is the relevance of expressed emotion in families with a member who has schizophrenia?
- Why are atypical antipsychotics the first-line treatment for schizophrenia?
- Define treatment-resistant schizophrenia and its management.
- What is the value of lorazepam in the treatment of schizophrenia?
- What types of symptoms in schizophrenia are associated with a good prognosis?

Suggested further reading

Birchwood M, Spencer E, McGovern D 2000 Schizophrenia: early warning signs. Advances in Psychiatric Treatment 6: 93–101

Clark A F 2001 Proposed treatment for adolescent psychosis. 1: Schizophrenia and schizophrenia-like psychoses. Advances in Psychiatric Treatment 7: 16–23

Seeman M V, Seeman P S 2002 Choosing an antipsychotic and why. Available on line at: http://www.medscape.com/viewprogram/2014

Spencer E, Birchwood M, McGovern D 2001 Management of first-episode psychosis. Advances in Psychiatric Treatment 7: 133–142

Zimbroff D L 2003 Clinical management of agitation. Available on line at: http://www.medscape.com/viewprogram/2311

15. The Anxiety and Somatoform Disorders

This chapter discusses the most important disorders associated with the presenting complaints in Chapters 5, 6, 7, and 8, which you might find helpful to read first.

Anxiety disorders

Epidemiology

The anxiety disorders are the most prevalent of all the psychiatric disorders, with a combined 1-year prevalence rate of 12–17%. Epidemiologic data collected from different countries have shown varying prevalence rates for the individual anxiety disorders (see Fig. 15.1 for the epidemiology of the anxiety disorders). It is important to remember that anxiety disorders are usually underdiagnosed in primary care settings, or only recognized years after onset.

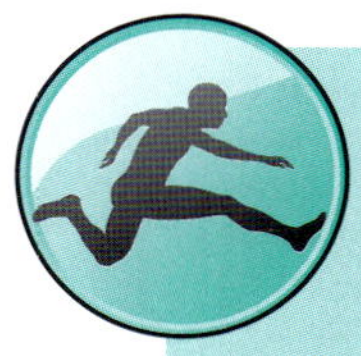

In clinical settings, over 95% of patients who present with agoraphobia also have a current diagnosis or a past history of panic disorder.

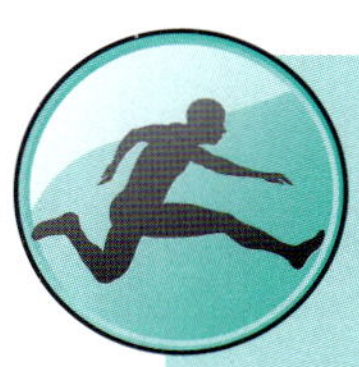

Anxiety disorders tend to be more common in women than men, apart from social phobia and obsessive-compulsive disorder, for which the prevalence is about equal.

Etiology

Genetic and biologic factors

Genetic factors are thought to play some role in the development of most anxiety disorders.

Panic disorder and obsessive-compulsive disorder appear to be the most heritable anxiety disorders, with more than a third of those affected having a first-degree relative who has had the same diagnosis. The genetic contribution to generalized anxiety disorder is less clearcut, but there is an association between this diagnosis and having relatives who abuse alcohol.

Biologic factors have been the subject of considerable interest in anxiety disorders. Defects in neurotransmitter systems such as abnormal receptors may contribute to the development of specific disorders (e.g., generalized anxiety disorder: serotonin or GABA systems; panic disorder: serotonin, norepinephrine, or GABA systems). Obsessive-compulsive disorder is associated with hypersensitivity of some serotonin receptors.

Social and psychological factors

Anxiety disorders have been linked to stressful life events. In posttraumatic stress disorder a significant traumatic event is essential to the diagnosis. Psychosocial stressors may also precede the onset of symptoms in other anxiety disorders.

Some psychiatrists take the view that anxiety disorders are predominantly psychological in origin. Cognitive-behavioral theories suggest that symptoms are a consequence of inappropriate thought processes and overestimation of dangers, as in the case of panic attacks:

- A cognitive model of the panic attack suggests that an attack may be initiated when a susceptible individual misinterprets a normal body stimulus. For example, a patient may become aware of their heart beating. Instead of dismissing this as normal, they may assume that it is under excessive pressure and that something could be physically wrong. This fear activates the sympathetic nervous system, producing a real increase in the rate and strength of the heart beat. A vicious cycle ensues in which the perception of increasing cardiac effort convinces the sufferer that they are on the point of collapse or a myocardial infarction. The resulting crescendo of symptoms may proceed to a full-blown panic attack involving several of the panic symptoms listed in Figure 5.2.

Epidemiology of the anxiety disorders			
Anxiety disorder	**One-year prevalence**	**Usual age of onset**	**Sex ratio (female: male)**
Generalized anxiety disorder	2.8%	Variable: childhood to late adulthood	2–3:1
Panic disorder (with or without agoraphobia	3.9%	Late adolescence to mid-30s	2–3:1
Social phobia	3.7%	Mid-teens	About equal
Specific phobia	4.4%	Childhood to adolescence	2:1
Posttraumatic stress disorder	3.6%	Any age – after trauma	2:1
Obsessive-compulsive disorder	2.1%	Adolescence to early adulthood	Equal

Fig. 15.1 Epidemiology of the anxiety disorders. (One-year prevalence rates from Narrow et al 2002. Revised prevalence estimates of mental disorders in the United States. Archives of General Psychiatry 59:115–123.)

- A psychoanalytical perspective may view anxiety as arising from unresolved conflicts from childhood psychosexual development.

Assessment, clinical features, investigations, and differential diagnosis

Discussed in Chapters 5, 6, and 7.

Management

Pharmacologic and psychological treatments are both effective in the treatment of anxiety disorders and should therefore be used in partnership wherever possible. Figure 15.2 summarizes the most important concepts in treating anxiety disorders. It is important that you familiarize yourself with this table, as anxiety disorders are common in primary care settings and can often be managed there.

Pharmacologic treatment

- Selective serotonin reuptake inhibitors (SSRIs) are considered first-line treatments for most anxiety disorders due to their proven efficacy and tolerable side-effect profile. Venlafaxine (SSNRI) has a similar side-effect profile and also has proven efficacy in generalized anxiety disorder and panic disorder.
- Despite their proven efficacy in anxiety disorders, tricyclic antidepressants (TCAs) are generally considered second-line treatments to the SSRIs because of their increased frequency of adverse effects (e.g., dry mouth, sedation, postural hypotension, tachycardia). Clomipramine has proven efficacy in obsessive-compulsive disorder (OCD).
- Restlessness, jitteriness, and an initial increase in anxiety symptoms may occur in the first few days of treatment with either the SSRIs or the TCAs, which may hamper compliance in already anxious patients. This can be managed by titrating the dose slowly upward or by using benzodiazepines in combination with antidepressants during the first few weeks of treatment. Also note that the anxiolytic effect of the benzodiazepines is immediate in comparison to the latency period of 2–4 weeks (up to 6 weeks in OCD) with the antidepressants.
- Benzodiazepines are used only in acute anxiety (e.g., panic attacks) and in treatment-resistant cases because of the risk of dependency and withdrawal reactions. They should not be used in patients with a history of benzodiazepine abuse.
- The monoamine oxidase inhibitors (MAOIs), despite being effective in some conditions, are not considered first-line agents because of the possibility of severe side effects and interactions with other drugs or food components (cheese reaction).

Psychological treatment

- Cognitive-behavioral therapy (CBT) has proven efficacy in most anxiety disorders and often has a synergistic effect with medication.
- CBT is the first-line treatment for specific phobias, mainly in the form of behavior therapy,

Treatment of anxiety disorders

Anxiety disorder	Pharmacotherapy	Psychotherapy
Generalized anxiety disorder	First line: SSNRI (venlafaxine) SSRI (paroxetine and escitalopram) Second line (as effective but less well tolerated): TCA (imipramine) Treatment-resistant cases: Consider benzodiazepines (clonazepam), hydroxyzine and buspirone	CBT Psychodynamic therapy Relaxation techniques
Panic disorder and agoraphobia	First line: SSRIs (citalopram, paroxetine, fluoxetine, sertraline, fluvoxamine) Second line (as effective but less well tolerated): TCA (clomipramine, imipramine) Treatment-resistant cases: Consider: benzodiazepines (diazepam, clonazepam, alprazolam), venlafaxine, and MAOIs (phenelzine) Acute panic attacks: Benzodiazepines (alprazolam, lorazepam)	CBT (including exposure therapy for agoraphobia)
Social phobia	First line: SSRIs (paroxetine, sertraline) Second line (as effective but less well tolerated): MAOI (phenelzine) – caution side effects Treatment-resistant cases: Consider benzodiazepines (clonazepam), venlafaxine, nefazodone, gabapentin	CBT (including exposure therapy)
Specific phobia	Pharmacotherapy is not standard treatment	CBT (desensitization, flooding, or modeling)
Obsessive-compulsive disorder	First line: SSRIs (fluvoxamine, sertraline, fluoxetine, paroxetine, citalopram) Second line (as effective but less well tolerated): Clomipramine Treatment-resistant cases: Consider antipsychotics, pindolol, clonazepam	CBT (including exposure therapy, and response prevention) Family therapy
Posttraumatic stress disorder	First line: SSRIs (sertraline, fluoxetine, paroxetine) Second line (as effective but less well tolerated): TCA (amitriptyline, imipramine) Treatment-resistant cases: Consider MAOI (phenelzine), lamotrigine	Systematic desensitization CBT Psychodynamic therapy

Note: psychological debriefing after the trauma is not effective and may be harmful.
Note: the first- and second-line drugs in parentheses are those that have proven efficacy from double-blind randomized control trials.
SSRI: selective serotonin reuptake inhibitor; TCA: tricyclic antidepressant; SSNRI: selective serotonin norepinephrine reuptake inhibitor; MAOI: monoamine oxidase inhibitor; CBT: cognitive-behavioral therapy.

Fig. 15.2 Treatment of anxiety disorders.

which may involve systematic desensitization, flooding, or modeling (see Ch. 28).

- In panic disorder, cognitive-behavioral therapy may involve helping the sufferer to understand that panic attacks may start from a misinterpretation of a normal stimulus, leading to a “vicious cycle” of spiraling fear and sympathetic activation. When the patient

understands this model, the therapist may encourage the patient to break the cycle by promoting rejection of the assumption that the original stimulus (e.g., palpitations) is indicative of impending physical dysfunction (e.g., heart attack).
- Effective treatments in posttraumatic stress disorder include systematic desensitization and psychodynamic therapy.
- Other therapies commonly used in anxiety disorders include supportive, psychodynamic, and family therapies (see Ch. 28).
- Counseling may be helpful for patients who are experiencing stressful life events, illnesses, or bereavements.

Inhibition of serotonin uptake seems to be the essential component of effective drug therapy for obsessive-compulsive disorder, as evidenced by the efficacy of the SSRIs and clomipramine. Clomipramine, which predominantly inhibits serotonin reuptake, is more effective than the other tricyclic antidepressants with predominant norepinephrine reuptake inhibition (e.g., desipramine, nortriptyline).

Beta blockers are sometimes used for anxiety because they reduce autonomic anxiety symptoms (e.g., palpitations, tremor). Although they have been shown to reduce performance anxiety (not the same as social phobia) in musicians, they should be used with caution in other anxiety disorders because of their propensity to lower blood pressure and induce postural hypotension (patients with anxiety disorders frequently suffer from postural hypotension anyway).

Course and prognosis

The prognoses of the anxiety disorders vary greatly between individuals.
- Generalized anxiety is likely to be chronic, but fluctuating, often worsening during times of stress.
- Depending on treatment, up to a half of panic disorder patients may be symptom-free after 3 years, but one-third of the remainder have chronic symptoms that are sufficiently distressing to significantly reduce quality of life. Panic attacks are central to the development of agoraphobia, which usually develops within 1 year after the onset of recurrent panic attacks.
- The course of social phobia is usually chronic, although adults may have long periods of remission. Life stressors (e.g., a job promotion) may exacerbate symptoms.
- The long-term prognosis of specific phobias is less well known, but it is thought that simple phobias that persist from childhood are less likely to remit than those that begin in response to distress in adulthood.
- Approximately half of patients with posttraumatic stress disorder will recover fully within 3 months. However, a third of patients are left with moderate to severe symptoms in the long term. The severity, duration, and proximity of a patient's exposure to the original trauma are the most important prognostic indicators.
- The majority of patients with obsessive-compulsive disorder have a chronic fluctuating course, with worsening of symptoms during times of stress. About 15% of patients show a progressive deterioration in functioning.

Somatoform disorders

The somatoform disorders – somatization disorder, hypochondriasis, body dysmorphic disorder, pain disorder, and factitious disorder and malingering – were discussed in Chapter 8. This section will focus on somatization disorder and hypochondriasis.

Epidemiology

Figure 15.3 presents the epidemiological data for somatization disorder and hypochondriasis.

Epidemiology of somatization disorder and hypochondriasis			
Anxiety disorder	**Lifetime prevalence**	**Usual age of onset**	**Sex ratio**
Somatization disorder	0.2–2%	Before age 25, often in adolescence	Far more common in women (about 10:1)
Hypochondriasis	1–5%	Early adulthood	Occurs in both men and women

Fig. 15.3 Epidemiology of somatization disorder and hypochondriasis.

Etiology

The etiology of somatoform disorders is poorly understood, although episodes often follow the appearance of a stressor.

Somatization disorder may, in part, be due to genetic factors, as up to one-fifth of sufferers' first-degree female relatives also have the condition. Theories of a biologic etiology include the suggestion that physical symptoms result from a failure to regulate cytokines (e.g., interleukins). Psychological models suggest that the symptoms are unconsciously produced as a substitute form of communication.

Patients with hypochondriasis may have a lower threshold for suspecting illness or may subconsciously covet the gains to be had from adopting the sick role.

Assessment, clinical features, investigations, and differential diagnosis

Discussed in Chapter 8.

Course and prognosis

Both somatization disorder and hypochondriasis tend to have a chronic episodic course, with waxing and waning symptoms often exacerbated by stress. Good prognostic features in hypochondriasis include acute onset, brief duration, mild hypochondriacal symptoms, the presence of genuine physical comorbidity, and the absence of a comorbid psychiatric disorder.

Treatment

Pharmacotherapy will only alleviate symptoms when the patient has an underlying drug-responsive condition such as an anxiety disorder or depression. Both individual and group psychotherapy may be useful in reducing symptoms by helping patients to cope with their symptoms and develop alternative strategies for expressing their emotions. Figure 15.4 summarizes the role of the family doctor in managing patients with somatoform disorders.

Role of the family doctor in managing patients with somatoform disorders

- Arrange to see patients at regular fixed intervals, rather than reacting to the patient's frequent requests to be seen
- Increase support during times of stress for the patient
- Take symptoms seriously, but also encourage patients to talk about emotional problems, rather than just focusing on physical complaints
- Limit the use of unnecessary medication, especially those that may be abused (e.g., benzodiazepines, opiates)
- Treat coexisting mental disorders, e.g., anxiety, depression
- Limit special investigations (especially invasive, costly investigations) to those absolutely necessary
- Have a high threshold of referral to specialists
- If possible, arrange that patients are only seen by one or two doctors in the practice to help with containment and to limit iatrogenic harm
- Help patients to think in terms of coping with their problem, rather than curing it
- Involve other family members and carers in the management plan
- Consider referral to a psychiatrist or psychotherapist

Fig. 15.4 Role of the family doctor in managing patients with somatoform disorders.

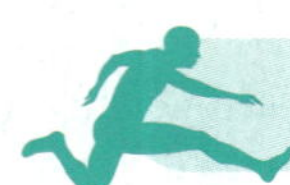

- What are the key epidemiologic differences between generalized anxiety disorder and obsessive-compulsive disorder (OCD)?
- How does the cognitive model account for panic attacks?
- When are benzodiazepines indicated in the treatment of anxiety?
- Which anxiety disorders are treated with SSRIs as a first-line pharmacologic option?
- Why is clomipramine effective in treating OCD?
- What are the treatment options for patients with a specific phobia?
- What is the role of medication in treating hypochondriasis and somatization disorder?

Suggested further reading

Bandelow B, Zohar J, et al 2002 World Federation of Societies of Biological Psychiatry (WFSBP). Guidelines for the pharmacological treatment of anxiety, obsessive-compulsive and posttraumatic stress disorders. World Journal of Biological Psychiatry 3: 171–199

Lingford-Hughes A, Potokar J, Nutt D 2002 Treating anxiety complicated by substance misuse. Advances in Psychiatric Treatment 8: 107–116

Rosenbaum J F, Fredman S 2002 Treatment of anxiety disorders with comorbid depression. Available on line at: http://www.medscape.com/viewprogram/1925

Sanderson W C, Rego S A 2000 Empirically supported psychological treatment of panic disorder and agoraphobia. Available on line at: http://www.medscape.com/viewprogram/350

16. Dementia and Delirium

This chapter discusses the disorders associated with the presenting complaints in Chapter 9, which you might find helpful to read first.

Dementia

Epidemiology

The overall prevalence of dementia is approximately 0.3% of the total US population, rising sharply with increasing age. Figure 16.1 illustrates the increasing prevalence of dementia with age. The prevalence in persons aged 65 or over is approximately 15–20% and in those over 80 up to 45%. The term senile or late-onset dementia is used if the onset of dementia is after age 65 and presenile or early-onset dementia if at or before age 65.

The relative proportions are:

- Alzheimer's disease, approximately 30–60% of cases
- Vascular dementia, approximately 10–30%
- Combined Alzheimer's and vascular dementia, approximately 10–30%
- Dementia with Lewy bodies, approximately 20%
- Frontotemporal dementia, which includes Pick's disease, is the most common form of primary degenerative dementia, after Alzheimer's disease, that affects the middle-aged, accounting for up to 20% of presenile dementia cases.

Etiology (each type of dementia is discussed separately)

Alzheimer's disease

Alzheimer's disease (AD) is classified as:

- Early-onset AD, or presenile AD, if the onset of dementia is before age 65
- Late-onset AD, or senile AD, if the onset of dementia is after age 65.

Some authors further divide AD into:

- Familial type: when numerous family members are affected
- Sporadic types: when no other family members are affected.

Late-onset sporadic AD is the most common form of AD and accounts for up to 90% of cases. Note that "familial" does not mean "genetic": there may be a genetic factor involved, or multiple family members may have been exposed to something in the environment that contributed to the development of dementia. Similarly "sporadic" does not mean "not genetic": strong evidence suggests that genetic factors play a significant role in "sporadic AD." Nevertheless, the onset of familial AD generally occurs earlier than the onset of sporadic AD.

At present, the cause of most cases of AD is unknown. It appears to be a combination of multifactorial genetic risk factors and, as yet, uncertain environmental factors. Increased production and deposition of β-amyloid appears to be the central pathological process in the so-called *amyloid cascade hypothesis*.

Genetic factors

Late-onset AD. It is not clear how much genetic factors contribute to the risk of developing late-onset AD (sporadic or familial). What is clear is that genetic factors are the largest single risk factor, and family studies have shown a threefold-increased risk of developing AD in the first-degree relatives of sufferers. The most important gene associated with late-onset AD is the gene that codes a protein involved in cholesterol metabolism called *apolipoprotein E (ApoE)*, which occurs in three different alleles. Individuals who inherit one copy of the ApoE4 allele are at an increased risk of developing AD, and those with two copies are at even greater risk. Also, individuals with increasing ApoE4 alleles tend to develop AD at a younger age. However, other environmental and genetic factors must be involved because having two ApoE4 alleles does not guarantee the development of AD, and many patients with AD have no copies of the allele at all.

Early-onset AD. Some forms of early-onset familial AD are inherited in an autosomal dominant fashion. From studies of the rare families affected, three genes have thus far been isolated:

- Amyloid precursor protein – chromosome 21
- Presenilin-1 – chromosome 14
- Presenilin-2 – chromosome 1.

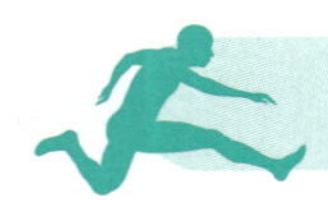

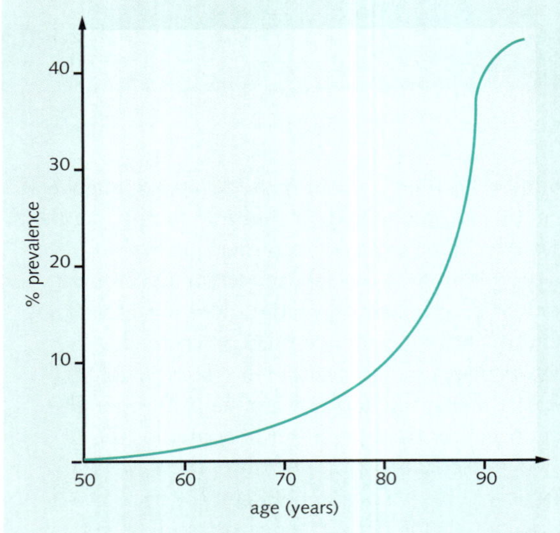

Fig. 16.1 Graph showing increasing prevalence of dementia with age.

Note that these genes that have been isolated thus far may only account for 30–50% of all autosomal dominant cases. These autosomal dominant dementias present between the ages of 30 and 60 years, sometimes as early as age 28 when there is a mutation at presenilin-1.

Note that adults with trisomy-21 (Down's syndrome) invariably develop neuropathologic changes similar to AD by middle age and many will develop dementia. This has been attributed to triplication and overexpression of the gene for amyloid precursor protein (APP).

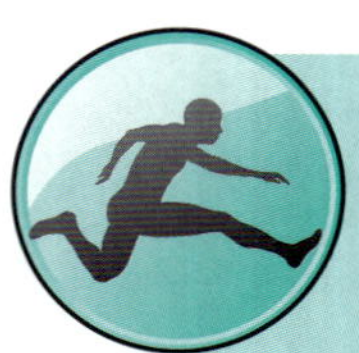

You should be aware of four genes in Alzheimer's disease – one in late-onset AD and three in early-onset autosomal dominant AD:

- In late-onset AD, the gene coding for the ApoE 4 allele increases an individual's susceptibility to develop AD.
- In early-onset AD, the possession of one of the three genes – amyloid precursor protein, presenilin-1, and presenilin-2 – virtually guarantees that an individual will develop AD.

Do not forget that late-onset sporadic AD accounts for the overwhelming majority of all AD cases.

Neurotransmitter abnormalities

The *cholinergic hypothesis* states that many of the cognitive, functional, and behavioral symptoms in AD are due to a reduction in brain acetylcholine activity, secondary to the degeneration of cholinergic neurons in the nucleus basalis of Meynert and other nuclei projecting to the hippocampus and mesial temporal region. Evidence for this theory comes from studies of physostigmine, a powerful inhibitor of acetylcholinesterase (acetylcholinesterase inactivates acetylcholine in the cholinergic synapse), which was shown to improve memory in healthy individuals. This led to the development of cholinesterase inhibitors in the symptomatic treatment of mild to moderate AD.

Environmental factors

There is no consistent evidence to confirm the role of toxins, viruses, and autoimmune factors in the etiology of AD. Aluminum is related to AD in dialysis patients but it has not been shown to increase the risk for the general population. Poor educational attainment appears to increase risk, but this relationship may equally be explained by other factors such as social class, nutrition, and delayed detection in the well educated. Postmenopausal hormone replacement therapy (HRT) appears to be a protective factor.

Neuropathology

The gross pathology is characterized by generalized atrophy of the brain, with widened sulci and enlarged ventricles – most marked in the frontal and temporal lobes.

The microscopic findings include:

- Intracellular *neurofibrillary tangles* resulting from abnormal phosphorylation of tau protein
- Granulovacuolar degeneration (intracellular cytoplasmic vacuoles)
- Extracellular senile plaques consisting of a central core of β-amyloid, aluminum, and silica
- *Amyloid deposition* in the walls of blood vessels.

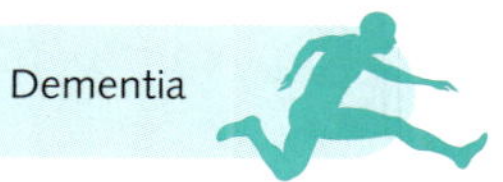

Vascular dementia

The cause of vascular dementia is presumed to be multiple cortical infarctions or many small infarctions in the white matter (Binswanger's disease) resulting from widespread cerebrovascular disease. On occasions, vascular dementia can arise from a single infarct. As with both Alzheimer's disease and cerebrovascular disease, vascular dementia is closely associated with increasing age. In rare cases, the disease is linked to a dominant gene on chromosome 19 (cerebral autosomal dominant arteriopathy). The risk factors for developing vascular dementia are the same as for cerebrovascular disease in general and are summarized in Figure 16.2.

Dementia with Lewy bodies (DLB)

Little is known about the cause of dementia with Lewy bodies. Allelic variation on the apolipoprotein E gene of chromosome 19 may be linked. Lewy bodies are neuronal inclusions composed of abnormally phosphorylated neurofilament proteins aggregated with ubiquitin and α-synuclein. The Lewy bodies found in the paralimbic and neocortical structures of patients with DLB are identical to those found in the basal ganglia of patients with Parkinson's disease. Lewy bodies are also found in the brains of patients with Alzheimer's disease and Down's syndrome. Remember from Chapter 9 that parkinson-like motor features may be a core feature of DLB.

Frontotemporal dementia

The cause of the frontotemporal dementias is unknown. They are associated with bilateral atrophy of the frontal and anterior temporal lobes (atrophied paper-thin gyri known as "knife-blade atrophy") and degeneration of the striatum. There are three main histologic types:

- Microvacuolar (60%)
- Pick's type (25%). Pick's bodies are intraneuronal masses of cytoskeletal elements
- Microvacuolar/Pick's type combined with histologic signs of motor neuron disease (15%).

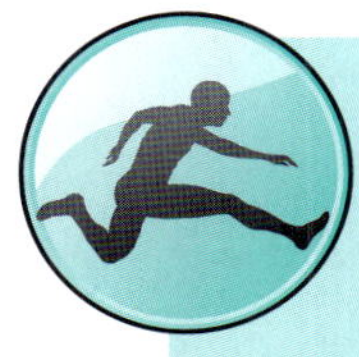

Only a minority of patients with frontotemporal dementia exhibit the Pick-type histologic changes; hence the term "frontotemporal dementia" is preferred to "Pick's disease."

Risk factors for vascular dementia

- Male
- Smoking
- Previous stroke
- Hypertension
- Diabetes
- History of myocardial infarct
- Carotid artery stenosis
- Valvular disease
- Hypercholesterolemia
- Hypercoagulation disorders

Fig. 16.2 Risk factors for vascular dementia.

Huntington's disease

Huntington's disease has autosomal dominant inheritance with complete penetrance. It is caused by a gene on the short arm of chromosome 4 that contains an excessive number of trinucleotide (CAG) repeat sequences, usually more than 40, which results in production of the abnormal protein "huntingtin." The length of the abnormal trinucleotide repeat sequence is inversely correlated to the age of onset of the disease.

Parkinson's disease

Like Huntington's disease, Parkinson's disease is also a disease of the basal ganglia and is often associated with a subcortical form of dementia (see Fig. 9.5). About 30% of patients with Parkinson's disease will develop dementia. The three classic symptoms of Parkinson's disease are resting tremor, rigidity, and bradykinesia (poverty of movement).

Creutzfeldt–Jakob disease (CJD) and other prion-related diseases

A prion is a proteinaceous particle that does not contain DNA or RNA. This agent, which seems to be infectious although structurally simpler than any virus, is able to cause a severe and invariably fatal disease of the brain. All the prion-related disorders result in a spongiform degeneration of the brain in the absence of an inflammatory immune response, associated with the deposition of the prion protein (PrP) in the form of amyloid sheets.

Most cases of CJD appear to be sporadic, affecting people in their 50s, although it can be transmitted iatrogenically (e.g., infected corneal transplants and surgical instruments). It presents with a rapidly progressing dementia with cerebellar ataxia and myoclonic jerks over a time course of 6–8 months. The EEG characteristically shows stereotyped sharp wave complexes.

New-variant CJD (nvCJD) is thought to be secondary to the ingestion of bovine spongiform encephalopathy (BSE)-infected beef products. It typically presents in young adults with mild psychiatric symptoms such as depression and anxiety before the development of ataxia, dementia, and finally death over a period of 18 months. There are no characteristic EEG changes, although nvCJD may have a characteristic MRI picture: a bilaterally evident high signal in the pulvinar (postthalamic) region.

Other prion diseases include kuru (prion transmitted by cannibalism of neural tissue, described in the highland tribes of New Guinea) and Gerstmann–Straussler syndrome (autosomal dominant condition caused by mutation of *PrP* gene on chromosome 20).

HIV-related dementia

Infection with the human immunodeficiency virus (HIV) is thought to cause direct damage to the brain in addition to the complications of HIV infection, such as opportunistic infections (cerebral cytomegalovirus infection, cryptococcosis, toxoplasmosis, tuberculosis, syphilis) and cerebral lymphoma. HIV encephalopathy presents clinically as a subcortical dementia and neuropathologic examination shows diffuse multifocal destruction of the white matter and subcortical structures.

Assessment, clinical features, investigations, and differential diagnosis

Discussed in Chapter 9.

Management

There is no cure for any of the neurodegenerative forms of dementia. Although the prognosis is invariably poor, considerable improvements in the quality of patients' lives are possible through a variety of psychosocial and pharmaceutical approaches. The principles of management are:

- Treating the underlying cause if possible (e.g., hypothyroidism, modifying vascular risk factors)
- Treating associated disorders or complications (e.g., aggression, chest infections, incontinence)
- Addressing functional problems that result (e.g., kitchen skills, financial management, social isolation)
- Providing advice and support for carers
- Symptomatic treatment with cholinesterase inhibitors when indicated.

Specific management strategies

- Family practitioners have a central role in the diagnosis and management of dementia. Dementia sufferers should, however, be referred as soon as possible to their local geriatric psychiatrist and neurologist, where appropriate management and support can be provided
- Assessment and treatment can usually be done in a primary care or outpatient setting. It may be necessary to admit patients with end-stage dementia or severe behavioral problems to a nursing home or specialist dementia unit.
- Disturbed behavior such as aggression or agitation may be treated with antipsychotics (especially atypical antipsychotics) or benzodiazepines. Psychotic and depressive symptoms may be treated with antipsychotics and antidepressants. Low doses are essential since the elderly may show greater susceptibility to parkinsonian side effects. All these drugs may worsen cognitive function, particularly those with strong anticholinergic effects. Be wary of treating a patient with dementia with Lewy bodies with antipsychotics because of the risk of a catastrophic parkinsonian reaction.
- The cholinesterase inhibitors donepezil, rivastigmine, and galantamine have been licensed in the US for use in the treatment of mild to moderate Alzheimer's disease and are recommended for patients with mild to moderate dementia. Up to half the patients given these drugs will show a slower rate of cognitive decline and possible improvement in neuropsychiatric symptoms (e.g., apathy, hallucinations, agitation) but they should be discontinued in those thought not to be responding. Cholinesterase inhibitors have also shown promise in the treatment of dementia with Lewy bodies (DLB) and may soon be licensed as first-line treatment.
- Memantine (Namenda), an N-methyl-D-aspartate (NMDA) receptor antagonist, belongs

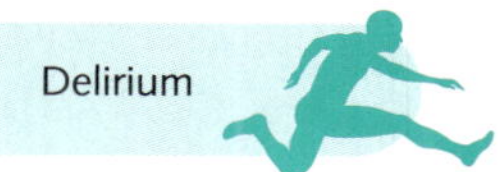

to a new class of anti-Alzheimer's drugs that have been shown to be effective in individuals with moderate to severe Alzheimer's disease. It protects against excess glutamate and subsequent high intracellular calcium by blocking NMDA receptors, thereby preventing the influx of calcium.
- Assessment of functioning in the form of activities of daily living (ADL) scales is useful in focusing on, and developing, patients' remaining skills and resources. Reality orientation and reminiscence therapies have been used to reduce confusion and stimulate remote memories. Practical social interventions such as memory aids (e.g. calendars, notebooks) may be helpful in the early stages of dementia.

- Benzodiazepines should be used with caution in patients with dementia, as they seem particularly vulnerable to their adverse effects such as sedation, with the risk of falls, and marked confusion.
- Remember that 50% of patients with dementia with Lewy bodies (DLB) will have a severe reaction to antipsychotics (even atypicals), precipitating irreversible parkinsonism, impaired consciousness, severe autonomic symptoms, and a two- to threefold increase in mortality.

Benzodiazepines and cholinesterase inhibitors are safer in this group of patients. This exemplifies the need to exercise caution when prescribing antipsychotics and the importance of differentiating the various types of dementia.

Course and prognosis

The course of dementia is invariably progressive and fatal. Successful treatment of medical causes such as hypothyroidism or hydrocephalus usually arrests rather than resolves the cognitive decline. The duration of survival from the time of diagnosis for the various forms of dementia is:
- Alzheimer's disease: 7–9 years
- Vascular dementia: variable, usually less than Alzheimer's disease
- Dementia with Lewy bodies: 1–2 years
- Frontotemporal dementia: 8–11 years
- Huntington's disease: 12–16 years
- Creutzfeldt–Jakob disease: 6–8 months (new variant CJD: 18 months).

Delirium

Epidemiology

Most research into the epidemiology of delirium concentrates on the elderly, who, along with infants and young children, are more vulnerable to this disorder. The prevalence in hospitalized, medically ill patients ranges from 10% to 30%. Between 10% and 15% of patients over the age of 65 are delirious on admission and 10–40% develop a delirium during hospitalization. Patients with dementia are at an increased risk of developing a delirium; in fact, up to two-thirds of cases of delirium occur in patients with dementia.

Etiology

An underlying medical or drug-related cause of delirium, as discussed in Chapter 9 (see Fig. 9.6) is usually identified. The exact pathophysiologic mechanisms for delirium remain unclear, but postulated mechanisms include:
- Alterations in cholinergic and noradrenergic neurotransmitter systems
- Interruption of the blood–brain barrier.

Assessment, clinical features, investigations, and differential diagnosis

Discussed in Chapter 9.

Management

Delirium can be highly distressing for patients and anxiety-provoking for medical ward staff who are not used to dealing with agitated patients. General principles of management are as follows:
- Hospitalization is essential.
- Vigorously investigate and treat any underlying medical condition.

- To limit confusion and foster trust, try to ensure that the patient is nursed by the same staff consistently.
- Merely the physical presence of a reassuring person is often enough to calm a distressed patient.
- Maximize visual acuity (e.g., glasses, appropriately lit environment) and hearing ability (e.g., hearing aid, quiet environment) to avoid misinterpretation of stimuli.
- Encourage a friend or family member to remain with the patient to help comfort and orientate them.
- Clocks, calendars, and familiar objects may be helpful with orientation.
- Typical antipsychotics, especially low-dose haloperidol, are generally effective in treating delirious symptoms, in part because of their sedative qualities, but perhaps also because of their effects on the dopamine–acetylcholine balance.
- Avoid sedative medication if possible, particularly drugs with a powerful anticholinergic effect (e.g., phenothiazines). The use of benzodiazepines requires caution, as they tend to be less effective at managing delirious symptoms than antipsychotics, except in alcohol- or substance-related delirium in which they are highly effective. They may be very effective in managing the common problem of insomnia.

The specific management of delirium tremens is outlined in Chapter 17.

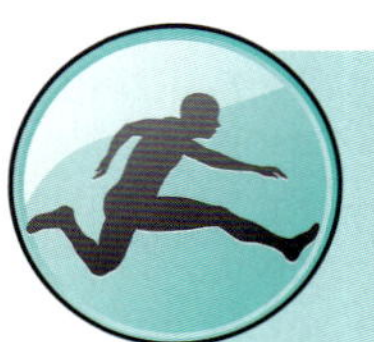

Remember that delirium is not a final diagnosis. This syndrome indicates the presence of a very serious medical condition that should be managed on a medical, not psychiatric, ward.

Course and prognosis

The average duration of a delirium is 7 days. Inpatients who develop delirium have an increased mortality, with elderly patients having up to a 75% chance of dying during that admission. This is unsurprising given the often serious nature of the underlying medical conditions.

- What is the prevalence of the three most common forms of dementia?
- Name four genes associated with Alzheimer's disease.
- Explain how cholinesterase inhibitors work with reference to the cholinergic hypothesis of Alzheimer's disease.
- What are the microscopic findings at autopsy in the brain of a patient with Alzheimer's disease?
- What are four modifiable risk factors for the development of vascular dementia?
- What is the genetic abnormality in Huntington's disease?
- Describe the clinical picture and give three examples of subcortical dementias.
- How does Creutzfeldt–Jakob disease (CJD) differ from new-variant CJD (nvCJD) in terms of age of onset, time course, and findings on special investigations?
- What are the advantages and potential dangers of using antipsychotics in dementia?
- In what sort of patients with dementia are cholinesterase inhibitors effective?
- How would you suggest the nurse in charge of a surgical ward manage a patient with delirium?
- What pharmacologic therapy is useful in delirium?

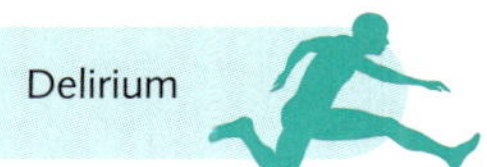

Suggested further reading

British Journal of Psychiatry 2002 Old age psychiatry papers. British Journal of Psychiatry 180: 116–167

McCullagh C D, Craig D, et al 2001 Risk factors for dementia. Advances in Psychiatric Treatment 7: 24–31

Meagher D 2001 Delirium: the role of psychiatry. Advances in Psychiatric Treatment 7: 433–443

Tangalos E G 2003 Transforming long-term care for Alzheimer's disease. Available on line at: http://www.medscape.com/viewprogram/2410

Treloar A, Beck S, Paton C 2001 Administering medicines to patients with dementia and other organic cognitive syndromes. Advances in Psychiatric Treatment 7: 444–450

17. Alcohol- and Substance-related Disorders

This chapter discusses the disorders associated with the presenting complaints in Chapter 10, which you might find helpful to read first. Alcohol-related disorders will be presented first, followed by other psychoactive substances.

Alcohol-related disorders

Epidemiology

Prevalence rates vary considerably, depending on the geographic location, the age group surveyed, and how drinking problems are defined.

- The prevalence of alcohol dependence in the US is approximately 6% for women and 12% for men.
- The percentage of current drinkers who had five or more drinks on at least one day in the past year: 32% (2003).
- According to data from the National Highway Traffic Safety Administration (NHTSA), 16,694 people were killed in alcohol-related crashes in 2004 – an average of one almost every half-hour. These deaths constituted approximately 39% of the 42,636 total traffic fatalities.
- Number of alcohol-induced deaths, excluding accidents and homicides: 19,928.
- Number of alcoholic liver disease deaths: 12,121.

Etiology

The causes of alcohol dependence are multifactorial and are determined by biologic, psychological, and sociocultural factors.

Genetic and biochemical factors

Strong evidence shows a genetic component to alcohol abuse. Family studies show an increased risk of dependence among relatives of dependent individuals. Twin studies indicate that monozygotic twins have a higher concordance rate than dizygotic twins, and adoption studies also indicate a heritable component. The nature of this influence is unclear. It may operate at the level of heritable personality characteristics, or it might relate to the body's inherited biochemical susceptibility to alcohol and its consequences. For example, 50% of east-Asian populations have a deficiency in one of the aldehyde dehydrogenase enzymes, leading to flushing and palpitations after small quantities of alcohol; this may explain reduced rates of consumption and dependence in these cultures.

From a biochemical perspective, chronic alcohol consumption produces decreasing activity of gamma-aminobutyric acid (GABA) systems and increasing activity of glutamate systems. Both of these changes increase the likelihood of neuroexcitability and withdrawal seizures on cessation of drinking.

Psychological factors

Behavioral models explain dependence in terms of operant conditioning:

- *Positive reinforcement* occurs when the pleasant effects of alcohol consumption reinforce drinking behavior, despite adverse social and medical consequences.
- *Negative reinforcement* occurs when continued drinking behavior is reinforced by the desire to avoid the negative effects of the alcohol withdrawal syndrome.

An alternative behavioral explanation is the observational learning theory (modeling), which suggests that patterns of drinking are modeled on the drinking behavior of relatives or peers. Family studies support the idea that drinking habits follow those of older relatives.

The presence of psychiatric (anxiety, mania, depression, and schizophrenia) or physical illness appears to increase the risk of problem drinking. There is also evidence linking alcohol dependence with antisocial and borderline personality traits.

Social and environmental factors

The cultural attitude towards alcohol affects the prevalence of alcohol-related problems (e.g., lower rates in Jewish societies as opposed to Mediterranean countries). Alcohol is also greatly affected by price; less alcohol is consumed and there are fewer alcohol-related illnesses in countries where it is expensive. There is also an association between certain occupations and deaths from alcohol-induced liver cirrhosis. The highest-risk professions are members of leisure and catering trades, doctors, journalists, and those involved with shipping and travel. Furthermore, higher rates of dependence are noted in unskilled workers and the unemployed compared to the higher social classes; this may be partly explained by the "social drift" caused by alcohol dependence (see Ch. 13).

The frequency of significant life events increases the risk of harmful drinking. Although the anxiolytic properties of alcohol are often used as a means of coping with stress ("tension reduction" hypothesis), the social and physical complications of heavy drinking often lead to even further stress.

Assessment, clinical features, investigations, and differential diagnosis

These are discussed in Chapter 10.

Management

The management of alcohol-related problems ranges from the early recognition of a drinking problem with subsequent advice concerning reduction of drinking, which can be undertaken by a primary care physician, to inpatient detoxification with subsequent long-stay rehabilitation, which usually takes place under the auspices of a psychiatrist and, if needed, a medical team.

The treatment of alcohol withdrawal

All clinicians working with problem drinkers need to be able to recognize alcohol dependence because the threat of experiencing withdrawal symptoms may be a barrier to the reduction of alcohol consumption and the withdrawal syndrome itself is associated with significant morbidity and mortality. Not all patients who are dependent will experience significant withdrawal symptoms. Therefore, a thorough assessment of the severity of potential withdrawal syndrome is required (see Ch. 10). The treatment of the withdrawal syndrome is commonly termed *detoxification*. The following points are important in this regard:

- Indications for inpatient detoxification include severe dependence, a history of withdrawal seizures or delirium tremens, an unsupportive home environment, and a previous failed community detoxification. In these cases, inpatient detoxification is advised.
- In order to ameliorate severe symptoms and reduce the risk of developing seizures or a delirium, a drug with cross-tolerance to alcohol is used if symptoms develop, usually in the form of the benzodiazepine chlordiazepoxide (diazepam and lorazepam are also effective).
- In order to avert a Wernicke's encephalopathy, it is wise to give thiamine (vitamin B_1) supplements orally (100mg daily).

Figure 17.1 summarizes the treatment of delirium tremens (and Wernicke's encephalopathy).

Management of delirium tremens

Emergency hospitalization essential
Vigorous search for a medical source, e.g.:
- Infection (especially pneumonia)
- Head injury
- Liver failure
- Gastrointestinal hemorrhage
- Wernicke's encephalopathy*

Medication:
- Treat withdrawal symptoms with a drug with cross-tolerance to alcohol e.g., benzodiazepines (oral chlordiazepoxide up to 400mg daily) – i.v. therapy seldom needed. Also treats seizures
- Only use antipsychotics (e.g., haloperidol) for severe psychotic symptoms (risk of lowering seizure threshold)
- Large doses of parenteral (intramuscular or slow intravenous) thiamine. Oral thiamine is not adequate*

Monitoring of temperature, fluid, electrolytes, and glucose:
- Risk of hyperthermia, dehydration, hypoglycemia, hypokalemia, hypomagnesemia

General principles for managing a delirium (see p. 121)

*Wernicke's encephalopathy can occur in the context of delirium tremens, or in isolation. Treatment is with large doses of parenteral thiamine (as listed under medication, above).

Fig. 17.1 Management of delirium tremens.

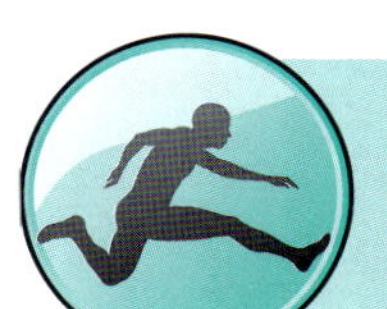

The treatment of alcohol dependence involves more than "detoxification." Detoxification treats the withdrawal syndrome (only one component of dependence), which involves ameliorating withdrawal symptoms and pre-empting or treating more serious complications such as withdrawal seizures or delirium. The management of dependence involves addressing all the psychological, biologic, and sociocultural factors that have led to its development.

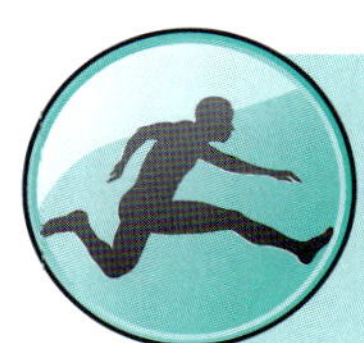

Delirium tremens is a medical emergency that is not uncommon on medical and surgical wards. It has a mortality of about 5%, emphasizing the need for prompt recognition and appropriate treatment. Make sure that you know the symptoms (Ch. 10) and management well.

Maintenance after detoxification

Pharmacologic therapy

- Disulfiram (Antabuse): blocks alcohol oxidation, leading to an accumulation of acetaldehyde. This causes unpleasant symptoms of anxiety, flushing, palpitations, headache, and a choking sensation within 20 minutes of alcohol consumption. The drug is usually taken orally, although surgical implants are available. It is contraindicated in patients with compromised cardiorespiratory function.
- Acamprosate (Campral): enhances GABA transmission and appears to reduce the likelihood of relapse after detoxification by reducing craving. Some patients find it helpful.

Psychosocial interventions

Not all interventions are suited to all patients, and the care package needs to be tailored accordingly. The various forms of psychosocial intervention that have been shown to be effective in managing alcohol problems include:

- Motivational interviewing (Miller and Rollnick) and the application of Prochaska and DiClemente's stages of change model, which moves patients through a cycle of change from "precontemplation" to "contemplation" to "preparation" to "action" to "maintenance."
- Cognitive-behavior therapy (cue exposure, relapse prevention work, behavioral contracting)
- Group therapy
- Alcoholics Anonymous: 12-step program (Al-Anon and Al-Ateen support the families and teenage children of alcoholics, respectively)
- Social support: social workers and probation officers may be able to help with homelessness, criminal charges, and debt
- Primary prevention: increasing the cost of alcohol through taxation appears to be the most effective strategy in reducing overall consumption. Limiting availability, curtailing advertising, and health education seem less effective measures.

Course and prognosis

Alcohol dependence has a variable course and is characterized by many relapses. However, the prognosis is not as poor as is often thought, as highly functioning individuals show a higher than 65% 1-year abstinence rate following treatment. Good prognostic indicators include being in a stable relationship, employment, having stable living conditions with good social supports, and having good insight and motivation. The studies that have followed up dependent drinkers for many years have demonstrated varying outcomes and indicated that there is no average outcome. Alcohol-dependent individuals have a 3.6-fold excess mortality compared with age-matched controls. The lifetime risk of suicide is 3–4%, which is 60–120 times greater than that of the general population.

Other psychoactive substances

Epidemiology

- According to the Substance Abuse and Mental Health Services Administration (SAMHSA) 2001 National Household Survey on Drug

Abuse, 15.9 million Americans aged 12 and over (7.1%) reported using an illicit drug in the month before the survey was conducted. More than 12% reported illicit drug use during the past year, and 41.7% reported some use of an illicit drug at least once during their lifetime.

- The most common illicit drugs used by current users over the age of 12 were marijuana (12.1 million users, or 5.4% of the population), cocaine (1.7 million users, or 0.7% of the population), and hallucinogens, which include LSD, PCP, and MDMA (1.3 million users, or 0.6% of the population).
- Approximately 37% of those over the age of 12 reported lifetime use of marijuana, 12.3% reported lifetime use of cocaine, and 12.5% reported lifetime use of hallucinogens.
- According to the 2002 Monitoring the Future Study by the National Institute on Drug Abuse, 53% of high school seniors reported using an illicit drug at least once in their lives, 41% within the past year, and 25.4% within the past month.
- During 2000, there were an estimated 2,707,000 chronic cocaine users and 3,035,000 occasional cocaine users in the US. Between 27% and 49% of male arrestees tested positive for cocaine.
- Estimate of the hardcore heroin addict population in the US places the number between 750,000 and 1,000,000.

Etiology

The etiologic factors for dependence on illicit drugs are not well understood, although they would appear to be related to a mixture of biopsychosocial factors. The operant conditioning model described in the alcohol section also applies to other psychoactive substances. Similarly, price, availability, and cultural attitudes appear to be key factors influencing the use of illicit substances. In addition, social deprivation, a family environment of substance abuse, conduct disorder in childhood, antisocial personality disorder, and severe mental illness all increase the likelihood of substance misuse problems.

The introduction of harsher legal penalties for suppliers and users of illicit drugs, and increased education about the effects of drug use, have not resulted in a decrease in illicit drug use over the last 30 years.

Assessment, clinical features, drug classification, and differential diagnosis

These were discussed in Chapter 10.

Management

As with the management of alcohol dependence, management involves more than treating physical dependence with detoxification but also concerns the maintenance of abstinence and the addressing of the psychological, biologic, and sociocultural factors that led to substance dependence in the first place.

A detailed management of substance abuse is beyond the scope of this book; however, specific key points on the treatment of some individual substances will be mentioned.

Opiates

- Patients should be given education about harm minimization, including the risks of using contaminated injecting equipment (e.g., HIV, hepatitis B and C, infective endocarditis) and unsafe sexual behavior.
- Clean needles and injecting equipment, hepatitis B vaccination, and condoms should be offered.
- Withdrawal is distressing, although not life-threatening, and may be attempted rapidly in mild to moderate dependence. The symptoms may be ameliorated by clonidine, a centrally acting α-adrenoceptor agonist that reduces sympathetic outflow.
- Maintenance treatment of opiate use can be offered to patients with severe dependence by converting to the longer-acting oral opiate methadone. It helps stabilize the user's life and prevents the complications of injecting. Serious respiratory depression may result if the patient is not already tolerant to opiates. Therefore, before prescribing potentially fatal doses of methadone, opiate dependence should be proven by a urine drug screen.
- Methadone may be prescribed indefinitely but the aim should be gradual reduction with long-term abstinence.
- Sublingual buprenorphine, a partial opiate agonist, is also used as substitution therapy for patients with moderate dependence. The dose is then gradually reduced to avoid a precipitous withdrawal syndrome. Note that, because it is

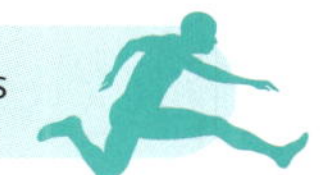

only a partial agonist, it may precipitate withdrawal in patients who are dependent on high doses of opiates (more than 30mg methadone daily).

- Psychological interventions are integral to good therapeutic outcomes and include motivational interviewing, cognitive-behavioural therapy (including relapse prevention), and social support.

Benzodiazepines

As with alcohol, caution must be exercised when attempting a withdrawal from benzodiazepines as it is potentially fatal and may include hallucinations, seizures, and delirium. Patients are initially converted from short-acting (e.g., lorazepam, temazepam) to long-acting compounds (usually diazepam). Doses are then reduced very slowly by a small amount every few weeks, depending on what the patient can tolerate.

Cocaine and amphetamine

Both cocaine and amphetamine can be stopped abruptly. Antidepressants may help the depressed mood that follows withdrawal from heavy use. Psychotic disorders induced by these drugs benefit from symptomatic treatment with short courses of benzodiazepines or antipsychotics.

- How does the operant conditioning model of behavioral theory explain alcohol and substance abuse?
- What does detoxification aim to treat? How does that differ from the treatment of dependence?
- What are the three most commonly encountered drug problems in patients presenting for treatment?
- What nondrug management strategies are employed in the treatment of intravenous heroin dependence?
- What is the role of methadone in the treatment of opiate dependence?
- How is benzodiazepine withdrawal similar to alcohol withdrawal?

Suggested further reading

Baigent M F 2003 Physical complications of substance abuse: what the psychiatrist needs to know. Current Opinion in Psychiatry 16(3): 291–296. Available online at: http://www.medscape.com/viewarticle/452724

British Journal of Psychiatry 2001 Substance misuse papers. British Journal of Psychiatry 178: 101–128

Edwards G, Marshall E J, Cook C C 1997 The treatment of drinking problems: a guide for the helping professions, 3rd edn. Cambridge University Press, Cambridge, UK

McIntosh C, Ritson B 2001 Treating depression complicated by substance misuse. Advances in Psychiatric Treatment 7: 357–364

Miller W R, Rollnick S 1991 Motivational interviewing: Preparing people to change addictive behavior. Guilford Press, New York

Prochaska J O, DiClemente C C, Norcross J C 1992 In search of how people change; applications to addictive behaviors. American Psychologist 47: 1102–1114

Raistrick D 2000 Management of alcohol detoxification. Advances in Psychiatric Treatment 6: 348–355

Swadi H 2000 Substance misuse in adolescents. Advances in Psychiatric Treatment 6: 201–210

18. The Personality Disorders

This chapter discusses the disorders associated with the presenting complaints in Chapter 11, which you might find helpful to read first. Personality disorders are classified into three groups in the DSM-IV-TR (Fig. 18.1)

Personality disorders

Epidemiology

Epidemiologic research in personality disorders is made difficult by poor case definitions and the lack of consensus regarding the correct diagnostic instruments. The prevalence of any personality disorder in community surveys ranges from 4% to 13%, although it varies according to the population group sampled. It is higher in patients consulting primary care practitioners (10–30%), even higher in psychiatric outpatient clinics (30–40%), and higher still in psychiatric inpatient (40–50%), parasuicidal samples (40–80%), and prisons (50–80%). Figure 18.2 describes the prevalence of the individual disorders and their relevant epidemiology.

Etiology

Although the etiology of personality disorders is unknown and many theories abound, both environmental and genetic factors seem to be important. The genetic evidence includes:

- Twin studies: monozygotic twins show a higher concordance for personality disorders than dizygotic twins.
- The cluster A personality disorders (especially schizotypal) are more common in the relatives of patients with schizophrenia.
- Depressive disorders are more common in the relatives of patients with borderline personality disorder.
- Individuals with XYY chromosomes show increased antisocial behavior independent of other variables.

Some authors have suggested that schizoid personality disorder might be a neurodevelopmental disorder, possibly within the autistic spectrum. There is also evidence that children with minimal brain damage are at risk for personality disorders, especially antisocial personality disorder, which may also be associated with electroencephalogram (EEG) abnormalities.

The finding of low levels of the serotonin metabolite 5-HIAA (5-hydroxyindoleacetic acid) in aggressive or suicidal patients as well as the observation that SSRIs can sometimes result in personality changes (e.g., increased threshold for rejection) indicates that neurotransmitters might have a significant influence on personality.

Early adverse social circumstances are associated with the development of dependent and borderline personality disorders (e.g., parental deprivation, impaired attachment). There is also an association between borderline personality disorder and childhood sexual abuse.

Psychoanalytical theory has attempted to explain personality disorders as arising from the failure to successfully progress through the stages of psychosexual development with the subsequent development of characteristic defense mechanisms (e.g., *projection* in paranoid personality disorder; *splitting* in borderline personality disorder).

Assessment, clinical features, classification, and differential diagnosis

These are discussed in Chapter 11. See also Figure 18.1.

Management

There is considerable debate concerning how personality disorders should be managed and by whom (see Suggested further reading). What is clear is that, at present, the management of personality disorders falls predominantly within the domain of the health-care establishment and to a lesser extent the criminal justice agencies.

A multidisciplinary approach is often essential as psychological, social, and biologic treatment modalities all have an important role. A comprehensive assessment should be made of sources of distress (thoughts, emotions, behavior,

Categorical classification of the personality disorders	
Cluster A: "odd or eccentric"	
Paranoid personality disorder	Suspects others are exploiting, harming, or deceiving them; doubts about spouse's fidelity; bears grudges; tenacious sense of personal rights; litigious
Schizold personality disorder	Emotional coldness; neither enjoys nor desires close or sexual relationships; prefers solitary activities; takes pleasure in few activities; indifferent to praise or criticism
Schizotypal personality disorder	Eccentric behaviour; odd beliefs or magical thinking; unusual perceptual experiences (e.g., "sensing" another's presence); ideas of reference; suspicious or paranoid ideas; vague or circumstantial thinking; social withdrawal
Cluster B: "dramatic, emotional, erratic"	
Borderline personality disorder	Unstable, intense relationships (fluctuating between extremes of idealization and devaluation); unstable self-image; impulsivity (sex, binge eating, substance abuse, spending money); repetitive suicidal or self-harm behavior, fluctuations in mood, frantic efforts to avoid abandonment (real or imagined), transient paranoid ideation or dissociation
Antisocial personality disorder	Repeated unlawful or aggressive behavior; deceitfulness; lying; reckless irresponsibility; lack of remorse or incapacity to experience guilt; often have *conduct disorder* in childhood – see p. 166
Histrionic personality disorder	Dramatic, exaggerated expressions of emotion; attention seeking; seductive behavior; labile, shallow emotions
Narcissistic personality disorder	Grandiose sense of self-importance, need for admiration
Cluster C: "anxious or fearful"	
Dependent personality disorder	Excessive need to be cared for; submissive, clinging behavior; needs others to assume responsibility for major life areas; fear of separation
Avoidant personality disorder	Hypersensitivity to critical remarks or rejection; inhibited in social situations; fears of inadequacy
Obsessive-compulsive personality disorder	Preoccupation with orderliness, perfectionism, and control; devoted to work at expense of leisure; pedantic, rigid, and stubborn; overly cautious

Fig. 18.1 Categorical classification of the personality disorders.

and relationships) to self and others, other comorbid mental illness, and specific impairments of functioning at work or home. If at all possible, a formulation of realistic goals of treatment should be discussed and agreed with patients.

Hospital admission may sometimes be helpful in times of crisis. However, it may be constructive to come to an agreement with the patient regarding the aims and duration of admission.

Psychosocial interventions include:

- Assistance with social problems such as housing, finances, employment, and disturbed relationships.
- Supportive psychotherapy provides patients with an authority figure during times of crisis and focuses on acceptance and helping patients with their dependence needs.
- Cognitive-behavioral therapy (CBT) may target specific symptoms or behaviors (e.g., depression, anxiety, anger, and deliberate self-harm).
- Dialectical behavior therapy (DBT) is a promising intervention for borderline personality disorder and has been shown to reduce parasuicidal behavior and time spent in hospital and to improve patient engagement and social and global functioning.
- Group or individual psychodynamic psychotherapy – see Chapter 28.
- Certain highly motivated patients derive benefit from treatment in a therapeutic community.

Epidemiology of personality disorders		
Personality disorder	**Prevalence in general population**	**Comments**
Paranoid	0.5–2.5%	More common in males and lower socioeconomic class individuals More common in relatives of patients with schizophrenia
Schizoid	0.5–1.5%	More common in males and offender populations May be more common in relatives of patients with schizophrenia
Schizotypal	3%	More common in relatives of patients with schizophrenia May be slightly more common in males
Borderline	2%	More prevalent in younger age groups and females Most severe in mid-20s with improvement in late 30s Associated with poor work history and single marital status Comorbid with depression, substance abuse, bulimia, and anxiety There is a 9% suicide rate High users of mental health services
Antisocial	3% males <1% females	Far more common in men Highest prevalence in 25–44-year-olds Associated with school drop-out, conduct disorder, and urban settings Very high prevalence in prisons and forensic settings Highly comorbid with substance abuse
Histrionic	2–3%	Recent research shows equal sex ratio (previously thought to be more common in women) Associated with parasuicide
Narcissistic	<1%	More common in males and forensic settings
Dependent	1–2%	Comorbid with borderline personality disorder
Avoidant (anxious)	1–5%	Equal sex ratio Comorbid with social phobia
Obsessive-compulsive	1–2%	More common in white, male, highly educated, married, and employed individuals

Fig. 18.2 Epidemiology of personality disorders.

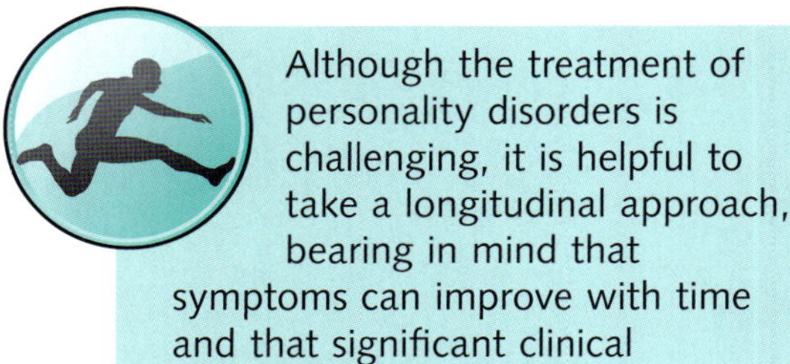

Although the treatment of personality disorders is challenging, it is helpful to take a longitudinal approach, bearing in mind that symptoms can improve with time and that significant clinical improvement is possible.

Pharmacologic treatments are used to treat specific symptoms as opposed to treating the underlying personality:

- Mood stabilizers such as lithium and carbamazepine may be useful in treating aggression, impulsivity and mood instability.
- Antipsychotics may be of some use in treating the psychotic symptoms that sometimes are experienced by schizotypal and borderline personality disorder patients. Antipsychotics are also sometimes used to help with impulsivity, agitation, and aggression.
- Antidepressants may be useful in treating depressive symptoms. SSRIs may help with obsessive-compulsive symptoms as well as impulsivity and self-harm behavior.
- Benzodiazepines should be used with caution as abuse may lead to dependence. They may, however, be used to alleviate acute anxiety or to sedate an acutely agitated or aggressive patient.

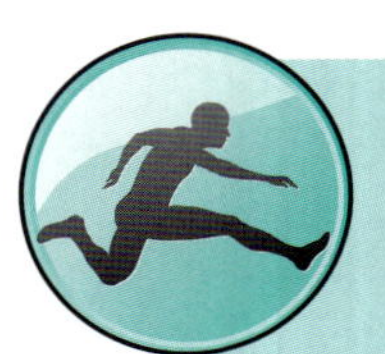

Although pharmacologic therapy may alleviate specific symptoms (e.g., depression, anxiety) in personality-disordered patients, it is unlikely to have any long-term effect on maladaptive personality traits.

Course and prognosis

It is important to remember that patients with personality disorder have a greater incidence of other mental illnesses such as depression, anxiety, and schizophrenia. Furthermore, these tend to be more severe and have a worse prognosis than if the personality disorder was not present. Patients with personality disorder (especially cluster B) also have higher rates of suicide and accidental death than the general population.

The course of personality disorders is not as dire as is often portrayed. Half of all borderline personality patients will show clinical recovery at 10–25-year follow-up. Patients with antisocial personality may also improve with time, especially if they have formed a relationship with a therapist. Schizotypal and obsessive-compulsive personality disorders tend to be stable over time, although schizotypal patients may go on to develop schizophrenia.

- What are the differences and similarities in epidemiology between borderline and antisocial personality disorders?
- Name three psychosocial interventions that are showing promise in the treatment of personality disorder.
- What are the roles of antipsychotics and benzodiazepines in the treatment of personality disorder?
- How are personality disorders and other mental illnesses related in terms of prognosis?

Suggested further reading

Adshead G 2001 Murmurs of discontent: treatment and treatability of personality disorder. Advances in Psychiatric Treatment 7: 407–415

British Journal of Psychiatry 2003 Ramifications of personality disorder in clinical practice. British Journal of Psychiatry 182(Suppl. 44): s1–s35

Davison S E 2002 Principles of managing patients with personality disorder. Advances in Psychiatric Treatment 8: 1–9

Palmer R L 2002 Dialectical behaviour therapy for borderline personality disorder. Advances in Psychiatric Treatment 8: 10–16

Winston A P 2000 Recent developments in borderline personality disorder. Advances in Psychiatric Treatment 6: 211–217

19. Eating Disorders

This chapter discusses the disorders associated with the presenting complaints in Chapter 12, which you might find helpful to read first.

Although this chapter focuses on anorexia and bulimia, binge eating disorder (BED) is another type of eating disorder. Briefly, BED is characterized by the following:

- Recurrent episodic binge eating (at least 2 days per week for at least 6 months) without compensatory measures to prevent weight gain, and
- Episodes are associated with significant distress or at least three of the following symptoms: eating abnormally rapidly; eating until uncomfortably full; eating larger amounts when not hungry; eating alone out of embarrassment; or feeling disgusted and guilty after eating.

Anorexia and bulimia nervosa

Epidemiology

Both anorexia and bulimia nervosa are far more common in women and have a male-to-female ratio of 1 : 10. Eating disorders typically affect young adult females, with 85–95% of cases of anorexia and bulimia occurring among females. Although more cases of both disorders have been identified over recent years, the evidence for a rising incidence is not conclusive. Figure 19.1 summarizes the epidemiology of both anorexia and bulimia nervosa.

Anorexia nervosa is 5–10 times less common, and tends to have an earlier age of onset, than bulimia nervosa. It was previously thought to have an increased prevalence in higher socioeconomic classes; however, a number of studies have produced conflicting results.

Etiology

The cause of neither anorexia nor bulimia has been clarified, but both biologic and psychosocial factors have been implicated.

Anorexia nervosa

Genetic/biologic factors

Twin studies have shown a higher concordance rate for monozygotic (55%) than dizygotic twins (24%). First-degree relatives have a higher incidence of eating disorders (5%), as well as mood disorders, which suggests an association between the two disorders. Abnormalities of serotonin metabolism have been implicated as serotonin suppresses food consumption, and one study found an increased concentration of a serotonin metabolite (5-HIAA) in anorectics.

Environmental/psychological factors

Western culture's obsession with thinness and the mass media's portrayal of the "ideal woman" influences young girls' perception of their own body image. Families of anorectics may be characterized by overprotection, enmeshment (overinvolvement, with lack of differentiation between parent and child), conflict avoidance, and rigidity (resistance to change). Another theory maintains that sexual maturity represents a conflict for anorectics, which results in them attempting to avoid menstruation and the changes in body shape that are associated with puberty.

Bulimia nervosa

Genetic/biologic factors

The role of genetic factors is unclear. Serotonin, norepinephrine, and plasma endorphins have all been implicated, although many neurotransmitter abnormalities occur secondary to weight loss and purging.

Environmental/psychological factors

A past history of dieting, which frequently triggers binge eating and increases the risk of developing

Epidemiology of anorexia and bulimia nervosa			
Disorder	**Prevalence**	**Age of onset**	**Socioeconomic class**
Anorexia nervosa	0.5–1% of schoolgirls/ university students; 4–6% of ballet dancers/models Increased prevalence in Western cultures	Mid- to late adolescence	Initially thought to be more prevalent in higher socioeconomic classes; however, several studies do not support this (still debated)
Bulimia nervosa	1–3% of young women	Late adolescence to early adulthood	Equal socioeconomic class distribution

Fig. 19.1 Epidemiology of anorexia and bulimia nervosa.

bulimia by eightfold, is always present. Up to half of bulimics have a history of anorexia. Family relationships seem to be more conflictual than in anorexia. Perfectionism, low self-esteem, and high neuroticism scores are common. Alcohol and substance abuse, personality disorders, and depression are associated conditions.

Assessment, clinical features, investigations, complications, and differential diagnosis

These are discussed in Chapter 12.

Management considerations in anorexia

Ambivalence toward treatment coupled with the psychological consequences of starvation (poor concentration, depression, lethargy) make patients with anorexia a difficult group to treat. Therefore treatment should be collaborative and a therapeutic alliance should be established early on. Motivational interviewing (Miller and Rollnick 1991) and the application of Prochaska and DiClemente's (1992) stages of change model are helpful in engaging patients and overcoming treatment resistance. The degree of severity of anorexia determines the level of care:

- Patients who simply diet excessively can be treated with education about nutrition and weight monitoring by a family doctor or nurse. Voluntary organizations and self-help groups may also be helpful.
- The treatment of choice in patients with anorexia nervosa is cognitive or interpersonal therapies with the encouragement of family involvement. Furthermore, weight should be monitored and medical complications (see Ch. 12) actively pursued. In these cases, a multidisciplinary approach is needed, involving the PCP, a general adult or child psychiatrist, and a psychotherapist. Figure 19.2 summarizes the various forms of psychosocial therapy interventions.
- There should be a low threshold for referral to a specialized eating disorder unit, especially in patients who are resistant to outpatient treatment and those who have severe anorexia or poor prognostic factors (see Fig. 19.3).
- Hospitalization is necessary for certain medical (e.g., estimated body weight [EBW] of less than 85%, rapid weight loss, severe electrolyte abnormalities, syncope) and psychiatric (risk of suicide, social crisis) indications. In rare cases, when patients lose insight into the dangerousness of their condition and the ability to make rational decisions about medical treatment, involuntary commitment for life-saving treatment may be necessary.

No medication has been shown to be useful for the primary symptoms of anorexia in randomized, double-blind trials. Once an anorexic's weight has stabilized, SSRIs may be useful for treating comorbid depression and obsessive-compulsive disorder. Fluoxetine may be helpful in maintaining weight gain and preventing relapse.

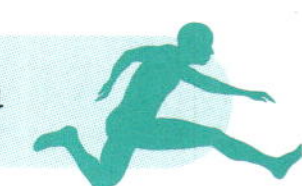

Psychosocial therapy options for anorexia nervosa	
Therapy type	**Comments**
Psychoeducation about nutrition and weight	Advice on balanced eating and dangers of excessive exercising Educate about the complications of starvation, binging, and purging Educate about the nature of anorexia (body image disturbance, starvation–hunger–binging relationship) Results of special investigations may be used to motivate
Nutritional management and weight restoration	Negotiation of target weight Eating plan: amount of calories per day; 3 meals/day with snacks in between to avoid hunger Teach shopping and cooking skills if necessary
Cognitive-behavioral therapy (CBT)	20–24 sessions with intermittent follow-up sessions as necessary May explore issues of control, low self-esteem, and perfectionism
Interpersonal therapy (IPT)	Focuses on improving social functioning and interpersonal skills
Family therapy	May be very effective for adolescents still living with parents, and for onset of illness before 18 years May expose attachment patterns and interpersonal difficulties
Psychodynamic psychotherapy	Reserved for specialists in eating disorders

Fig. 19.2 Psychosocial therapy options for anorexia nervosa.

Poor prognostic factors in anorexia nervosa
Long duration of illness A late age of onset Very low weight Associated bulimic symptoms Personality difficulties A poor family relationship Poor social adjustment

Fig. 19.3 Poor prognostic factors in anorexia nervosa.

Although patients with anorexia frequently have depression and obsessive-compulsive disorder as comorbid illnesses, starvation-induced malnutrition itself may lead to depression, obsessional symptoms, sleep disturbances, and a lack of concentration. The use of medication should be restricted to severe symptoms and those that do not improve with weight gain.

Management considerations in bulimia

Patients with bulimia tend to be more motivated to improve and are usually of a healthy weight. The treatment is predominantly psychological, ranging from psychoeducation, self-help manuals, and self-help groups in mild cases to cognitive-behavioral therapy or interpersonal psychotherapy in more serious cases. Specialist eating disorder input or inpatient care may be necessary in severe cases. Tricyclic antidepressants and SSRIs (fluoxetine licensed at 60 mg) have been shown to reduce binging and purging behavior, but psychotherapy remains the treatment of choice. Comorbid substance abuse and depression is common and should be managed as indicated.

Prognosis

Anorexia

The course of anorexia is variable. Up to 50% of patients recover and return to normal weight, eating, and menstruation. Note that studies have shown that up to 25% of patients go on to develop normal-weight bulimia. About a third of patients fail to recover. The mortality from anorexia is over 10%; half of these deaths are due to the complications of starving and about a third to suicide. The factors that are associated with a poorer prognosis are described in Figure 19.3, and indicate that the more severe the illness the poorer the outcome.

Bulimia

The course of bulimia is also variable, although generally better than anorexia, with 50–70% of patients recovering after 2–5 years. There is no increased mortality. Poor prognostic factors include severe binging and purging behavior, low weight and comorbid depression.

- In which population groups is anorexia nervosa more prevalent?
- How does anorexia nervosa differ from bulimia nervosa in terms of prevalence and age of onset?
- What observations have been made about the families of patients with anorexia and bulimia nervosa?
- What is the role of SSRIs in the treatment of patients with anorexia and bulimia nervosa?
- What is the treatment of choice in patients with anorexia?
- What are the indications for hospitalization in patients with anorexia?
- What are the poor prognostic factors in anorexia and bulimia nervosa?

Suggested further reading

Connan F, Treasure J 2000 Working with adults with anorexia nervosa in an out-patient setting. Advances in Psychiatric Treatment 6: 135–144

Daee A, Robinson P, Lawson M, et al 2002 Psychologic and physiologic effects of dieting in adolescents. Southern Medical Journal 95(9): 1032–1041. Available on line at: http://www.medscape.com/viewarticle/442892

Miller W R, Rollnick S 1991 Motivational interviewing: preparing people to change addictive behavior. Guilford Press, New York

Prochaska J O, DiClemente C C, Norcross J C 1992 In search of how people change; applications to addictive behaviors. American Psychologist 47:1102–1114

Sharp C W, Freeman C P L 1993 The medical complications of anorexia nervosa. British Journal of Psychiatry 162: 452–462

Tamburrino M B, McGinnis R A 2002 Anorexia nervosa: a review. Panminerva Medica 44: 301–311

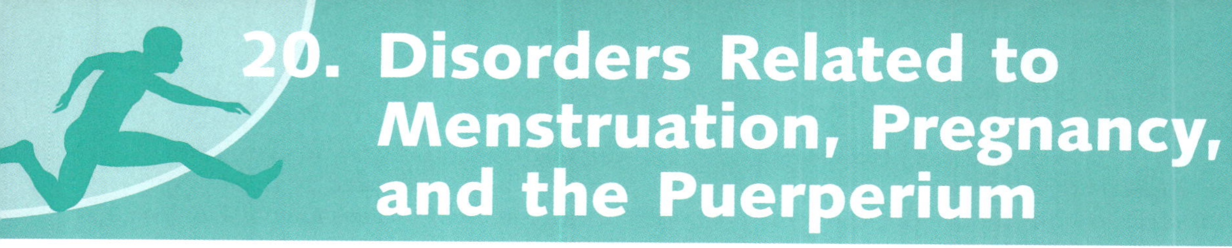

20. Disorders Related to Menstruation, Pregnancy, and the Puerperium

This chapter will discuss disorders specific to the female reproductive cycle and include:

- Premenstrual syndrome
- Psychiatric considerations in pregnancy
- Puerperal disorders, including postnatal blues, depression, and psychosis
- Mental illness in menopause.

Premenstrual syndrome

Clinical features

Premenstrual syndrome (PMS) has been defined as the recurrence of symptoms during the luteal phase (i.e., between ovulation and menses) with complete remission after menses (Dalton 1984). The symptoms of PMS tend to occur in the 10 days prior to menstruation and remit in the 2 weeks following menstruation. Over 150 symptoms have been implicated, but mood symptoms in the form of depression (71%), irritability (56%), and tiredness (35%) predominate. Physical symptoms such as headache (33%), abdominal bloating (31%), and breast tenderness (21%) are also fairly common.

Epidemiology/etiology

Up to 80% of women report experiencing some symptoms of PMS. However, only about 5% of women have PMS symptoms severe enough to meet the criteria for premenstrual dysphoric disorder (PMDD). The prevalence is higher in women over the age of 30 years, multiparous women (prevalence increases with parity), women who do not use oral contraception, and women who experience significant degrees of psychosocial stress. Genetic, hormonal/biologic, and psychosocial factors have been implicated in the etiology (good relationships have a protective effect).

Management

The management of PMDD involves both nonpharmacologic and pharmacologic treatment. Anecdotally, women may benefit from decreasing salt intake to reduce bloating and decreasing caffeine intake to reduce breast tenderness. Consuming more complex carbohydrates during the late luteal phase may also improve PMS symptoms by increasing synthesis of serotonin in the brain. Both calcium (1200 mg/day) and magnesium (360 mg/day) supplements have been shown to be helpful in decreasing symptoms of PMDD.

Other interventions, such as aerobic exercise, light therapy, cognitive therapy, and relaxation techniques, may also be helpful. At this time, no definitive statements can be made regarding the efficacy or safety of various hormone treatments for PMDD. The efficacy of SSRIs (including fluoxetine, sertraline, paroxetine, and citalopram) in treating PMDD has been demonstrated in several randomized controlled trials. Unlike major depression, SSRIs may decrease symptoms of PMDD within days rather than weeks. Trials of fluoxetine, sertraline, and citalopram have shown that luteal-phase dosing is both effective and well tolerated for treating PMDD.

Psychiatric considerations in pregnancy

- Despite early assumptions that pregnancy has protective effects on women's psychological health, approximately 10% of women experience significant depressive symptoms during pregnancy.
- There is evidence of an increased incidence of adverse life events in the weeks and months prior to a spontaneous abortion (miscarriage). At a month following miscarriage, up to 50% of women have a diagnosable depressive disorder (four times normal) with features typical of a bereavement (see Ch. 6).
- There appears to be no significant increase in the rates of mental illness following a termination of pregnancy (TOP), especially since society's attitude toward abortion has become more accepting.

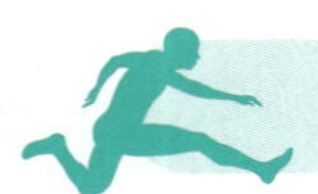

- With the help of their psychiatrists and obstetricians, patients must weight the risks of prenatal exposure against the risk of unmedicated psychiatric illness. Data continue to accumulate, and many unanswered questions remain.
- Lithium use during the first trimester has been associated with a 10–20 times greater risk for Ebstein's anomaly. First-trimester use of valproic acid and carbamazepine involves risks of neural tube defects of 5% and 1%, respectively. Benzodiazepine use during pregnancy has been associated with case reports of perinatal toxicity and increased risk of cleft palate. However, the extent of this risk remains controversial. There is limited information about the reproductive safety of atypical antidepressants.

Pseudocyesis is the rare condition in which a nonpregnant woman has the signs and symptoms of pregnancy (e.g., abdominal distention, breast enlargement, cessation of menses, slight enlargement of the uterus). *Couvade syndrome* describes the condition in which men develop typical pregnancy-related symptoms during their partner's pregnancy, ranging from morning sickness and vague abdominal pains in mild cases to experiencing the pain of labor and childbirth in severe cases. Both these conditions are psychosomatic and should be distinguished from *delusion of pregnancy*, which is the delusion of being pregnant, without the physical symptoms. Pseudocyesis and delusion of pregnancy may occur together.

Menopause

Menopause is defined as the cessation of menses for 12 consecutive months. Women usually enter menopause between the ages of 41 and 59 years, with an average age of 51 years. Psychological symptoms may understandably accompany the changes that occur with menopause. However, no specific psychiatric disorder has been associated with menopause itself. There is no clear psychiatric indication for hormone replacement therapy (HRT), and its use for psychological symptoms is still controversial. HRT should never substitute for treatment with recognized antidepressants for genuine depression. In addition to the potential role of estrogen withdrawal, psychosocial theories suggest that life changes may also contribute to perimenopausal depression. These psychosocial factors may include changing family roles, loss of reproductive potential, and aging.

Puerperal disorders

The puerperium, unlike pregnancy, is a relatively high-risk period for the relapse of a pre-existing mental illness as well as for the development of a new mental illness. There are three conditions that you should consider when evaluating the woman with psychological symptoms in the puerperium:

- Postpartum blues (PPB)
- Postpartum depression (PPD)
- Postpartum psychosis (PPP).

Postpartum blues

This very common condition, which occurs in 50–85% of all postpartum women, is also called "maternity blues," "baby blues," and "third day blues." It occurs within the first 10 days after delivery and is characterized by crying spells associated with mild depression or emotional lability, anxiety, and irritability that peak between the third and fifth day. The absence of a link between postpartum blues and life events, demographic factors, or obstetric events suggests an underlying biologic cause (e.g., a precipitous fall in progesterone after delivery). Postpartum blues is a self-limiting condition that resolves spontaneously and usually requires only reassurance. However, an apparent bad case of postpartum blues may herald the onset of postpartum depression. About 20% of mothers with postpartum blues will progress to postpartum depression.

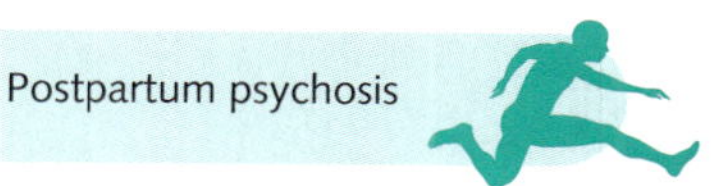

Postpartum depression

Clinical features

Postpartum depression usually develops within 3 months after delivery and typically lasts between 3 and 14 months. The DSM-IV-TR classifies PPD as major depression that occurs within 4 weeks after delivery. The symptoms are similar to a depressive episode, that is, low mood, loss of interest or pleasure, fatigability, and suicidal ideation (although suicide is rare). Note, however, that sleeping difficulties, weight loss, and decreased libido can be normal for the first few months following delivery. Additional features of PPD may include:

- Anxious preoccupation with the baby's health, despite a relatively healthy baby, often associated with feelings of guilt and inadequacy
- Reduced affection for the baby, with possible impaired bonding
- Obsessional phenomena, which often involve recurrent, intrusive thoughts of harming the baby (note that it is crucial to ascertain whether these are regarded as repugnant (ego-dystonic), as obsessions usually are, or whether they pose a potential risk)
- Infanticidal thoughts (thoughts of killing baby), which are different from obsessions in that they are not experienced as repugnant (i.e., they are ego-syntonic), may be seriously entertained, and, worryingly, may involve planning.

Epidemiology

The prevalence of depression in postpartum women is about 12–13%. Studies have shown that this is similar to that found in the general population of women. There is no association with socioeconomic class or parity.

Etiology

Psychosocial factors are strongly linked to the development of PPD, with recent stressful life events, lack of close confiding relationships, young maternal age, and marital strife all implicated. A previous history of depression, particularly PPD and postpartum blues, is an important risk factor. Among women with a history of depressive disorder, obstetric complications during delivery are associated with an increased rate of PPD. Evidence indicates that biologic factors are not as important as they are in postpartum blues and postpartum psychosis.

It is important to diagnose any coexisting medical conditions, including anemia, diabetes, and thyroid disease.

Management

The treatment of choice in most cases of PPD is counseling (e.g., supportive counseling, mother-and-baby groups, relationship counseling). For more severe cases, antidepressant medication is necessary. For women with prior episodes of depression, prevention with medications is recommended in the first few days after delivery.

Antidepressants may be transmitted in small quantities to the baby via breast milk; however, unless bottle-feeding is preferred (e.g., to allow the duty of feeding to be shared), breast-feeding need not necessarily stop. As in pregnancy, a judgment needs to be made, in conjunction with the patient, regarding the risks versus benefits of medication. Depression during pregnancy is associated with an increased risk of preterm delivery and a low birth weight infant. In addition, there is a high risk of relapse among pregnant women who discontinue antidepressant medication during pregnancy. Figure 20.1 summarizes the information available about the use of psychotropic medication in breast-feeding mothers.

Mothers with severe PPD with suicidal/infanticidal ideation may require hospital admission and, in these cases, admission with the baby to a mother-and-baby unit is preferable. Electroconvulsive therapy (ECT) may be a highly effective treatment when indicated and usually results in a rapid improvement, which is important when mother and baby are separated. Remember that the assessment of the infant's well-being is an additional part of the comprehensive psychosocial and risk assessment.

Prognosis

Most women respond to standard treatment; however, some patients have a protracted course. They should be followed up closely and may need long-term treatment. Postpartum depression tends to reoccur. Nearly 80% of women with one or more episodes of PPD spontaneously relapse to depression over the next five years. Approximately 50% will do so after a subsequent delivery.

Psychiatric medication in breast-feeding mothers	
Drug group	**Comments**
Tricyclic antidepressants	Amounts transmitted in breast milk are too small to be harmful Low-dose nortriptyline appears safe Clomipramine may be used for obsessional phenomena Avoid doxepin – accumulation of metabolite
SSRIs Fluoxetine and citalopram have the maximum transmission to infants during breast-feeding Sertraline, fluvoxamine, and paroxetine have the least transmission to the infant	Paroxetine now contraindicated for use during pregnancy. The FDA has recently revised safety labeling for paroxetine: its use past the 20th week of pregnancy has been linked to an increased risk of persistent pulmonary hypertension of the newborn (PPHN) as well as cardiac abnormalities in the fetus.
Lithium	Risk of neonatal lithium toxicity as breast milk contains 40% of maternal lithium concentration Avoid if possible
Antipsychotics	Only small amounts excreted but possible effects on developing nervous system Avoid high doses because of risk of lethargy in infant Only use when benefit outweighs risk; consider bottle-feeding
Benzodiazepines and other hypnotics	Avoid. May cause lethargy in infant

Fig. 20.1 Psychiatric medication in breast-feeding mothers.

- The incidence of psychiatric illness in the puerperium is exceptionally high. In primiparous women, there may be up to a 35-fold increased risk of developing a psychotic illness and needing hospital admission within the first month of child birth. This emphasizes the importance of close vigilance in the postpartum period, especially in women with a prior, or family, history of mental illness.
- Despite the increased rate of depression, postnatal suicide is rare. The suicide rate in the year following childbirth is one-sixth the rate for a matched control group. Note, however, that suicide is far more common than infanticide and, therefore, becomes a particular concern when infanticidal thoughts are present.

Note that PPD is associated with disturbances in the mother–infant relationship, and studies have shown that this can lead to problems with the child's cognitive and emotional development.

Postpartum psychosis

Clinical features

The postpartum period is an extremely high-risk period for the development of a psychotic episode. These episodes characteristically have a rapid onset, usually between day 4 and 3 weeks after delivery and almost always within 8 weeks. They often begin with insomnia, restlessness, and perplexity, later progressing to suspiciousness and marked confusion, with psychotic symptoms. These symptoms often fluctuate dramatically in their nature and intensity over a short space of time. There is some debate as to whether the postpartum psychoses represent a separate disease entity, a mood disorder with psychotic features, a schizophrenic episode, an organic psychosis, or a combination of the aforementioned. In 80% of cases, the clinical presentation resembles a mood disorder (depression or mania) with delusions and

Risk factors for postpartum psychosis
Previous postpartum psychosis
History of mood disorder
Family history of psychotic illness or mood disorder
Primiparous mother
Delivery associated with cesarean section or perinatal death

Fig. 20.2 Risk factors for postpartum psychosis.

hallucinations. Even when typical schizophrenic symptoms are present, patients often have associated mood symptoms.

Epidemiology

Postpartum psychosis develops in about two in 1000 childbirths.

Etiology

The evidence seems to indicate that postpartum psychosis is most closely related to bipolar affective disorder. The relatives of patients with postpartum psychosis have a similar incidence of mood disorders to the relatives of patients with mood disorders. Patients with postpartum psychosis are also more likely to have a past psychiatric history of a mood disorder or have a family history of mental illness. Psychosocial factors seem less important, unlike in postnatal depression. Occasionally, a postpartum psychosis may be due to an obstetric complication (e.g. pre-eclampsia, puerperal infection) or medication. Figure 20.2 summarizes the risk factors for postpartum psychosis.

Management

As with postnatal depression, the assessment of risk of infanticide and suicide on mental state examination is crucial. Concerning symptoms include:

- Thoughts of self-harm or harming the baby
- Severe depressive delusions (e.g., belief that the baby is, or should be, dead)
- Command hallucinations instructing the mother to harm herself or her baby.

Hospitalization is invariably necessary, with joint admissions to a mother-and-baby unit being indicated when the mother is able to look after her infant with some supervision. Involuntary commitment may be necessary. The pharmacologic treatment is the same as for other psychotic episodes, with antipsychotics, antidepressants, and lithium, depending on the clinical presentation. Benzodiazepines may be needed in cases of severe behavioral disturbance. All psychotropic drugs should be used with caution in breast-feeding mothers (see Fig. 20.1); it is often advisable to bottle-feed. ECT is particularly effective in severe or treatment-resistant cases, regardless of the clinical presentation.

Psychosocial interventions are similar to those for other psychotic episodes but also include providing support for the father.

Prognosis

Most cases of postpartum psychosis will have recovered by 3 months – 75% within 6 weeks.

There is about a 30% chance of experiencing a recurrence after future childbirths. Women who have had both postpartum and nonpostpartum depressive or manic episodes (i.e., have an established mood disorder) have a 50–85% chance of future postpartum episodes.

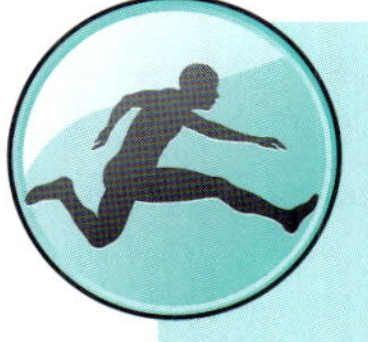

The prevalence of postpartum blues, postpartum depression, and postpartum psychosis is inversely related to their severity:

- Postpartum blues develops after one in two childbirths.
- Postpartum depression develops after one in eight childbirths.
- Postpartum psychosis develops after about one in 500 childbirths.

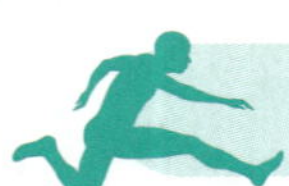

- What types of psychiatric symptoms occur in the premenstruum, pregnancy, the puerperium, and menopause?
- What types of symptoms occur in PMS? When do they occur in the menstrual cycle?
- What is the risk of mental illness following miscarriage and termination of pregnancy?
- What is the difference between pseudocyesis and couvade syndrome?
- What are the symptoms and management of postpartum blues?
- How does the etiology of postpartum depression differ from the etiology of postpartum blues and postpartum psychosis?
- How would you manage a woman with postpartum depression who wanted to continue breast-feeding?
- What factors on mental state examination would concern you when assessing risk in a woman with postpartum psychosis?
- How is postpartum psychosis related to bipolar affective disorder (with reference to clinical features and etiology)?

Suggested further reading

Burt V K, Stein K 2002 Epidemiology of depression throughout the female life cycle. Journal of Clinical Psychiatry 63(Suppl. 7): 9–15

Connolly M 2001 Premenstrual syndrome: an update on definitions, diagnosis and management. Advances in Psychiatric Treatment 7: 469–477

Cooper P J, Murray L 1998 Fortnightly review: postnatal depression. British Medical Journal 316(7148): 1884–1886

Misri S, Kostaras X 2000 Reproductive psychiatry: an overview. Available on line at: http://www.medscape.com/viewprogram/138

21. The Sleep Disorders

Sleeping is intimately related to mental health. Not only can psychiatric illnesses such as depression and schizophrenia disturb the quantity and quality of sleep, but certain psychiatric drugs can also have the same effect. Furthermore, persistent primary sleep disturbances, which are common, can result in significant psychological consequences in an otherwise mentally healthy individual.

Definitions and classification

Sleep is divided into five distinct stages as measured by polysomnography (see later), which includes four stages of non-rapid eye movement (stages 1, 2, 3 and 4) and a rapid eye movement stage (REM). Figure 21.1 summarizes the key characteristics of the stages of sleep.

The DSM-IV organizes the sleep disorders into four sections according to their causes:

1. Primary sleep disorders
2. Sleep disorders secondary to another mental illness
3. Sleep disorders secondary to another medical condition
4. Sleep disorders secondary to the use of a substance.

This chapter will focus principally on primary sleep disorders, which by definition are not caused by another medical condition (e.g., arthritis) or mental illness (e.g., depression) and do not occur secondary to the use of a substance (e.g., alcohol). These disorders are presumed to arise from some defect of an individual's endogenous sleeping mechanism (mainly hypothalamus) coupled with unhelpful learned behaviors (e.g., worrying about not sleeping).

The primary sleep disorders, in turn, are divided into the dyssomnias and the parasomnias:

- The *dyssomnias* are characterized by abnormalities in the amount, quality, or timing of sleep. They include primary insomnia, primary hypersomnia, narcolepsy, circadian rhythm sleep disorders, and breathing-related sleep disorders.
- The *parasomnias* are characterized by abnormal episodes that occur during sleep or sleep–wake transitions. They include nightmares, night terrors, and sleepwalking.

Insomnia

Insomnia describes sleep of insufficient quantity or poor quality due to:

- Difficulty in falling asleep
- Frequent awakening during the course of sleep
- Early morning awakening with subsequent difficulty getting back to sleep
- Sleep that is not refreshing despite being adequate in length.

In addition to daytime tiredness, persistent insomnia can have significant effects on mood, behavior, and performance. Some researchers have suggested that insomnia may play a contributing or even causal role in some cases of depression. It has been shown that insomnia can also lead to an impairment of health-related quality of life similar to congestive cardiac failure or depression.

Primary insomnia is diagnosed when patients present with insomnia for at least a month not attributable to a medical condition, psychiatric disorder, use of a substance, or other dyssomnia (e.g., circadian rhythm sleep disorder) or parasomnia.

The numerous causes of insomnia summarized in Figure 21.2 include primary sleep disorders, medical and psychiatric illness, and substance use.

Assessment of insomnia

The assessment of insomnia involves excluding a medical, psychiatric, or substance-related cause of insomnia. Many cases of primary insomnia are related to poor sleep hygiene (Fig. 21.3). Therefore, it is essential to inquire about sleeping times, daytime sleeping, drinking of coffee, erratic sleeping hours, etc. It is also useful to obtain collateral information from the patient's sleeping partner regarding sleeping patterns, snoring, and movements during the night.

The following questions might be helpful in eliciting the key symptoms of insomnia:

Stage of sleep	Duration spent in this phase during night	Characteristics and electroencephalogram (EEG) findings
Stage 1	5%	• Transition from wakefulness to sleep **EEG: theta waves** 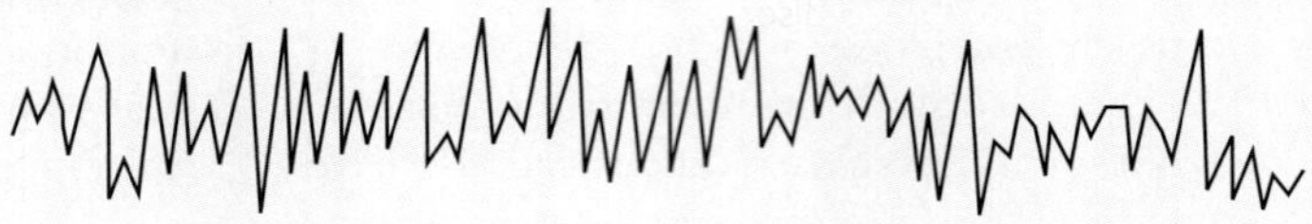 Theta waves: low amplitude, spike-like waves, 4–7Hz
Stage 2	45%	**EEG: sleep spindles and K-complexes** 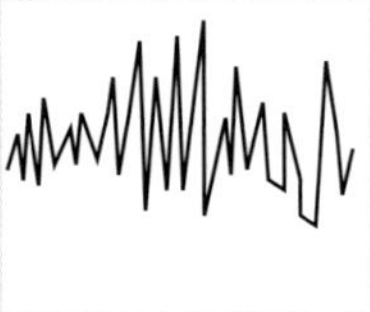 Sleep spindles: short rhythmic waveform clusters of 12–14Hz 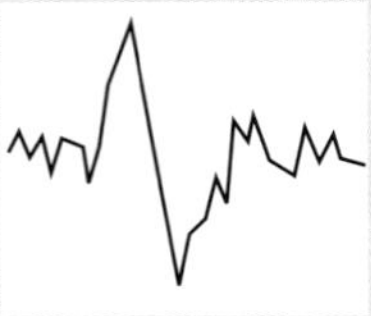 K-complex: sharp negative wave followed by a slower positive component
Stages 3 and 4 (Slow wave sleep)	25%	• Deep sleep • Unusual arousal characteristics: disorientation, sleep terrors, sleepwalking • Occur in first third to half of night **EEG: delta waves** *Stage 3 – delta waves <50%* *Stage 4 – delta waves >50%* 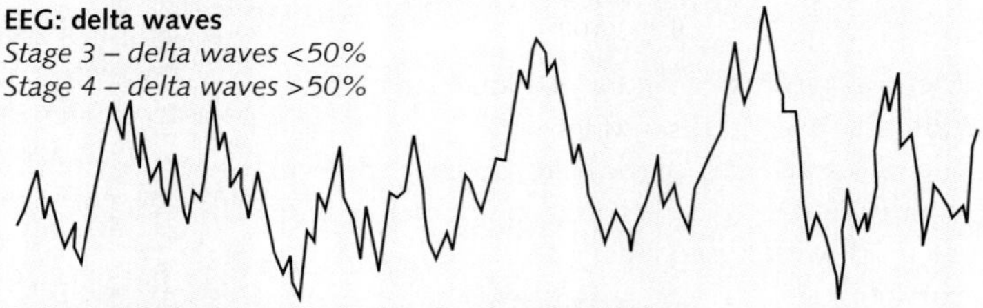 Delta waves: high amplitude, low frequency (<4Hz)
REM	25%	• Occurs cyclically through the night, every 90 minutes alternating with non-REM sleep • Each episode increases in duration – most episodes occur in last third of night • Features penile erection, skeletal muscle paralysis, and surreal dreaming (including nightmares) **EEG: low amplitude, high frequency, with saw-tooth waves** 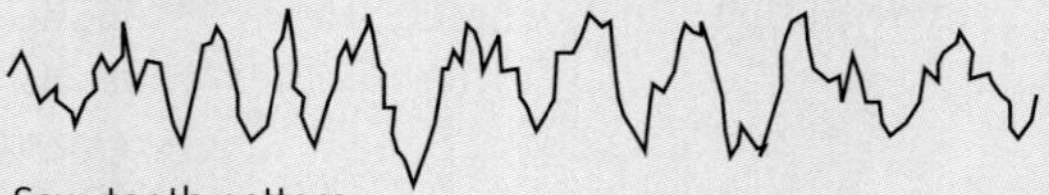 Saw-tooth pattern

Fig. 21.1 Stages of sleep.

Common causes of insomnia

Primary sleep disorders
- Dyssomnias
  a. Primary insomnia
  b. Circadian rhythm sleep disorders (jet-lag, shift-work)
  c. Breathing-related sleep disorders (sleep apnea syndromes)
- Parasomnias (all)

Psychiatric
- Anxiety
- Depression
- Mania
- Schizophrenia

Medical
- Painful conditions (malignancies, arthritis, reflux disease)
- Cardiorespiratory discomfort (dyspnea, coughing, palpitations)
- Nocturia (prostatism, urinary tract infections)
- Metabolic or endocrine conditions (thyroid disease, renal or liver failure)
- Central nervous system lesion (especially brainstem and hypothalamus)

Substances
- Caffeine and other stimulants
- Alcohol
- Prescribed drugs (e.g. SSRIs, some antipsychotics)
- Substance withdrawal syndrome

Fig. 21.2 Common causes of insomnia.

Correct sleep hygiene

- Avoid sleeping during the day
- Exercise during the day and maintain a healthy diet
- Eliminate the use of stimulants (e.g., caffeine, nicotine, alcohol), especially around bedtime
- Condition the brain by only using the bed for sleeping and sex – not for reading, watching TV, etc.
- Go to bed and awaken at the same time each day
- Avoid stimulating activities before bedtime (e.g., television, games). Instead, engage in relaxation techniques or reading
- Try having a hot bath or drinking a cup of warm milk near bedtime
- Avoid large meals near bedtime
- Ensure that the bed is comfortable and that the bedroom is quiet
- Do not lie in bed awake for longer than 15 minutes. Get up and do another relaxing activity and try sleeping later

Fig. 21.3 Correct sleep hygiene.

- Do you fall asleep quickly or do you find yourself tossing and turning for some time before dropping off?
- Do you wake up repeatedly in the night, or can you sleep through once you have managed to get to sleep?
- Do you sometimes awaken too early in the morning and then find that you are unable to get back to sleep?
- Is your sleep refreshing, or do you still feel tired in the morning?

In treatment-resistant cases it might be necessary to refer the patient to a sleep specialist for further investigation. Polysomnography is the simultaneous process of monitoring multiple electrophysiologic parameters during sleep. Tests include the electroencephalogram (EEG), electrocardiogram (ECG), electromyogram, electrooculogram (eye movement), blood oxygen saturation, chest and abdominal excursion, mouth and nose air entry rates, and the loudness of snoring.

Management of primary insomnia

It follows that the most important aspect of management is providing education about correct sleep hygiene. Sleep hygiene, which is described in Figure 21.3, includes a number of nonspecific, nonpharmacologic measures that should lead to an improvement in sleep.

There is a limited role for medication in the treatment of primary insomnia. Insomnia associated with depression may be helped by an antidepressant with sedative properties (e.g., mirtazapine, trazodone, amitriptyline). Hypnotics may help with sleep in the short term, but the development of tolerance to their effects (usually within 2 weeks), possible dependence, and their propensity to cause rebound insomnia limit their use. Therefore, they should be prescribed only on a time-limited basis, ideally for use on alternate or occasional nights rather than every night. Short-acting benzodiazepines (e.g., temazepam) are preferred, as they do not leave patients feeling drowsy the next day and do not accumulate with repeated doses. The related short-acting compounds – zopiclone, zolpidem, and zaleplon, which act on receptors similar to the benzodiazepines – are also very effective in the short term. Note, however, that they can be associated with the development of tolerance and possible dependence.

Hypersomnia and narcolepsy

Hypersomnia describes excessive sleepiness that manifests as either a prolonged period of sleep or sleep episodes that occur during normal waking hours.

Primary hypersomnia is diagnosed when patients present with hypersomnia for at least a month not attributable to a medical condition, psychiatric disorder, use of a substance, or other dyssomnia (especially narcolepsy and sleep apnea), or parasomnia.

> There is a considerable interindividual variation in normal sleep duration. Some individuals, termed "short sleepers," require less sleep than average. They fall asleep quickly and do not suffer from intermittent awakening or daytime fatigue. Some of them may attempt to prolong their sleeping time, which may resemble a primary insomnia.

Narcolepsy is seen as a neurological condition, mainly due to an abnormality of the REM-inhibiting mechanism, and is characterized by a tetrad of:

1. Irresistible attacks of refreshing sleep that may occur at inappropriate times (e.g., driving)
2. Cataplexy (sudden, bilateral loss of muscle tone usually precipitated by intense emotion, leading to collapse and lasting for seconds to minutes)
3. Hypnagogic or hypnopompic hallucinations (see p. 27)
4. Sleep paralysis at the beginning or end of sleep episodes.

Patients usually have 2–6 episodes of sleep per day, which usually last 10–20 minutes. Hypnagogic/hypnopompic hallucinations and the paralysis of voluntary muscles occur as a result of elements of REM sleep intruding into the transition between sleep and wakefulness. All four symptoms occur in less than 50% of cases and the diagnosis is usually made with evidence of sleep attacks and cataplexy. Other features may include persistent tiredness (narcoleptics often experience broken sleep) and problems with memory and concentration.

The numerous causes of hypersomnia summarized in Figure 21.4 include primary sleep disorders, medical and psychiatric illness, substance use, and sleep deprivation.

The *treatment* of primary hypersomnia is usually with stimulants such as dexamphetamine and methylphenidate. The treatment of narcolepsy includes taking forced naps at regular times. In some cases, stimulants are needed to reduce daytime sleepiness; tricyclic antidepressants increase muscle tone and may help to control cataplexy and sleep paralysis.

> Insomnia is a common complaint in depression; however, early morning awakening is the most common somatic syndrome (see Ch. 1) of depression. A fifth of depressed patients may experience hypersomnia. Increased appetite or weight gain and hypersomnia may be referred to as atypical depressive features.

Common causes of hypersomnia

Primary sleep disorders
- Dyssomnias
  - a. Primary hypersomnia
  - b. Narcolepsy
  - c. Breathing-related sleep disorders (sleep apnea syndromes)
  - d. Circadian rhythm sleep disorders (jet-lag, shift-work)
- Parasomnias (all)

Psychiatric
- Depression with atypical features

Medical
- Encephalitis and meningitis
- Stroke, head injury, space-occupying lesion
- Degenerative neurologic conditions
- Toxic, metabolic or endocrine abnormalities
- Kleine–Levin syndrome

Substances
- Alcohol
- Prescribed drugs (e.g., antipsychotics, benzodiazepines, tricyclic antidepressants)
- Substance withdrawal syndrome

Secondary to insomnia or sleep deprivation

Fig. 21.4 Common causes of hypersomnia.

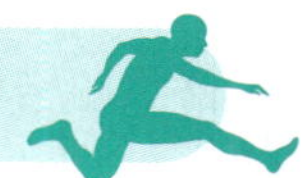

Circadian rhythm sleep disorders

Circadian rhythm sleep disorder (sleep–wake schedule disorder) is characterized by a lack of synchrony between an individual's endogenous circadian rhythm for sleep and that demanded by their environment, resulting in their being tired when they should be awake (hypersomnia) and being awake when they should be sleeping (insomnia). This disorder results from either a malfunction of the internal "biological clock" that regulates sleep or from an unnatural environmental change (e.g., jet-lag, night-shift work). Individuals with delayed sleep phase syndrome (DSPS) have a normal length of sleep but the timing of sleep and wakefulness is set later than other individuals from the same environment. DSPS often occurs in adolescents when a pattern of going to bed late is established (late-night social activities combined with caffeine, nicotine, alcohol), which resets the biological clock to a later time. Awakening at a time to meet daily commitments becomes excruciatingly difficult and daytime drowsiness ensues.

Breathing-related sleep disorders

These disorders feature a repeated disruption of sleep due to abnormalities of ventilation during sleep. This results in unrefreshing sleep and excessive sleepiness during the day. Obstructive sleep apnea syndrome, the most common breathing-related sleep disorder, is characterized by obstruction of the upper airways during sleep, in spite of an adequate respiratory effort. Typically, an individual will have noisy breathing during sleep with loud snoring interspersed with apneic episodes lasting from 20 to 90 seconds, sometimes associated with cyanosis. It is not an uncommon condition, affecting 4% of middle-aged men, 2% of adult women, and 1% of children. The prevalence is much higher in obese, elderly, or hypertensive individuals and is also prominent in some forms of mental retardation (e.g., Down's syndrome). This illness has significant cardiovascular and neuropsychiatric morbidity and should be actively excluded when an at-risk patient presents with hypersomnia, impairment of concentration, and memory or other psychiatric symptoms. Collateral history from a bed-partner, who is often aware of the sleeping difficulties, can be extremely useful in this regard.

Many primary sleep problems often present with psychiatric symptoms that are misdiagnosed as primary psychiatric illnesses and treated symptomatically. For example, depression is one of the conditions for which patients are sometimes treated before obstructive sleep apnea syndrome is correctly diagnosed.

Sleep terrors (night terrors)

Sleep terrors are episodes that feature an individual (usually a child) abruptly waking from sleep, usually with a scream, appearing to be in a state of extreme terror and panic. These episodes are associated with:

- Autonomic arousal (e.g., tachycardia, dilated pupils, sweating, and rapid breathing)
- A relative unresponsiveness to the efforts of others to comfort the person, who appears confused and disorientated.

Upon full awakening, there is amnesia for the episode and no recall of any dream or nightmare. Sleep terrors last from 1 to 10 minutes, usually occur during slow wave sleep (stages 3 and 4), and are therefore predominant in the first third of the night. Sleep terrors are seen in up to 6% of children aged 4–12 and usually resolve by adolescence. Sleepwalking and sleep terrors seem to be related conditions as they share clinical and etiologic similarities. Sleep terrors should be distinguished from nightmares and epileptic seizures, although seizures seldom occur during sleep.

Nightmares

Between 10% and 50% of children aged 3–5 experience repeated nightmares, although they occur occasionally in up to 50% of adults. Nightmares are characterized by an individual waking from sleep because of an intensely frightening dream involving threats to survival, security, or self-esteem. Nightmares are distinguished from sleep terrors by the observation that the individual is not only alert and oriented immediately after awakening but is also able to recall the dream in vivid detail. Furthermore, nightmares tend to occur during the second half of the night because they arise almost exclusively during REM sleep, which tends to be longer and have more intense, surreal dreaming during the latter part of the night.

Sleepwalking (somnambulism)

Sleepwalking is characterized by an unusual state of consciousness in which complex motor behavior, including walking around, occurs during sleep. While sleepwalking, the individual has a blank, staring face and is relatively unresponsive to the communicative efforts of others and is difficult to awaken. When sleepwalkers do wake up, either during an episode or the following morning, they have no recollection of the event ever having occurred and have no impairment of cognition or behavior, although they may have an initial brief period of disorientation subsequent to waking up from a sleepwalking episode. Sleepwalking usually occurs during slow wave sleep (stages 3 and 4) and is therefore predominant in the first third of the night. The peak prevalence of sleepwalking occurs at the age of 12, with an onset between the age of 4 and 8 years. About 2–3% of children and about 0.5% of adults have regular episodes. Sleepwalking runs in families, with 80% of sleepwalkers having a positive family history for sleepwalking or sleep terrors.

- What are the differences between slow wave (stages 3 and 4) and REM sleep and what parasomnias are they associated with?
- What are the three main causes of secondary sleep disorders?
- What nonpharmacologic strategies may be used to treat primary insomnia?
- What is the role of the benzodiazepines in treating primary insomnia?
- What are the four characteristic symptoms of narcolepsy?
- How do circadian rhythm sleep disorders cause hypersomnia?
- Name four risk factors for obstructive sleep apnea syndrome.
- How do you distinguish between nightmares and night terrors (sleep terrors)?

Suggested further reading

Doghramji K 1999 Clinical frontiers in the sleep/psychiatry interface. Available on line at: http://www.medscape.com/viewprogram/689

Doghramji K 2000 Sleepless in America: diagnosing and treating insomnia. Available on line at: http://www.medscape.com/viewprogram/347

Stores G 2003 Misdiagnosing sleep disorders as primary psychiatric conditions. Advances in Psychiatric Treatment 9: 69–77

22. The Psychosexual Disorders

Healthy sexual functioning requires a healthy body and, perhaps more importantly, a healthy mind and relationship. Physical or psychological problems or, as is often the case, a combination of the two can cause a wide variety of sexual problems. Mental health workers may be consulted about sexual problems that are largely due to intrapsychic or interpersonal conflicts (not predominantly due to a biologic problem) – i.e., psychosexual problems.

The psychosexual disorders can be classified into three groups:

- Sexual dysfunction
- Disorders of sexual preference (paraphilias)
- Gender identity disorders.

Women have a large interindividual variability in the type and duration of stimulation that results in orgasm. The diagnosis of female orgasmic disorder should be made only if the ability to achieve orgasm is less than would be reasonably expected for a woman's age, sexual experience, and quality of sexual activity – and then only if the orgasmic dysfunction results in marked distress or relationship difficulties.

Sexual dysfunction

Clinical features

Following the original description by Masters and Johnson, the DSM-IV-TR describes the sequence of psychological and physiologic responses to sexual stimulation in a four-phase sexual response cycle, which is summarized in Figure 22.1.

Sexual dysfunctions describe abnormalities of the sexual response cycle or pain associated with sexual intercourse that lead to difficulties in participating in sexual relationships. Although this chapter is focused on psychosexual or psychogenic sexual dysfunction, the sexual response cycle consists of both psychological and biologic processes, and it is rarely possible to identify cases with a purely organic or purely psychogenic etiology. Nevertheless, the DSM-IV-TR stipulates that a sexual dysfunction disorder should only be diagnosed when there is a suspected psychogenic component to the problem, i.e., it should not be due exclusively to a medical condition or use of a substance. Figure 22.2 summarizes the sexual dysfunction disorders.

Epidemiology

A comprehensive survey was conducted in the US on a representative sample of 3159 people between the ages of 18 and 59. The findings indicate that sexual dysfunction is very common, with a prevalence of about 43% in women and 31% in men. The reported frequency of specific sexual dysfunction is shown in Figure 22.3. Further findings from the same study include:

- The prevalence of sexual problems in women tends to decrease with increasing age except for those who report trouble lubricating.
- Men, in contrast, have an increased prevalence of erectile problems and lack of interest in sex with increasing age.
- Sexual dysfunction is more likely among people with poor physical and emotional health.
- Sexual dysfunction is highly associated with negative experiences in sexual relationships.
- Married individuals and those with high educational attainment are at a lower risk of experiencing sexual dysfunction.

Etiology

There are many, often interrelated, psychosocial factors that may result in psychogenic sexual dysfunction:

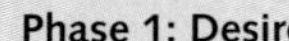

Phase 1: Desire
Consists of sexual fantasies and the desire to have sexual activity

↓

Phase 2: Excitement
Consists of the subjective sense of sexual pleasure and the accompanying physiologic changes (e.g., erection in the man; vaginal lubrication in the woman)

↓

Phase 3: Orgasm
Consists of the peaking of sexual pleasure, release of sexual tension, and rhythmic contraction of the perineal muscles and pelvic reproductive organs (men: sensation of ejaculatory contractions inevitably followed by ejaculation; women: contractions of outer third of vagina)

↓

Phase 4: Resolution
Consists of a sense of muscular relaxation and general well-being. Men are refractory to further erection and orgasm for a period of time. Women may be able to have multiple orgasms.

Fig. 22.1 The DSM-IV-TR's four-phase sexual response cycle.

Sexual dysfunction disorders

Phase of cycle	Dysfunction	Description
Desire	Hypoactive sexual desire disorder	Loss of desire to have or fantasize about sex – not due to other sexual dysfunction (e.g., erectile dysfunction, dyspareunia)
	Sexual aversion disorder	Avoidance of sex due to negative feelings (fear, anxiety, repulsion), or lack of enjoyment
Excitement	Male erectile disorder, female sexual arousal disorder	Inability to attain or maintain sexual intercourse due to an inadequate erection in men or poor lubrication–swelling response in women
Orgasm	Male/female orgasmic disorder	Recurrent absence of delay of orgasm or ejaculation despite adequate sexual stimulation
	Premature ejaculation	Recurrent ejaculation with minimal sexual stimulation before the man wishes
Sexual pain	Dyspareunia not due to a general medical condition	Genital pain during sex in men or women – not due to other sexual dysfunction (e.g., poor lubrication–swelling response, vaginismus) or medical condition (e.g., atrophic vaginitis)
	Vaginismus not due to a general medical condition	Recurrent, involuntary spasm of the muscles that surround the outer third of the vagina, causing occlusion of the vaginal opening

Fig. 22.2 Sexual dysfunction disorders.

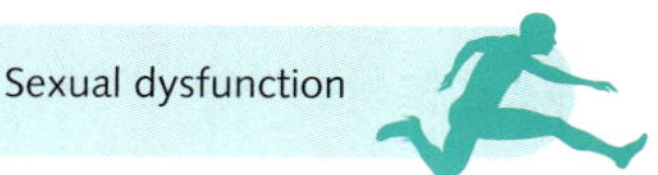

Reported frequency of sexual dysfunction in Americans aged 18–59 years		
Men	Premature ejaculation Lack of sexual interest Erectile difficulties Unable to achieve orgasm	31% 15% 10% 10%
Women	Lack of sexual interest Unable to achieve orgasm Trouble lubricating Dyspareunia	32% 26% 21% 16%

Fig. 22.3 Reported frequency of sexual dysfunction in Americans aged 18–59 years. (Data from Laumann E O et al 1999 Sexual dysfunction in the United States: prevalence and predictors. Journal of the American Medical Association 281: 537–544.)

- Ambivalent attitude about sex or intimacy (anxiety, fear, guilt, shame)
- History of rape or childhood sexual abuse
- Fears of consequences of sex (e.g., pregnancy, sexually transmitted diseases)
- A poor or deteriorating relationship. This includes feeling undesirable or finding the partner undesirable; lack of trust; feelings of resentment or hostility, lack of respect, fear of rejection, etc.
- Anxiety about sexual performance or physical attractiveness
- Fatigue, stress or difficult psychosocial circumstances.

Frequently, there is more than one psychosocial problem that can affect more than one of the phases of the sexual response cycle. For example, the belief that sex is inherently sinful, in the context of an abusive relationship may lead to a lack of desire, a poor lubrication–swelling response, and difficulty in reaching orgasm.

Differential diagnosis

Other causes of sexual dysfunction should be excluded when assessing a patient with sexual dysfunction. These include:

- Medical conditions (e.g., diabetes mellitus, vascular disease, vaginitis, endometriosis, trauma or radical surgery [pelvic fractures, spinal cord injuries, prostatectomy], multiple sclerosis, thyroid disease, hyperprolactinemia)
- Prescribed or illicit drugs (Fig. 22.4).
- Psychiatric illness: mental disorders such as depression, anxiety, and alcohol dependence are frequently associated with sexual dysfunction. In addition, psychiatric medication often results in sexual dysfunction as a side effect. However, sexual functioning frequently improves as the patient's mental illness (e.g., depression) improves, even though the medication (e.g., antidepressants) may have adverse sexual effects.

Prescribed and recreational drugs associated with sexual dysfunction

Psychiatric drugs
- Antidepressants (tricyclics, SSRIs and MAOIs)
- Antipsychotics (especially typical antipsychotics)
- Benzodiazepines
- Lithium

Recreational drugs
- Alcohol
- Amphetamines
- Cannabis
- Cocaine
- Opiates

Medical drugs
- Anticonvulsants
- Antihistamines
- Antihypertensives (including beta-blockers)
- Digoxin
- Diuretics

Fig. 22.4 Prescribed and recreational drugs associated with sexual dysfunction.

The finding that patients have a clear biologic component to their sexual dysfunction does not rule out a psychogenic sexual dysfunction, as the two are often interrelated. For example, a 55-year-old man with diabetes and advanced atherosclerosis notices a weakened erection; he subsequently becomes anxious during sex, fearing that he is losing his virility. This leads to a complete loss of erectile potency.

Assessment considerations

- The wide differential diagnosis requires a comprehensive history, including medical, psychiatric, sexual, and relationship histories as

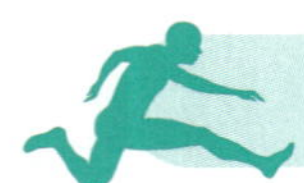

well as current medication and recreational substance use.
- In addition to a thorough physical examination, including genitalia, the investigation of dyspareunia or vaginismus in women requires specialist gynecologic examination (e.g., endometriosis, atrophic vaginitis).
- In addition to indicated blood tests (e.g., thyroid functions, fasting glucose, liver and renal functions, prolactin, testosterone, sex hormone-binding globulin), special investigations are performed to exclude medical causes of sexual dysfunction (e.g., monitoring of nocturnal penile tumescence to exclude organic causes of impotence if the man is able to have erection during REM sleep and monitoring of penile blood flow [internal pudendal artery] with Doppler ultrasonography).

Management considerations

- Many patients may need no more than reassurance, advice, and sex education. Furthermore, patients who have significant relationship difficulties may be advised to engage in relationship counseling or marital therapy before attempting specific treatment for sexual dysfunction.
- Some couples with minor problems benefit from self-help instruction manuals (bibliotherapy) and videotapes, particularly those with no major relationship difficulties.
- Urology clinics deal mainly with organic sexual dysfunction, particularly erectile problems.
- Sexual dysfunction clinics have multidisciplinary teams that focus on both psychological and physical aspects of sexual dysfunction and are best equipped to deal with cases that do not respond to nonspecific measures.
- Some couples benefit from sex therapy, in which partners are treated together and are taught to communicate freely about sex, in addition to receiving education about sexual anatomy and the physiology of the sexual response cycle. They also take part in graded assignments, beginning with caressing of their partner's body, without genital contact, for their own and then their partner's pleasure (Sensate Focus: Masters and Johnson 1970). These behavioral tasks progress through a number of stages with increasing sexual intimacy, with the focus remaining on pleasurable physical contact as opposed to the monitoring of sexual arousal or preoccupation with achieving orgasm. Couples suitable for sex therapy include those with a significant psychological component to their problem, those with reasonable motivation, and those with a reasonably harmonious relationship.
- Figure 22.5 summarizes some of the specific exercises often used in the context of sex therapy that may be helpful with particular problems.
- Biologic treatments may be very effective, especially for erectile problems (e.g., oral sildenafil [Viagra], intracavernosal injections [prostaglandin E_1], vacuum devices, prosthetic implants, and surgery for venous leakage). Testosterone may increase sexual drive in

Specific exercises useful in sexual dysfunction

Sexual dysfunction	Exercise
Female orgasmic disorder	Exercises in sexual fantasy and masturbation, sometimes with a vibrator
Premature ejaculation	Squeeze technique: woman squeezes the glans of her partner's penis for a few seconds when he feels that he is about to ejaculate Start–stop method: stimulation is halted and arousal is allowed to subside when the man feels that ejaculation is imminent. The process is then repeated Quiet vagina: man keeps penis motionless in vagina for increasing periods before ejaculating
Vaginismus	Desensitization, first by finger insertion followed by dilators of increasing size

Fig. 22.5 Specific exercises useful in sexual dysfunction.

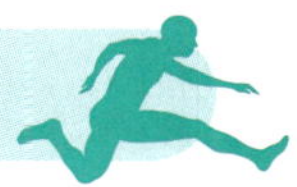

patients with low levels. SSRIs and tricyclic antidepressants may delay ejaculation, but this is rarely a long-term solution.

Prognosis

Vaginismus has an excellent prognosis. Premature ejaculation and psychogenic erectile dysfunction also respond fairly well to treatment. Problems associated with poor sexual desire, especially in men, seem more resistant to treatment.

Disorders of sexual preference (paraphilias)

The DSM-IV-TR describes the essential features of a paraphilia as recurrent, intensely sexually arousing fantasies, sexual urges, or behaviors involving (1) nonhuman objects; (2) the suffering or humiliation of oneself or one's partner; or (3) children or other nonconsenting individuals. It is useful to divide the paraphilias into two groups:

1. Abnormalities of the object of sexual interest (e.g., pedophilia, fetishism, transvestic fetishism)
2. Abnormalities of the sexual act (e.g., exhibitionism, voyeurism, sexual sadism, sexual masochism).

Figure 22.6 summarizes the specific paraphilias.

The paraphilias are mostly seen in men (with the exception of sexual masochism), usually begin in late adolescence or early adulthood, and tend to be chronic. Pedophilia and exhibitionism are frequently seen in a forensic setting and account for the majority of sexual offenders referred for a psychiatric opinion.

The etiology is unknown, but there is often an impaired capacity for affectionate sexual activity, and paraphilics frequently have diagnosable personality disorders.

Treatment options include behavior therapy (e.g., covert sensitization), in which patients attempt to pair paraphilic thoughts with humiliating consequences, and aversion therapy, which involves pairing paraphilic thoughts with a noxious stimulus such as an unpleasant odor or taste. Individual psychodynamic and group therapies are also used. Cognitive-behavioral therapy programs and antiandrogens (e.g., cyproterone acetate) have shown some efficacy in

The paraphilias	
Abnormalities of the object of sexual interest	
Pedophilia	Sexual fantasies, urges, or behaviors involving prepubertal children
Fetishism	Sexual fantasies, urges, or behaviors involving inanimate objects or parts of the body that are not directly erogenous
Transvestic fetishism	Sexual fantasies, urges, or behaviors involving cross-dressing (wearing of clothes of the opposite sex). Rare in women
Zoophilia (bestiality)	Sexual fantasies, urges, or behaviors involving animals
Necrophilia	Sexual fantasies, urges, or behaviors involving corpses
Abnormalities of the sexual act	
Exhibitionism	Sexual fantasies, urges, or behaviors involving the exposure of genitals to unsuspecting strangers
Voyeurism	Sexual fantasies, urges, or behaviors involving the act of observing unsuspecting people engaging in sexual activity or undressing
Sexual sadism	Sexual fantasies, urges, or behaviors involving the infliction of acts of physical or psychological suffering or humiliation on others
Sexual masochism	Sexual fantasies, urges, or behaviors involving the infliction of acts of humiliation or suffering on oneself

Fig. 22.6 The paraphilias.

the treatment of some pedophiles and exhibitionists; however, there is little evidence that any treatment is consistently effective in either condition.

Paraphilias associated with a young age of onset, a high frequency of acts, no remorse about acts, and a lack of motivation for change have a particularly poor prognosis.

Gender identity disorders

Gender identity describes an individual's inner sense of being male or female. This usually corresponds to an individual's *sexual identity*, which comprises all an individual's biologic and anatomic sexual characteristics, i.e., external genitalia, internal genitalia, chromosomes, sex hormones, and secondary sex characteristics. *Sexual orientation* describes the preferred gender of an individual's sexual desires, i.e., heterosexual (opposite sex), homosexual (same sex), and bisexual (both sexes).

An individual whose gender identity does not correspond to his or her sexual identity has a *gender identity disorder*. This is the DSM-IV-TR term. Gender identity disorder or transsexualism is characterized by:

- A desire to live and be accepted as a member of the opposite sex (may include cross-dressing and attempts at passing as the opposite sex)
- A strong sense of discomfort with, or inappropriateness of, one's own anatomic sex (may include attempts to minimize or remove one's primary and secondary sexual characteristics, such as hormone therapy, surgery).

Gender identity disorder in children may manifest as a strong desire to participate in the typical games that are played by the opposite sex, cross-sex roles in make-believe play, and a preference for playmates of the opposite sex.

At clinic centers the male-to-female ratio is about 3 : 1. The cause of this condition is unknown. There is no convincing evidence of abnormalities in genetic make-up, upbringing, or endocrine function. However, a minority of men with transvestic fetishism may progress to transsexualism after many years, coinciding with diminishing sexual arousal from cross-dressing.

The treatment of gender identity disorder requires specialist care. Patients who are committed to gender change may be helped with hormones and surgery, usually after they have completed a "real life test," which involves living as the opposite sex for at least a year. The success of gender reassignment surgery in terms of long-term outcome is not conclusive.

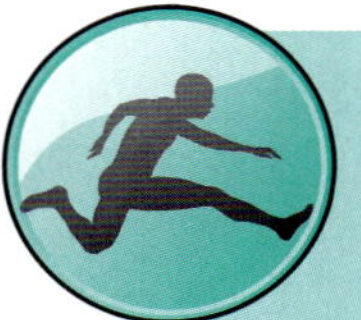

Do not confuse transsexualism with transvestic fetishism. In transsexualism, individuals cross-dress in an attempt to live and be accepted as a member of the opposite sex; whereas in transvestic fetishism, individuals are sexually aroused by cross-dressing but are content with their gender identity. Note that, in a small minority of cases, transvestic fetishism may progress to transsexualism.

- How is sexual dysfunction classified in relation to the four-phase sexual response cycle?
- What are the three most common sexual dysfunctions in men and women respectively?
- How do age, physical and relationship health, and educational achievement affect sexual functioning?
- How may antidepressants worsen and improve sexual functioning?
- What are the principles of sex therapy and which type of couples are most suitable?
- What three techniques may be useful in treating premature ejaculation?
- What biologic treatments may be very effective in erectile dysfunction?
- Which sexual dysfunctions have the best prognosis?
- Which two paraphilias are most often seen in forensic settings? How do they differ in terms of their classification?
- Which interventions have shown limited efficacy in the treatment of paraphilias?
- How does transsexualism differ from transvestic fetishism? How may they be associated?

Suggested further reading

Baldwin D, Mayers A 2003 Sexual side-effects of antidepressant and antipsychotic drugs. Advances in Psychiatric Treatment 9: 202–210

Di Ceglie D 2000 Gender identity disorder in young people. Advances in Psychiatric Treatment 6: 458–466

Hawton K 1995 Treatment of sexual dysfunctions by sex therapy and other approaches. British Journal of Psychiatry 167: 307–314

Padma-Nathan H 2001 Challenges and solutions in the treatment of erectile dysfunction. Available on line at: http://www.medscape.com/viewprogram/603

Phanjoo A L 2000 Sexual dysfunction in old age. Advances in Psychiatric Treatment 6: 270–277

23. Child and Adolescent Psychiatry

Children are often not able to verbalize any psychological symptoms they might have in explicit terms. In fact, "the problem" is usually brought to the psychiatrist's attention by someone else, such as a parent, schoolteacher, or pediatrician. Therefore the presenting problem is invariably a complaint about the child's abnormal behavior or performance rather than psychological symptoms. Inevitably, this means that the clinician is presented with a nonspecific presentation (e.g., "being disruptive in the classroom").

Furthermore, problems need to be seen in the context of a child's developmental stage; for example, "temper tantrums" are normal for a 2-year-old child but should have subsided by age 5.

Considerations in the assessment of children

- Parents or caregivers usually accompany children and young adolescents. It is often useful to first interview them, with or without the child present, to obtain a full description of the current concerns as well as complete psychiatric, neurodevelopmental, educational, and medical history. An indirect evaluation of the parents' personalities, marital relationship, and style of parenting often creates another perspective from which to understand the context of the "presenting complaint."
- An interview with the child usually follows. The explicit information gathered from this interview will depend on the age of the child. Younger children may not be able to articulate their inner experiences; therefore, it is often necessary to observe them in play situations.
- The obtaining of collateral information is extremely important in fully understanding the development of the presenting problem and the child's premorbid functioning. It includes obtaining academic, educational, or psychological reports, as well as discussions with teachers and any other involved agencies.
- Further information can be obtained from structured and semistructured interviews (e.g., Kiddie Schedule for Affective Disorders and Schizophrenia [K-SADS-P]) and parent/teacher rating scales.

Classification

The DSM-IV-TR essentially divides psychiatric disorders in childhood and adolescence into two broad categories:

1. Disorders first diagnosed in infancy, childhood, or adolescence (Fig. 23.1).
2. "Adult" disorders that may begin in childhood or adolescence.

The latter refers to most axis I diagnosis, such as mood disorders, anxiety disorders, eating disorders, substance abuse disorders, etc. The DSM-IV-TR sometimes uses modifying criteria to apply the adult disorders to children and adolescents – for example, irritable mood instead of sadness for depression criteria, anxiety expressed as crying, tantrums, freezing, or clinging rather than panic attacks, decreasing the number of criteria needed for a disorder to be diagnosed in a child (even dropping an adult criterion all together in some cases).

Figure 23.2 provides another conceptual framework for the disorders of childhood and adolescence.

Mental retardation

Definition and diagnosis

Mental retardation is the umbrella term used to describe a group of individuals who have suffered an interruption in the normal development of the brain, from any possible cause, that leads to *subaverage intellectual functioning* and thus an *impaired ability to adapt* to the normal demands of daily living. Mental retardation usually presents in early childhood and is a lifelong condition.

Disorders first diagnosed in infancy, childhood, or adolescence

Mental retardation
Learning disorders
Motor skills disorders
Communication disorders
Pervasive developmental disorders
Attention deficit and disruptive behavioral disorders
Feeding and eating disorders of infancy or early childhood
Tic disorders
Elimination disorders
Other disorders of infancy, childhood, or adolescence
- Separation anxiety disorders
- Selective mutism
- Reactive attachment disorder of infancy or early childhood
- Stereotypic movement disorder
- Disorders of infancy, childhood, or adolescence not otherwise specified (NOS)

Fig. 23.1 Disorders first diagnosed in infancy, childhood, or adolescence.

Intellectual functioning is usually defined by the intelligence quotient (IQ), which is assessed by standardized intelligence tests (e.g., Wechsler Intelligence Scales for Children). An IQ of 70 or below, which is about two standard deviations below the mean, is said to represent subaverage intellectual functioning.

Adaptive functioning is a measure of how patients cope with tasks of living such as communication, self-care, social skills, and academic and vocational skills. This is assessed by a thorough developmental, psychiatric, and medical history from the patient's parents in addition to reports from teachers and other care providers. Standardized scales measuring adaptive functioning should be used whenever possible (e.g., Vinelands Adaptive Behavior Scale).

It is important to remember the limitations of using standardized testing instruments and scales. Differences in sociocultural background and native language as well as sensory, motor, or communication handicaps may lead to patients obtaining falsely low IQ scores. Therefore, patients obtaining IQ scores lower than 70 should not be diagnosed as having mental retardation if there is no evidence of significant impairments in adaptive functioning.

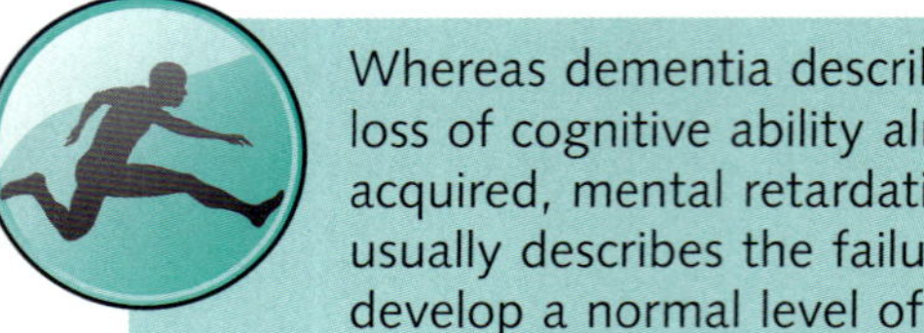

Whereas dementia describes a loss of cognitive ability already acquired, mental retardation usually describes the failure to develop a normal level of cognitive functioning in the first place. Note that individuals with mental retardation due to Down's syndrome are at very high risk for developing Alzheimer's disease in later life.

Classification and clinical features

Mental retardation is the only axis II diagnosis in the DSM-IV-TR section on disorders usually first diagnosed in infancy, childhood, or adolescence. All other disorders are classified as axis I. The DSM-IV-TR specifies mental retardation as mild, moderate, severe, and profound, according to the degree of intellectual and adaptive impairment. Figure 23.3 summarizes the clinical features of the degrees of mental retardation. In addition to the impairment of adaptive functioning, patients may have clinical features associated with the specific cause of their mental retardation (e.g., Down's syndrome: epicanthic folds with oblique palpebral fissures, broad hands with single transverse palmar crease, flattened occiput, cardiac septal defects). Other features associated with mental retardation include aggression, self-injurious behaviors, repetitive stereotypical motor movements, and poor impulse control.

Epidemiology and etiology

- The prevalence of mental retardation in the general population is about 1–3%.
- The male-to-female ratio is approximately 1.5 : 1.
- 85% of cases are mild (see Fig. 23.3).

In 30–40% of cases of mental retardation no clear etiology can be determined and patients with mild mental retardation may represent the lower end of a normal distribution curve for intellectual functioning. Specific causes,

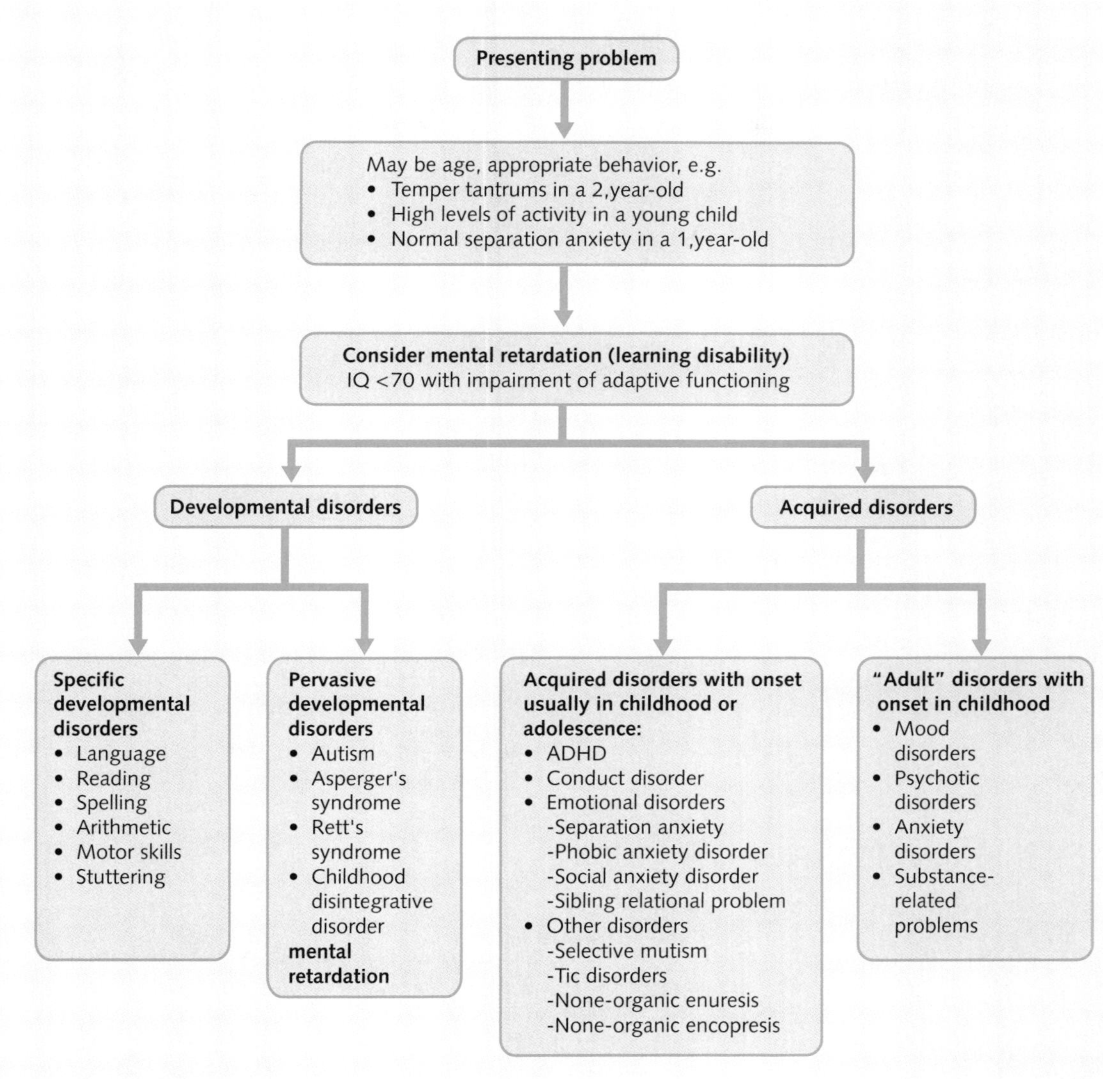

Fig. 23.2 Conceptual framework for the disorders of childhood and adolescence.

however, are likely to be found in patients with severe or profound mental retardation. Remember that mental retardation is a descriptive term and should still be used regardless of whether patients have a specific psychiatric or physical cause for their intellectual impairment or not (e.g., autism, Down's syndrome). Figure 23.4 lists the potential identifiable causes of mental retardation.

> The DSM-IV-TR uses a multiaxial diagnostic system that separates axis I conditions (major mental illnesses, such as psychotic and mood disorders), axis II conditions (personality disorders and mental retardation), and axis III conditions (general medical conditions) so that all three areas potentially requiring clinical attention are considered.

Degrees of mental retardation		
Degree of mental retardation	**Intelligence quotient (IQ) range**	**Adaptive functioning**
Mild (85% of cases)	50–69	Often only identified at a later age Delayed, but usually adequate use of language and self-care Difficulties in academic work (reading and writing) but greatly helped by educational programmes Usually capable of unskilled or semiskilled manual labor May be able to live independently
Moderate (10% of cases)	35–49	Language and comprehension limited Self-care and motor skills retarded, may need supervision May be able to do simple practical work with supervision Completely independent living rarely achieved, usually settle in supervised accommodation
Severe (3–4% cases)	20–34	Marked degree of motor impairment Little or no speech during early childhood; may learn to talk in school-age period Capable of only elementary self-care skills May be able to perform simple tasks under close supervision Usually settle in group homes, family settings
Profound (1–2% of cases)	<20	Severely limited in ability to understand or comply with requests or instructions Often severe motor impairment with restricted mobility and incontinence Little or no self-care Usually require residential care

Fig. 23.3 Degrees of mental retardation.

Causes of mental retardation	
Genetic	Chromosomal: Down's syndrome, fragile X syndrome, Prader-Willi syndrome Other: phenylketonuria, neurofibromatosis, tuberous sclerosis, Lesch-Nyhan syndrome, Tay-Sachs disease, other enzyme deficiency diseases.
Prenatal	Congenital infections (TORCH infections): toxoplasmosis, rubella, cytomegalovirus, herpes simples and zoster (chicken pox), also syphilis and acquired immune deficiency syndrome (AIDS) Substance use during pregnancy (including alcohol: fetal alcohol syndrome) or prescribed drugs with teratogenic effects Complications of pregnancy: pre-eclampsia, intrauterine growth retardation, antepartum hemorrhage
Perinatal	Birth trauma (intracranial hemorrhage) and hypoxia Prematurity: intraventricular hemorrhage, hyperbilirubinemia (kernicterus) infections
Environmental	Malnutrition, poor linguistic and social stimulation Abuse
Psychiatric conditions	Prevasive developmental disorders (e.g. autism, Rett's syndrome)
Medical conditions in childhood	Infections: meningitis, encephalitis Head injury Toxins (e.g. lead)

Fig. 23.4 Causes of mental retardation.

Management and prognosis

Prevention of mental retardation includes:

- Improved perinatal and child health care
- Early detection of metabolic abnormalities, which, if left untreated, can lead to mental retardation (e.g., neonatal hypothyroidism, phenylketonuria)
- Genetic counseling, amniocentesis, and chorionic villus sampling with the option of therapeutic abortion in pregnant women over the age of 35 or those with a family history of genetic disorders.

Intellectual functioning does not improve in most cases of mental retardation. However, adaptive functioning may improve with:

- Comprehensive educational and vocational programs
- Family education and support
- Behavior therapy for behavioral difficulties (aggressive and destructive behaviors)
- In some cases, medication may be helpful in managing aggressive and destructive behavior (antipsychotics, benzodiazepines, lithium, carbamazepine)
- Appropriate residential placement
- Treatment of comorbid psychiatric and medical conditions.

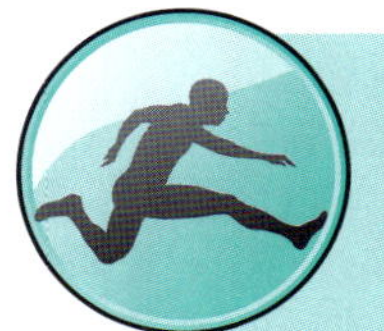

The prevalence of other psychiatric disorders (e.g., schizophrenia, depression) is 3–4 times higher in patients with mental retardation than in the general population. Therefore, it is important to exclude these whenever there is a change in a patient's behavior pattern.

Developmental disorders

The developmental disorders are a heterogeneous group of disorders whose defining characteristic is an inherent impairment in the development of the brain resulting in an impaired acquisition of (or loss of, in the case of the pervasive developmental disorders) expected cognitive, motor, social, or adaptive skills. The onset of these disorders is usually in infancy or early childhood, and they tend to follow a chronic, steady course (see Fig. 23.2)

Specific developmental disorders

These disorders are marked by the disturbed acquisition of a *specific* cognitive or motor function during a child's development, such as language, reading, spelling, arithmetic ability, and motor skills. Other areas of cognitive functioning are average or can even be above average; therefore, a child may have a specific reading disorder (developmental dyslexia) but be of normal intelligence and have no problem with writing or mathematics. These disorders are not simply the consequence of a lack of opportunity to learn, sensory impairment, or neurologic disease but are thought to arise from some specific biologic abnormality in cognitive processing. Compared with mental retardation, patients have less difficulty with overall social and personal functioning, although the consequences of the delay (e.g., school problems, teasing) might lead to emotional or behavioral problems.

Pervasive developmental disorders

The pervasive developmental disorders are characterized by:

- Severe impairments in social interactions and communication skills
- Restricted, stereotyped interests and behaviors.

These behavioral abnormalities pervade all areas of patient functioning and are usually evident within the first few years of life. Although they are often associated with mental retardation, this is not essential for the diagnosis, the emphasis being on deviant *behavior* regardless of intellectual functioning. The pervasive developmental disorders include autism, Asperger's syndrome, Rett's syndrome, and childhood disintegrative disorder.

Autism (childhood autism, autistic disorder)

Diagnosis and clinical features

The three characteristic features of autism manifest within the first 3 years of life and include:

1. *Impairment in social interaction* as evidenced by the poor use of nonverbal behaviors (e.g., eye contact, facial expression, gestures) and a failure to develop and share in the enjoyment of peer relationships
2. *Impairment in communication* as evidenced by poor development of spoken language; extreme

difficulty in initiating or sustaining conversation; repetitive use of idiosyncratic language, and lack of imitative or make-believe play
3. *Restricted, stereotyped interests and behaviors* as evidenced by intense preoccupations with interests such as dates, phone numbers, and timetables; inflexible adherence to routines and rituals; repetitive, stereotyped motor movements such as clapping, rocking, or twisting; and an unusual interest in parts of hard or moving objects.

In addition to these diagnostic features, patients may also exhibit behavioral problems such as aggressiveness, impulsivity, and self-injurious behavior. Although autistic children can be of normal intelligence, 75% have significant mental retardation. Epilepsy may develop in about 25–30% of cases.

Epidemiology and etiology

- The prevalence of autism in the general population is about 0.05% (5 cases per 10,000 people).
- The male-to-female ratio is approximately 3–5 : 1, but girls are more seriously affected.
- The exact cause of autism has not been clarified, but genetic, prenatal, perinatal, and immunologic factors have been implicated. Phenylketonuria, tuberous sclerosis, and congenital rubella are associated conditions. Notwithstanding the turbulent speculation in the mass media, there is no good evidence to indicate that the MMR vaccine (mumps, measles, rubella) results in autism.

Management and prognosis

- Prognosis is poor: only 1–2% achieve full independence; 20–30% achieve partial independence.
- Autistic children with IQs above 70 and those who have good language development by age 5–7 have the best prognosis.
- Prognosis is improved if the home environment is supportive – family education and support are crucial.
- Treatment approach is similar to mental retardation.

Asperger's syndrome

Asperger's syndrome is similar to autism in that there is impairment in social interaction coupled with restricted, stereotyped interests and behaviors. However, there are no significant abnormalities in language acquisition and ability or in cognitive development and intelligence. Asperger's syndrome is far more prevalent in boys, and schizoid and anankastic personality traits are common (see Ch. 11). Many authors conceptualize Asperger's syndrome as a disorder on the so-called *autistic spectrum*.

Rett's syndrome (disorder)

Rett's syndrome, which has almost only been seen in girls, is initially characterized by an apparently normal antenatal development with a normal head circumference at birth, followed by an apparently normal psychomotor development in the first 5 months to 2 years after birth. Then a progressive and destructive encephalopathy results in a deceleration of head growth; loss or lack of development of language; and loss of purposeful hand movements and fine motor skills, with subsequent development of stereotyped hand movements (e.g., midline hand-wringing). After a decade, most girls are bound to a wheelchair with incontinence, muscle wasting and rigidity, and almost no language ability.

Childhood disintegrative disorder (Heller's syndrome)

This disorder, which is more common in boys, is characterized by about 2 years of normal development, followed by a loss of previously acquired skills (language, social and adaptive skills, play, bowel and bladder control, and motor skills) before age 10. It is also associated with an autism-like impairment of social interaction and communication as well as repetitive, stereotyped interests and mannerisms. Thus, after the deterioration, these children may resemble autistic children.

Acquired disorders

The *acquired disorders* of childhood are illnesses "superimposed" on a relatively normally developing child, implying that if the illness were "removed," a more or less normally developed child would remain. They tend to follow a fluctuating course and are often amenable to treatment. Acquired disorders can further be divided into those disorders developing specifically in childhood and the "adult" psychiatric disorders that have their onset in childhood (see Fig. 23.2).

Acquired disorders with onset usually in childhood or adolescence

Attention-deficit/hyperactivity disorder – DSM-IV-TR

Diagnosis and clinical features

Attention-deficit/hyperactivity disorder (ADHD) usually has its onset before the age of 6 or 7 and is characterized by: (1) *impaired attention*; and/or (2) *hyperactivity or impulsivity*:

1. Impaired attention ability includes difficulty sustaining attention in work or play tasks; not listening when being spoken to; being highly distractible – moving from one activity to another; reluctance to engage in activities that require a sustained mental effort (e.g., schoolwork), and being forgetful or regularly losing things.
2. Hyperactivity includes restlessness; incessant fidgeting; running and jumping around in inappropriate situations; excessive talkativeness or noisiness; and difficulty engaging in quiet activities. Impulsivity includes difficulty awaiting turn, interrupting others' conversations or games, and prematurely blurting out answers to questions.

These symptoms should be evident in more than one situation (e.g., at school and at home) and should have been present for at least 6 months.

It is important to distinguish ADHD from:

- Age-appropriate behaviors in young, active children. ADHD is usually not recognized until the child has started school because of the normal variation of behaviors in preschool children. However, ADHD is diagnosed and treated in clear cases in young children.
- Children placed in academic settings inappropriate to their intellectual ability. This includes children with learning disabilities and highly intelligent children in an understimulating environment.
- Other mental illnesses (e.g., pervasive developmental disorders, depression).

Restlessness, overactivity, impaired concentration, and inattention may also arise in children with agitated depression or anxiety. ADHD should not be diagnosed in these cases unless there is clear evidence that these symptoms were present before, or persist after the resolution of, the depression or anxiety.

Epidemiology and etiology

- The prevalence of ADHD in the US is 3–7% in school-age children.
- The male-to-female ratio is approximately 3–9 : 1.
- The cause of ADHD is not known. Genetic factors, anatomic variations, dietary factors, and psychosocial factors (prolonged emotional deprivation) have all been implicated.

Management and prognosis

- Pharmacologic: central nervous system stimulants such as methylphenidate (Ritalin) and dexamphetamine have been shown to be highly effective in up to three-quarters of children, improving ability to sustain attention and academic efficiency. Antidepressants (e.g.,

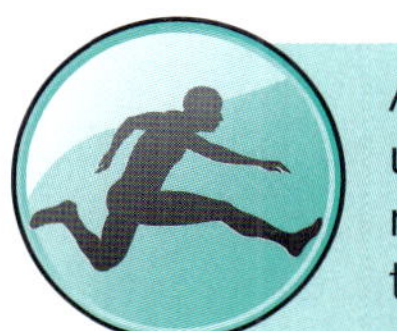

A particular concern with the use of stimulants such as methylphenidate (Ritalin) is that they may cause transient growth suppression with prolonged use. They are therefore prescribed in specialist settings where growth and weight can be monitored. However, studies show that final height and weight are not significantly affected. Drug-free periods (so-called drug holidays) are no longer recommended.

Wellbutrin, Strettera), clonidine, and Tenex are second-line options.

- Psychotherapy: behavior modification in a structured environment, family education and support (parental permissiveness is not helpful).
- Improvement usually occurs with development and remission of symptoms may occur between the ages of 12 and 20, although 15% of patients have symptoms persisting into adulthood.
- Unstable family dynamics and coexisting conduct disorder are associated with a worse prognosis.

Conduct disorder

The onset of conduct disorder is usually before the age of 18. Most affected boys meet the criteria by age 10–12 years and most affected girls by age 14–16 years. The disorder is characterized by a repetitive and persistent pattern of:

- Aggression to people and animals
- Destruction of property (including fire-setting)
- Deceitfulness or theft
- Major violations of age-appropriate societal expectations or rules (e.g., truancy, staying out at night, running away from home).

Etiologic factors include genetic factors, parental psychopathology (mental illness, substance abuse, antisocial personality traits), child abuse and neglect, poor socioeconomic status, and educational impairment. Prevalence estimates vary from 5% to 15% of adolescent boys and from 2% to 10% of adolescent girls. More boys than girls are affected, with a male-to-female ratio of approximately 3–12 : 1. Many adolescents improve by adulthood; however, a substantial proportion develop antisocial personality disorder and substance-related problems, especially children with an early age of onset of symptoms. Management strategies include behavior, cognitive, family, and group therapy.

Oppositional defiant disorder describes a persistent pattern of negativistic, defiant, hostile, and disruptive behavior *in the absence* of behavior that violates the law or the basic rights of others as occurs in conduct disorder (e.g. theft, cruelty, bullying, assault). Children with this disorder deliberately defy requests or rules, are angry and resentful, and annoy others on purpose.

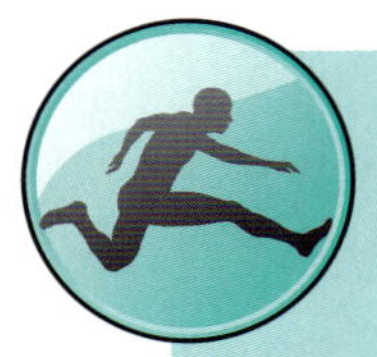

The risk of developing conduct disorder is increased in children with a biologic or adoptive parent with antisocial personality disorder or a sibling with conduct disorder.

Anxiety disorders specific to childhood

The anxiety disorders in childhood are marked by anxiety or depression and often seem to be exaggerations of normal developmental trends rather than discrete illnesses in themselves. They seldom persist into adult life and tend to have a good prognosis. The treatment of these disorders is focused on behavioral and family therapy. They include:

- *Separation anxiety disorder:* inappropriate and excessive anxiety about separation from those to whom the child is attached. Normal separation anxiety occurs in well-adjusted children from 6 months to 2 years. This disorder is diagnosed only when the anxiety is of such a severity that it is markedly different from other children of a similar age or when it persists beyond the usual age period.
- *Phobic anxiety disorder:* a developmental phase-specific fear or phobia (e.g., fear of animals in preschool children) that features a degree of anxiety that is clinically abnormal. Note that nondevelopmental phobias (e.g., agoraphobia) do not fall under this category but fall under the adult phobia category (see Ch. 5).
- *Social anxiety disorder:* a persistent and recurrent fear or avoidance of strangers. Normal stranger anxiety occurs in well-adjusted children from 8 months to 1 year. This disorder is diagnosed only when the anxiety is of such a severity that it is markedly different from other children of a similar age or when it persists beyond the usual age period.
- *Sibling relational disorder:* abnormal levels of sibling rivalry or jealousy following the birth of a younger sibling. Some emotional disturbance or jealousy is normal after the birth of a sibling. This disorder is diagnosed when the disturbance is excessive or persistent.

School refusal is the refusal to go to school because of anxiety in spite of parental pressure. It may be caused by separation anxiety (younger children) or be a symptom of another mental illness, such as depression, adjustment disorder (change from junior to secondary school), or social phobia. Truancy, on the other hand, is an absence from school by choice and is associated with conduct disorder, poor academic performance, family history of antisocial behavior, and large family size.

Other disorders with onset usually in childhood or adolescence

Selective mutism

Selective mutism is a condition characterized by a marked selectivity in speaking depending on the specific social situation. The child will typically speak normally in certain situations (e.g., at home) but is mute in others (e.g., at school). These children have adequately developed language comprehension and ability, although a minority may have speech delay or articulation problems. It usually presents before the age of 5, is slightly more common in girls, and is associated with psychological stress, social anxiety, and oppositional behavior.

Tic disorders

Tics are sudden, involuntary, rapid, recurrent, nonrhythmic motor movements or vocalizations that are experienced as irresistible. They are divided into:

- Simple motor tics: eye-blinking, neck-jerking, facial grimacing
- Simple vocal tics: grunting, coughing, barking, sniffing
- Complex motor tics: jumping, touching or hitting oneself, echopraxia (see Ch. 4), copropraxia (use of obscene gestures)
- Complex vocal tics: senseless repetition of words, coprolalia (use of obscene words or phrases), palilalia, echolalia (see Ch. 4).

Gilles de la Tourette's syndrome is characterized by the presence of *both* multiple motor tics and one or more vocal tics for more than 1 year. The motor tics usually present by age 7 years, although tics can present as early as 2 years of age. Obsessions and compulsions (OCD) and attention difficulties and impulsivity (ADHD) are associated conditions that may require treatment (see Ch. 7).

Pharmacotherapy is the most effective treatment for tics, but behavior therapy may reduce the stress that aggravates them. Dopamine antagonists, such as haloperidol and pimozide, as well as atypical antipsychotics are most commonly used, but side effects are a concern. SSRIs and clomipramine may be useful in treating associated obsessions and compulsions.

Other tic disorders include *transient tic disorder* (motor and/or vocal tics lasting no longer than 12 months) and *chronic motor or vocal tic disorder* (either motor or vocal tics, but not both).

Tics may be aggravated by anxiety, stressful situations or stimulants (e.g., caffeine, methylphenidate, and amphetamines). In contrast, sleep, relaxation or concentration on absorbing activities reduces their frequency.

Nonorganic enuresis

This condition is characterized by the involuntary voiding of urine into the bed or clothes in children who, according to their mental age, should have established consistent bladder control (therefore ordinarily not diagnosed before the age of 5). It may occur day or night and is not directly caused by any medical condition (e.g., seizures, diabetes, urinary tract infection, structural abnormalities of the urinary tract) or use of a substance (e.g., diuretic). Two types of enuresis have been described: *primary enuresis* means that urinary continence has never been established, and *secondary enuresis* means that continence has been achieved in the past.

Prevalence

- 5–10% of 5-year-olds.
- 3–5% of 10-year-olds.
- 1% of adolescents over age 15.
- Male-to-female ratio 1 : 1 in 5-year-olds; 2 : 1 in adolescents.

Etiology

Genetic factors, developmental delays, psychosocial stressors (moving house, birth of a sibling, start or change of school, divorce, bereavement), inadequate toilet training.

Treatment

- Exclude a physical problem (e.g., urinary tract infection).
- Parental education about appropriate toilet training (especially in primary enuresis).
- Behavior therapy (pad and buzzer apparatus, star chart, bladder training).
- Pharmacotherapy as a last resort: imipramine, nasal desmopressin (DDAVP).

Prognosis

Most cases resolve by adolescence.

About 75% of children with nonorganic enuresis have a first-degree biologic relative who has had the same problem.

Nonorganic encopresis

This condition is characterized by the deposition of normal feces (i.e., not diarrhea) in inappropriate places in children who, according to their mental age, should have established consistent bowel control (therefore ordinarily not diagnosed before the age of 4). It may be due to unsuccessful toilet training in which bowel control has never been achieved (primary encopresis) or may occur after a period of normal bowel control (secondary encopresis). Encopresis may result from a developmental delay, coercive or punitive potty training, emotional, physical, or sexual abuse, a disturbed parent–child relationship, marital conflict, or feature as a symptom of another psychiatric disturbance (e.g., autism). About 1% of 5-year-olds have the condition, and it is more common in males. Management includes ruling out an organic cause (constipation with overflow incontinence, anal fissure, gastrointestinal infection), assessing and treating disturbed family dynamics (ruling out child abuse), parental guidance regarding toilet training, and behavior therapy (e.g., star chart). Stool softeners may be used for constipation. The prognosis is good, with 90% of cases improving within a year.

"Adult" disorders with onset in childhood

All psychiatric disorders that usually present in adulthood can also develop in childhood (e.g., mood disorders, psychotic disorders, anxiety disorders, substance-related problems). The diagnostic criteria are essentially the same as for adults (see relevant chapters); although a diagnosis in a child may require fewer criteria be met and/or there may be minor variations.

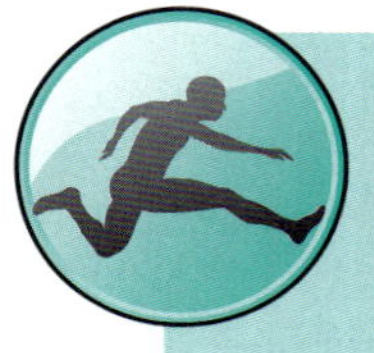

Depression in childhood may present with irritable rather than depressed mood and with failure to make expected weight gains rather than weight loss.

Child abuse

Child abuse includes the overlapping concepts of physical (nonaccidental injury), sexual and emotional abuse, as well as neglect or deprivation of the child. Figure 23.5 lists the risk factors associated with child abuse.

In addition to the physical manifestations of abuse, children who have been abused may present with failure to thrive and symptoms of depression, anxiety, aggression, precocious sexual behavior, posttraumatic stress disorder, and suicidal behavior. They are also at an increased risk for the development of a substantial range of psychiatric problems in later life. It is often difficult making the diagnosis, so a high index of suspicion is needed. Remember that the child's safety is always the main priority, and health-care professionals should have a low threshold for informing social services when their suspicions are raised.

Risk factors for child abuse	
Parent/environmental factors	**Child factors**
Parents who were abused Parental substance abuse Parental mental illness (mental retardation, depression, schizophrenia, personality disorders) Step-parent Young, immature parents Parental criminality Poor socioeconomic status and overcrowding	Low birth weight or prematurity Early maternal separation Unwanted child Mental retardation or physical disability Challenging behavior Hyperactivity Excessive crying

Fig. 23.5 Risk factors for child abuse.

- How are psychiatric disorders in children classified?
- What are the two essential characteristics of mental retardation?
- How is mental retardation classified?
- What prenatal factors are associated with mental retardation?
- What environmental and physical conditions should you exclude before diagnosing a child with a specific reading disorder?
- What are the three main characteristics of autism?
- What is the difference between Rett's syndrome and childhood disintegrative disorder?
- What common conditions should attention-deficit/hyperactivity disorder (ADHD) be distinguished from?
- What is the pharmacologic treatment of ADHD?
- How does conduct disorder differ from oppositional defiant disorder?
- What are the causes of school refusal? How does it differ from truancy?
- What types of tic occur in Gilles de la Tourette's syndrome? With what other conditions is it associated?
- What is the treatment of nonorganic enuresis?
- How may depression present in children?
- What are the risk factors for child abuse?

Suggested further reading

Coghill D 2003 Current issues in child and adolescent psychopharmacology. Part 1: Attention-deficit hyperactivity and affective disorders. Advances in Psychiatric Treatment 9: 86–94

Coghill D 2003 Current issues in child and adolescent psychopharmacology. Part 2: Anxiety and obsessive-compulsive disorders, autism, Tourette's and schizophrenia. Advances in Psychiatric Treatment 9: 289–299

Fitzgerald M, Corvin A 2001 Diagnosis and differential diagnosis of Asperger syndrome. Advances in Psychiatric Treatment 7: 310–318

Kramer T, Garralda M E 2000 Child and adolescent mental health problems in primary care. Advances in Psychiatric Treatment 6: 287–294

Scott S 2002 Classification of psychiatric disorders in childhood and adolescence: building castles in the sand? Advances in Psychiatric Treatment 8: 205–213

24. Geriatric Psychiatry

Patients arbitrarily come under the care of geriatric psychiatrists at the age of 65 years, as it is the average age of retirement. The number of people over the age of 65 has more than doubled since the 1930s. As life expectancy continues to increase, this percentage is likely to rise. Between 1995 and 2025 the number of people aged 80 and over should increase by nearly half, and the number of people aged 90 and over should double.

Mental illness in the elderly

The psychosocial consequences of aging

Not only is aging associated with a decline in physical health but also psychological and social changes. The psychological changes with aging include a decline in intellectual functioning as evidenced by:

- Cognitive slowing: there is slowing of the speed of processing of new information and an increase in reaction times. There tends to be no impairment of well-rehearsed (e.g., verbal comprehension) and knowledge-based skills.
- Impaired long-term remote memory, although memory for events of personal significance remains intact. There tends to be no impairment of short-term memory (as measured by digit span).

Important social challenges include coming to terms with retirement; income reduction; living alone, or being separated from family; death of spouse, siblings. and peers; and coping with deteriorating physical health and mobility.

Epidemiology of mental illness in the elderly

The prevalence of all mental illness tends to increase with age and is about 25–30% in people over the age of 65. The prevalence of mental illness tends to be higher in residential homes. Figure 24.1 summarizes the prevalence of the individual psychiatric disorders in the elderly.

Depressive disorders

Depression in the elderly presents similarly to that in younger people, although certain features seem more prevalent:

- Severe psychomotor agitation or retardation
- Apparent cognitive impairment (depressive pseudodementia)
- Poor concentration
- Generalized anxiety
- Excessive concerns about physical health (hypochondriasis)
- When psychotic, the elderly may have hypochondriacal delusions, delusions of poverty, and nihilistic delusions (see Ch. 4).

Depression is often underdiagnosed in the elderly, so a high index of suspicion is needed. This is important considering that the elderly are at high risk for completed suicide, even though the prevalence of parasuicide in this group is lower than in adults.

The principles of treatment are the same as for younger adults, although medication should be introduced cautiously as the elderly have an increased risk of developing adverse side effects and generally need lower doses; postural hypotension is a particular problem with tricyclic antidepressants. Electroconvulsive therapy (ECT) is a very effective treatment for depression in this population group and should be considered for severe depression, suicidal ideation, severe psychomotor retardation, failure to respond to or tolerate medication, and previous good response to ECT. Lithium augmentation may be used in treatment-resistant cases, although the dose is generally half that used in younger adults. Patients in this age group often need lifelong antidepressant treatment to reduce the chance of relapse. Psychosocial intervention in the form of social support and possibly cognitive-behavioral therapy are also important.

Poor prognostic factors include comorbid physical illness, late detection of illness, and poor compliance with antidepressant medication. Elderly depressed patients have a higher mortality than the nondepressed do, even when physical illness is taken into account.

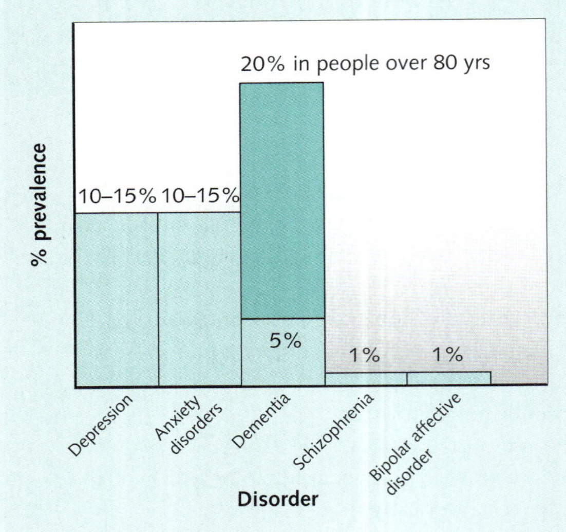

Fig. 24.1 Prevalence of mental illness in people over the age of 65.

Cotard's syndrome describes the presence of nihilistic and hypochondriacal delusions as part of a depressive psychosis and is typically seen in the elderly.

Mania

Unlike depression, the incidence of bipolar affective disorder does not increase with age, although late-onset cases seem to be less influenced by genetic factors (fewer of these patients have positive family histories for mood disorders). In a fifth of cases, mania is precipitated by an acute medical condition (e.g., stroke or myocardial infarction). The presentation and treatment is similar to that of younger adults.

Dementia and delirium

See Chapters 9 and 16.

Late-onset schizophrenia

Geriatric psychiatrists use the term *late-onset schizophrenia* to denote a group of patients who develop psychotic symptoms late in life, usually over the age of 60. Late-onset schizophrenia is characterized predominantly by delusional thinking, usually of a persecutory or grandiose nature. These delusions tend not to be as fantastic as they sometimes are in earlier-onset schizophrenia; for example, rather than believing that secret agents are monitoring them by satellite, patients will assert that the neighbors have been poisoning their water supply. Hallucinations may occur but disorganized thinking, inappropriate affect, and catatonic features rarely are present.

The etiology of late-onset schizophrenia seems different from that of early-onset schizophrenia, especially as regards genetic loading: the risk of schizophrenia in first-degree relatives is highest for a young schizophrenic, intermediate for a late-onset schizophrenic, and lowest for an unaffected person in the general population. Also, late-onset schizophrenia is far more common in women than men, whereas early-onset schizophrenia has a more equal sex ratio. Sensory deprivation, particularly hearing loss and social isolation, is also implicated in its etiology.

The treatment is with antipsychotics, but some work is needed in building up a therapeutic relationship as these patients are often difficult to engage and poor compliance is associated with a poor treatment response. Note that, although late-onset schizophrenia does seem to be a distinct entity, it is not a term used by the DSM-IV-TR or the ICD-10; here, these patients would be classified as having schizophrenia or delusional disorder.

Diogenes syndrome or "senile squalor" is the term used to describe an elderly recluse who lives in a state of perpetual filth and gross self-neglect, often with the hoarding of rubbish. This is purely a descriptive term and may occur in individuals with alcohol abuse, frontal lobe dysfunction, personality disorder, or chronic psychotic illness. It may also occur at a younger age.

Assessment considerations in the elderly

- Home assessments are a very important part of geriatric psychiatry. Patients can be assessed in their normal environment and collateral information can be obtained from family members. It is important to ascertain whether the patient can be managed at home (e.g., risk of harm to self and others; ability to carry out activities of daily living, drive, and manage financial affairs) or whether additional community support or hospitalization is needed.

- Collateral information from the patient's physician, family, and neighbors is an important part of history taking.
- The mental state examination follows the same format as for younger adults, although extra consideration should be given to the assessment of cognitive functioning, and it is advisable to always do a Mini-Mental State Examination (see Fig. 9.10, p. 71).
- A thorough physical examination is very important. Do not forget to assess hearing and vision as well as tremors and involuntary movements.
- Routine investigations in the newly diagnosed or hospitalized elderly include complete blood count, BUN and electrolytes, liver function tests, thyroid function tests, calcium, glucose, serum proteins, midstream urine microscopy and culture, chest X-ray, ECG, and CT scan when indicated. Remember that the chances of a physical illness causing or aggravating a mental deterioration are significant in the elderly.

Treatment considerations in the elderly

Physiologic changes with aging

There are a number of physiologic changes that occur with aging, which may affect the handling of certain drugs. Figure 24.2 describes the most important changes and their effects. The net result of these changes is that the tissue concentration of a drug may be increased by over 50%, especially in malnourished, dehydrated, and debilitated patients. Therefore the adage "start low and go slow" applies especially to the use of psychotropic drugs in the elderly.

Polypharmacy

The elderly receive almost a third of all prescriptions issued in the US, and 15% of these are for four drugs or more. This increases the risk of adverse reactions, drug interactions, and poor compliance. The practice of prescribing psychotropic drugs for common symptoms such as insomnia and headache should be avoided as they may lead to further nonspecific symptoms

Age-related changes in drug-handling and effects	
Physiologic change	**Effect**
Reduction in renal clearance (glomerular filtration rate and tubular function)	Drugs excreted by filtration (e.g., lithium) need lower doses Drug concentrations may rise rapidly with dehydration, heart failure, etc.
Decreased lean body mass and total body water and increased body fat	Volume of distribution increases for lipid-soluble drugs (most psychotropic drugs), and reduces for water-soluble drugs (e.g., lithium)
Decreased plasma albumin	Reduced drug binding resulting in increased physiologically active unbound fraction
Reduced hepatic metabolism and first-pass metabolism	May increase the bioavailability and elimination of some drugs
Increased sensitivity to central nervous system drugs	Sedating drugs may result in drowsiness, confusion, falls, and delirium Sensitive to anticholinergic, postural hypotensive, and parkinsonian effects of tricyclic antidepressants and conventional antipsychotics
Decreased total body mass	Lower doses of drugs needed (think in terms of "mg/kg" as opposed to standard dose for all)

Fig. 24.2 Age-related changes in drug-handling and effects.

(e.g., confusion, drowsiness, and light-headedness). Medication should not be a substitute for adequate social care, the lack of which often underlies many of these symptoms.

Compliance

Compliance is often a problem with the elderly, especially with those who are visually impaired, confused, take numerous drugs, and live alone. This may be improved by simplifying medication regimens, taking time to explain dosing schedules, and labeling prescriptions clearly. Organizing supervision of medication taking by a relative, friend, or visiting nurse may be necessary.

Psychosocial interventions

Psychological treatment, such as supportive and cognitive behavior therapy, has been applied with success in the elderly. Reality orientation and reminiscence therapies have been used to reduce confusion and stimulate remote memories in patients with dementia. Practical psychosocial interventions such as memory aids (e.g., notebooks, calendars) and assistance with mobility and daily activities by a support worker should not be underestimated. Activities of daily living (ADL) scales, which assess skills such as washing, dressing, eating, shopping, etc., provide caregivers with an indication of patients' strengths and weaknesses and enable them to tailor a package that caters specifically to these.

- What are the three most prevalent mental illnesses in people over the age of 65?
- What features are particularly prominent in depression in the elderly?
- What are the dangers of prescribing tricyclic antidepressants to the elderly considering age-related changes in physiology?
- How does late-onset schizophrenia differ from early-onset schizophrenia in terms of etiology and clinical presentation?
- What is the role of home assessments in old age psychiatry?
- What factors should be considered before prescribing a benzodiazepine to an elderly patient on numerous cardiac drugs who lives alone?

Suggested further reading

Bouman W P, Pinner G 2002 Use of atypical antipsychotic drugs in old age psychiatry. Advances in Psychiatric Treatment 8: 49–58

British Journal of Psychiatry 2002 Old age psychiatry papers. British Journal of Psychiatry 180: 116–167

Cattell H 2000 Suicide in the elderly. Advances in Psychiatric Treatment 6: 102–108

Evans M, Mottram P 2000 Diagnosis of depression in elderly patients. Advances in Psychiatric Treatment 6: 49–56

25. Forensic Psychiatry

Forensic psychiatry, in its narrowest sense, is concerned with assessment and treatment of mentally ill offenders as well as with the assessment of the dangerousness of individuals who may not yet have committed an offense. Certain patients may require treatment and rehabilitation in a secure environment, such as a special hospital or regional secure unit.

Mental illness and crime

The vast majority of patients suffering from a mental illness have never committed an offense, and most offenses are not committed by people with a mental illness. However, there is a significantly higher prevalence of mental illness among prisoners than in the general population. Yet this does not mean that mental illness causes people to offend. In fact, most evidence indicates that crime and mental illness are only weakly associated.

Certain mental disorders, however, have shown some association with both violent and nonviolent crime. These are summarized in Figure 25.1.

- Note that the mental disorders associated with violent crime – personality disorders (especially antisocial personality disorder), alcohol and substance dependence, and paranoid psychotic disorders – may have an additive effect to the risk of future violence when they occur in combination.
- Remember that delusions of jealousy (Othello syndrome) are common with alcohol abuse and are linked to violent crime such as battering and homicide.

Personality disorder and crime

The German clinician Koch first used the term "psychopathy" in 1891. At that time it included all forms of personality disorder. However, the term was later used to describe individuals who exhibited antisocial behavior. Unfortunately, the term "psychopathic personality" and the related term "psychopath" have been misused in both the medical and tabloid press. They were, for the most part, superseded by the term sociopathic personality disorder for a time and subsequently by the favored, and currently used term, antisocial personality disorder (see Ch. 11).

Assessing dangerousness

The key principle in assessing dangerousness concerns an ethical conflict between protecting the community from a potentially violent offender and respecting the human rights of the individual in question. Despite much research on this very complex subject, the ability of experts to predict whether an individual will behave violently in the future is still not completely reliable. The approaches to the prediction of violence include:

- Unaided clinical risk assessment: assessment on an individual patient basis using unaided clinical judgment
- Actuarial methods: time-consuming assessment using predetermined static actuarial or statistical variables (e.g., demographic factors)
- Structured clinical judgment: assessment utilizing both empirical actuarial knowledge and clinical expertise.

Figure 25.2 summarizes some of the factors that have been associated with the risk of violence.

A clinician confronted with an individual who poses a serious risk of violent behavior should discuss the case with colleagues, including psychiatrists, psychologists, and forensic specialists. Involuntary commitment may be required in serious cases. Clinicians may, and indeed have a duty to, breach confidentiality considerations to warn potential victims of serious

Mental disorders associated with crime	
Mental disorder	**Associations with crime**
Personality disorder	Associated with violent crime. Antisocial and borderline personally disorders are frequently diagnosed in forensic settings, often in association with comorbid substance abuse
Alcohol and substance use	Alcohol leads to disinhibition and is strongly associated with violent crime. Alcohol intoxication may also lead to driving offenses and public drunkenness. Drug intoxication is also associated with violent crime and offenses may be committed to fund drug habits
Schizophrenia	There is conflicting evidence concerning schizophrenia and crime, but it appears that schizophrenic patients commit more violent crimes than the general population. These crimes are associated with command hallucinations and paranoid delusions accompanied by strong affect. However, most offenses committed by schizophrenics are minor and are manifestations of social incompetence
Mood disorders	Depression is associated with shoplifting and, in rare cases, homicide, or infanticide in psychotic postpartum depression. These cases are usually due to mood-congruent delusions (e.g., everyone would be better off dead) and are often followed by suicide. Offenses by manic patients usually reflect financial irresponsibility or acts of aggression, which are usually not serious
Mental retardation	There is an association between mental retardation and sexual offenses (especially indecent exposure), as well as arson

Fig. 25.1 Mental disorders associated with crime.

threats that have been made, in consultation with the police.

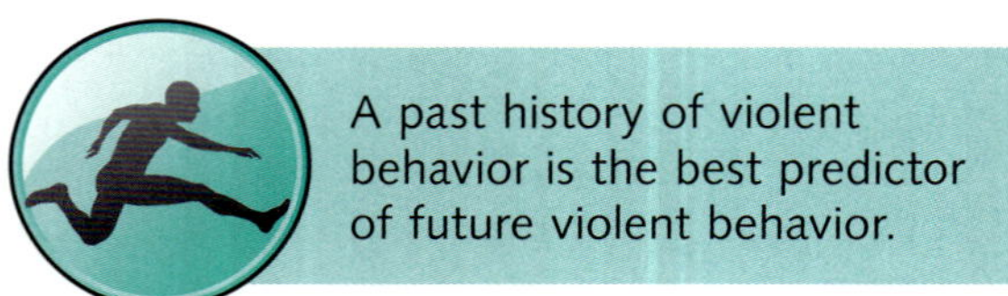

Considerations in court proceedings

Competence to stand trial

Individuals with severe mental illness are not exempt from taking responsibility for their actions. However, defendants should be competent to stand trial and mount a defense against their charges. In order to be found competent, the defendant must demonstrate "significant present ability to consult with his lawyer with a reasonable degree of rational understanding, and . . . a rational as well as factual understanding of the proceedings against him" (*Dusky v. United States* [US 1960]).

Clinicians may offer opinions about competence. The judge will consider these opinions and ultimately rule whether a patient is competent or incompetent.

Criminal responsibility

Before a defendant can be convicted, criminal responsibility needs to be determined. For an objectionable act to be considered a crime, two components must be present:

1. Voluntary conduct (actus reus) and
2. Evil intent (mens rea).

The person must be able to control his/her own behavior and make the choice to commit the act, *and* the individual must intend to commit the act and understand the nature of it.

In a tiny fraction of cases, a defendant may be found not guilty by reason of insanity. The precedent for the insanity defense was established in the English courts in 1843. The so-called M'Naghten Rule states the following: *"at the time of committing the act, the party accused was laboring under such a defect of reason, from disease of the mind, as to not know the nature and quality of the act he was doing, or, if he did know it, that*

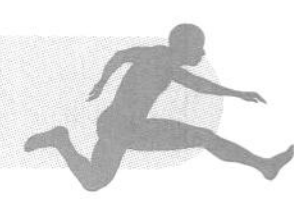

Factors associated with risk of violence	
Demographic factors	Male Young age Poor socioeconomic status Poor social support • Relationship instability • Employment difficulties
History and background	Previous episodes of violence/convictions • Numerous serious offenses • Young age at first violent offense • Sadistic, unprovoked or bizarre offenses • Lack of remorse Alcohol or substance misuse Antisocial personality disorder; conduct disorder Presence of major psychiatric illness Continued presence of precipitants of previous offenses Impulsivity/poor self-control Poor compliance with psychiatric care or recent discontinuation of treatment Drug use by father History of parental fighting Abuse in childhood
Mental state examination	Violence ideation • Violent fantasies • High degree of intent • Repeated threats • Presence of a victim • Planning of violence • Access to weapons Paranoid beliefs/psychosis • Persecutory delusions/ideas • Delusions of external control • Delusions/ideas of jealousy (morbid jealousy) • Command auditory hallucinations Irritability, hostility, psychomotor agitation

Fig. 25.2 Factors associated with risk of violence.

he did not know what he was doing was wrong." If found "not guilty by reason of insanity," an offender is detained in a psychiatric hospital.

A more common defense is the alternative option of *diminished capacity.* This defense can be applied if the defendant suffers from a mental illness or cognitive deficit that does not meet the criteria for the insanity defense but nonetheless provides a basis for not holding the defendant completely responsible for his/her behavior. In this defense, the defendant's impairment (usually but not always mental illness) interferes with the ability to formulate a specific element (e.g., forethought) of the particular crime. This defense is most commonly used to reduce the level of the conviction (e.g., from first-degree to second-degree murder).

Self-induced intoxication with alcohol or other drugs is not considered to be a defense to those crimes for which "specific intent" need not be proved (e.g., rape, manslaughter, indecent assault). It may, however, indicate lack of intent in crimes for which "specific intent" must be proved (e.g., murder, theft).

- What is the association between mental illness and crime?
- What psychiatric disorders are associated with violent crime?
- What is the difference between psychopathy, psychopathic disorder, and antisocial personality disorder?
- What factors on mental state examination are associated with a future risk of violence?
- Name circumstances in which a person may be found to be lacking mens rea.

Suggested further reading

Birmingham L 2003 The mental health of prisoners. Advances in Psychiatric Treatment 9: 191–199

Humphreys M 2000 Aspects of basic management of offenders with mental disorders. Advances in Psychiatric Treatment 6: 22–30

Rice M E, Harris G T, Quinsey V L 2002 The appraisal of violence risk. Current Opinion in Psychiatry 15: 559–589. Available on line at: http://www.medscape.com/viewarticle/444153

Snowden P 2001 Substance misuse and violence: the scope and limitations of forensic psychiatry's role. Advances in Psychiatric Treatment 7: 189–197

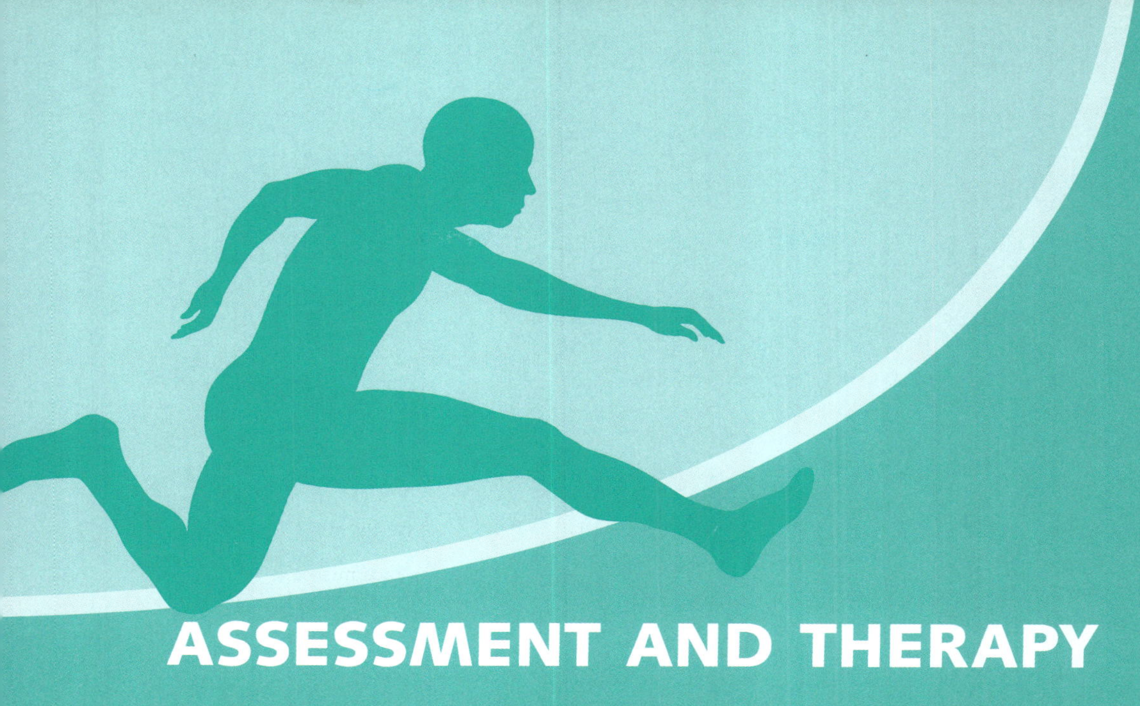

ASSESSMENT AND THERAPY

26. Psychiatric Assessment and Diagnosis

The psychiatric assessment is different from a medical or surgical assessment in that (1) the history taking is longer and is aimed at understanding psychological problems that develop in patients, each with a unique background and social environment; and (2) a mental status examination is performed. Figure 26.1 provides an outline of the psychiatric assessment, which includes a psychiatric history, mental status examination, physical examination, and formulation.

Interview technique

- Whenever possible, patients should be interviewed in settings where privacy can be ensured. A patient who has just attempted suicide will be put more at ease in a quiet office than in an emergency department cubicle.
- Establishing rapport is an immediate priority and requires the display of genuineness, empathy, and sensitivity by the interviewer.
- Notes may be taken during the interview; however, explain to patients that you will be doing so. Make sure that you still maintain good eye contact.
- Ensure that you are seated near the door. This allows an unobstructed exit for you if you feel threatened.
- Introduce yourself to the patient and ask how the patient would like to be addressed. Explain how long the interview will last. In examination situations it may prove helpful to explain to patients that you may need to interrupt them due to time constraints.
- Keep track of, and ration, your time appropriately.
- Flexibility is essential. For example, it may be helpful to put very anxious patients at ease by talking about their background before zooming in on the presenting complaint.

Make use of both closed and open-ended questions when appropriate:

Closed questions limit the scope of the response to one or two word answers. They are used to gain specific information and can be used to control the length of the interview when patients are being over-inclusive. For example:

- Are you low in mood? (Yes or no answer)
- What time do you wake up in the morning? (Specific answer).

Note that closed questions can be used at the very beginning of the interview as they are easier to answer and help to put patients at ease. Examples include "Do you live locally?" and "Are you married?" See "identifying information" below.

Open-ended questions encourage the patient to answer freely with a wide range of responses and should be used to elicit the presenting complaint, as well as feelings and attitudes. For example

- How have you been feeling lately?
- What led you to feel this way?

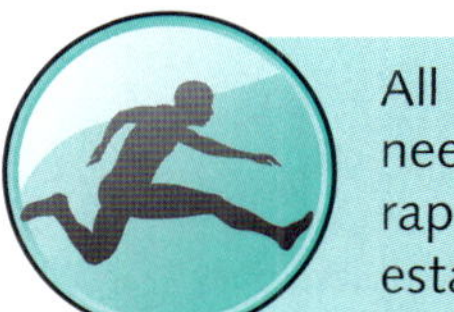

All mental health workers need to work on being expert rapport-builders. Failure to establish rapport should be due to patient, not interviewer, factors, as the failure to establish rapport may be an important sign of mental illness. For example, patients with persecutory delusions may believe that the interviewer is trying to harm them; or patients with paranoid personality traits may mistrust the interviewer's motives.

Psychiatric history

The order in which you take the history is not as important as being systematic, making sure you cover all the essential subsections. A typical format for taking a psychiatric history is outlined in Figure 26.1 and will now follow in more detail.

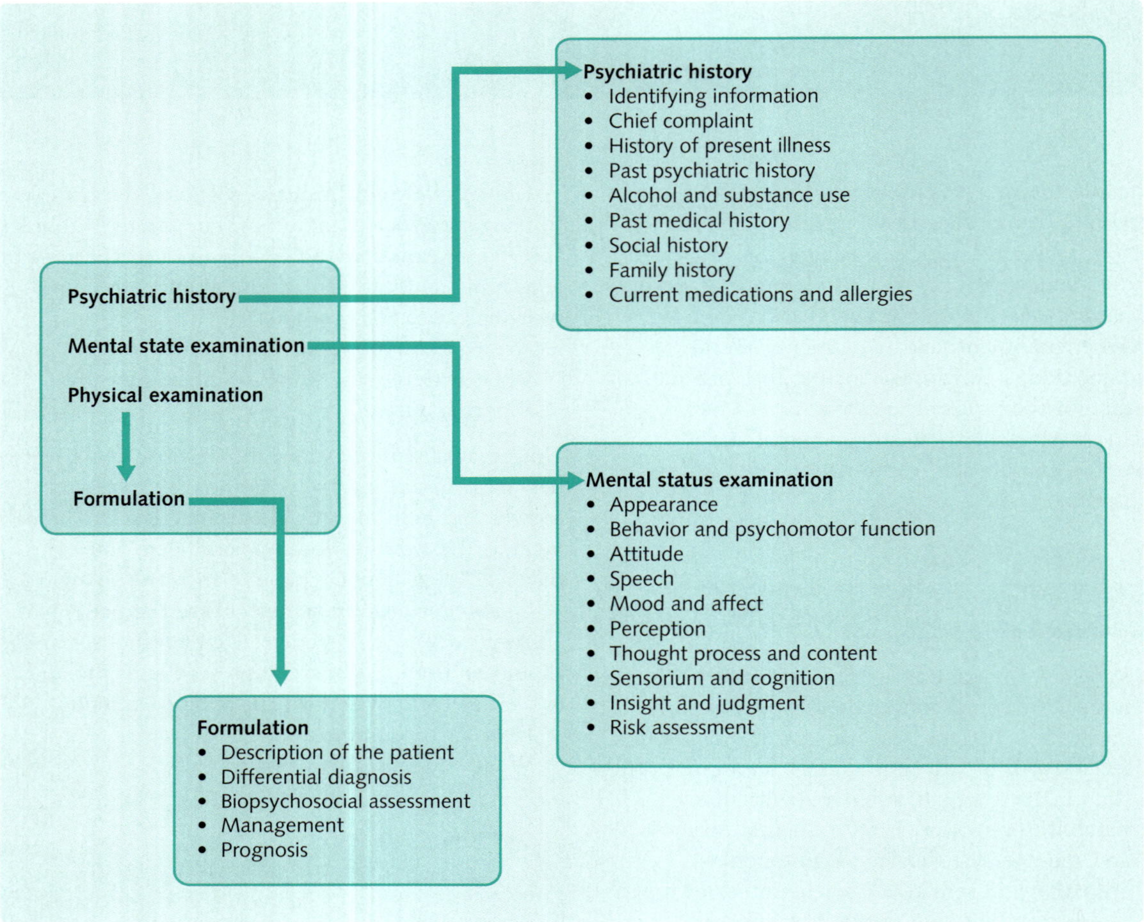

Psychiatric history
Mental state examination
Physical examination
Formulation

Psychiatric history
- Identifying information
- Chief complaint
- History of present illness
- Past psychiatric history
- Alcohol and substance use
- Past medical history
- Social history
- Family history
- Current medications and allergies

Mental status examination
- Appearance
- Behavior and psychomotor function
- Attitude
- Speech
- Mood and affect
- Perception
- Thought process and content
- Sensorium and cognition
- Insight and judgment
- Risk assessment

Formulation
- Description of the patient
- Differential diagnosis
- Biopsychosocial assessment
- Management
- Prognosis

Fig. 26.1 Outline of the psychiatric assessment.

Identifying information

- Name
- Age
- Marital status and children
- Occupation
- Reason for the patient's presence in a psychiatric setting (e.g., referral to outpatient clinic by family doctor or admitted to ward informally having presented at casualty).

For example:

> Mrs LM is a 32-year-old married housewife with two children aged 4 and 6 years, who was referred by her family doctor to a psychiatric outpatient clinic.

Chief complaint

Open-ended questions are used to elicit the chief complaint. Whenever possible, record the main problems in the patient's own words, in one or two sentences, instead of using technical psychiatric terms. For example:

> Mrs LM complains of "feeling as though I don't know who I am, like I'm living in an empty shell."

Patients frequently have more than one complaint, some of which may be related. It is helpful to organize multiple presenting complaints into groups of symptoms that are related. For instance, "low mood," "poor concentration," and "lack of energy" are common features of depression:

Mrs LM complains firstly of "low mood," "difficulty sleeping," and "poor self-esteem" as well as "increased alcohol consumption" associated with withdrawal symptoms of "shaking, sweating, and jitteriness" in the morning.

History of present illness

This section is concerned with eliciting the nature and development of the chief complaint. The following headings may be helpful in structuring your questioning:

- Duration: when did the problems start?
- Development: how did the problems develop?
- Mode of onset: suddenly or over a period of time?
- Course: are symptoms constant, progressively worsening, or intermittent?
- Severity: how much is the patient suffering? To what extent are symptoms affecting the patient's social and occupational functioning?
- Associated symptoms: certain complaints are associated with certain symptoms that should be inquired about if patients don't mention them spontaneously. For example, when "feeling sad" is a presenting complaint, biologic, cognitive, and psychotic features of depression as well as suicidal ideation should be asked about. Also, certain symptoms are common to many psychiatric conditions and these should be screened for. For example, a primary complaint of insomnia may be a sign of depression, mania, psychosis, or a primary sleep disorder.
- Precipitating factors: psychosocial stress frequently precipitates episodes of mental illness (e.g., bereavement, moving house, relationship difficulties).
- The premorbid personality is an indication of the patient's personality and character before the onset of mental illness. Patients may be asked directly about their personality before they became ill, or it may be useful to ask a close family member or friend about a patient's premorbid personality. For example: a young schizophrenic man, with prominent negative symptoms of lack of motivation and interest, and poverty of thought, was described by his mother as being outgoing, intelligent, and ambitious before becoming ill.

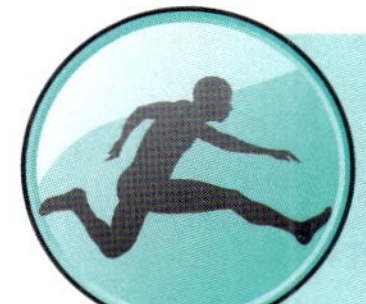

Because patients are not always forthcoming with all of their symptoms, it is wise to briefly screen all patients for the most common psychiatric disorders to ensure that you do not miss an important condition. Symptoms worth asking about include:

- Low mood (depression)
- Elevated mood and increased energy (hypomania and mania)
- Delusions and hallucinations (psychosis)
- Free-floating anxiety, panic attacks, or phobias (anxiety disorders)
- Obsessions or compulsions (obsessive-compulsive disorder)
- Alcohol or substance abuse.

Past psychiatric history

This is an extremely important section as it may provide clues to the patient's current diagnosis. It should include:

- Dates and duration of previous mental illness episodes
- Details of previous treatments, including medication, psychotherapy, electroconvulsive therapy, and hospitalizations
- Details of previous contact with psychiatric services.

Alcohol and substance use

This section should never be overlooked, as alcohol/substance-related psychiatric conditions are not uncommon.

The CAGE questionnaire (see Ch. 10) is a useful tool to screen for alcohol dependence. If patients answer affirmatively to two or more questions, regard the screen as positive and go on to check if they meet the definitive criteria for the alcohol dependence syndrome (see Ch. 10). Try to elicit a patient's typical drinking day, including daily intake of alcohol in units, type of alcohol used, time of first drink of the day, and places where drinking occurs (e.g., at home alone or in a bar).

If illicit drugs have been or are being used, record the drug names, routes of administration (intravenous, inhaled, oral ingestion), and the years and frequency of use. Also inquire about possible dependence (see Ch. 10).

Past medical history

Inquire about medical illnesses, surgical procedures, and hospitalizations. Past head injury or surgery, neurologic conditions (e.g., epilepsy), and endocrine abnormalities (e.g., thyroid problems) are especially relevant to psychiatry. Include a developmental history:

- Pregnancy and birth complications (e.g., prematurity, fetal distress, cesarean section)
- Developmental milestones (age of crawling, walking, speaking, bladder and bowel control)
- Childhood illnesses.

Social history

This includes living situation, social supports and relationships, employment and financial circumstances, and hobbies or leisure activities. This section is important in order to understand the social context in which the patient's problems developed.

The social history includes a brief description of the patient's life. Time constraints will not allow an exhaustive biographical account but you should attempt to include significant events, perhaps under the following useful headings:

Infancy and early childhood (until age 5)

- Unusually aggressive behavior.
- Impaired social interaction.

Later childhood and adolescence (until completion of higher education)

- School record (academic performance, number and type of schools attended, age on leaving, and final qualifications).
- Relationships with parents, teachers, and peers. History of physical, sexual, or emotional abuse. Victim or perpetrator of bullying.
- Behavioral problems, including antisocial behavior, drug use, or truancy.
- Higher education and training.

Occupational record

- Details of types and duration of jobs.
- Details of and reasons for unemployment and/or dismissal

Relationship, marital, and sexual history

- Puberty: significant early relationships and experiences, as well as sexual orientation.
- Details and duration of significant relationships. Reasons for break-ups.
- Marriage/divorce details. Children.
- Ability to engage in satisfactory sexual relationships. Sexual dysfunction, fetishes, or gender identity problems (inquire if problem is suspected).

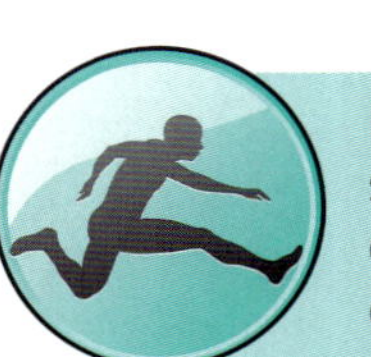

Inquiring about a history of sexual abuse is important, especially in patients who exhibit personality traits suggestive of a personality disorder or in those who regularly self-harm. Tact and discretion are clearly essential. A useful question to screen for sexual abuse is: "Have you ever had an unpleasant sexual experience?"

Forensic history

Inquire about the details and dates of previous offenses and antisocial behavior, including prosecutions, convictions, and prison sentences. It is important to ask specifically about violent crime and the age of the patient's first violent offense.

Family history

- Inquire about the presence of psychiatric illness (including suicide and substance abuse) in family members, remembering that genetic factors are implicated in the etiology of many psychiatric conditions – a family tree may be useful to summarize information.
- Inquire whether parents are still alive and, if not, causes of death. Also ask about significant physical illnesses in the family.
- Inquire about the quality of the patient's relationships with close family members.

Current medications and allergies

Note all the medication patients are using, including psychiatric, nonpsychiatric, and over-the-counter drugs. Also inquire how long patients have

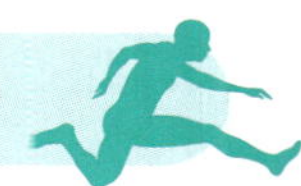

been on specific medication and whether it has been effective. Noncompliance as well as reactions and allergies should be recorded.

Mental status examination

The mental status examination (MSE) describes an interviewer's impression of many aspects of a patient's mental functioning at a certain period of time. Whereas the psychiatric history remains relatively constant, the MSE may fluctuate from day to day or hour to hour. It is useful to try and gather as much evidence as possible about the MSE while doing the psychiatric history, instead of viewing this as a separate section. In fact, the MSE begins the moment you meet the patient. In addition to noting their appearance, you should observe how patients first behave on meeting you. This includes their body language and the way that they respond to your attempts to establish rapport.

By the time you have finished the psychiatric history, you should have completed many aspects of the MSE, and you should just need to ask certain key questions to finish this process. The individual aspects of the MSE, which are summarized in Figure 26.1, are now discussed in more detail.

You should not just be recording patients' answers to questions while doing the psychiatric history section of the assessment. You should also be observing the way they speak, their posture, their facial expressiveness, their state of relaxation, and their movements as well as displays of emotion such as tearfulness, smiling, anger, and anxiety, all of which contribute to the mental state examination.

Appearance

- Physical state: how old does the patient appear? Does the patient appear physically unwell? Is he or she sweating? Is he or she too thin or obese?
- Clothes and accessories: are clothes clean? Do clothes match? Are clothes appropriate to the weather and circumstances, or are they bizarre? Is the patient carrying strange objects?
- Self-care and hygiene: does the patient appear in a state of self-neglect (e.g., unshaven, dirty tangled hair, malodorous, disheveled)? Is there any evidence of injury or self-harm (e.g., multiple cuts to wrists or forearms)?

Behavior and psychomotor function

This section focuses on all motor behavior, including abnormal movements such as tremors, tics, and twitches, as well as displays of suspiciousness, aggression, or fear, and catatonic features. Documenting patients' behavior at the start of, and during, the interview is an integral part of the mental state examination and should be done in as much detail as possible. For example:

> Mrs LM introduced herself appropriately, although only made fleeting eye contact. She sat rigidly throughout the first half of the interview, mostly staring at the floor and speaking very softly. She became tearful halfway through the interview when

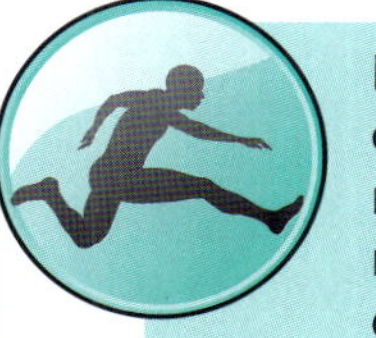

Remember that patients on conventional antipsychotics may display abnormal movements due to extrapyramidal side effects (EPS):

- Parkinson-like symptoms – muscular rigidity, bradykinesia (lack of or slowing of movement) and resting tremor
- Acute dystonia – involuntary sustained muscular contractions or spasms
- Akathisia – subjective feeling of inner restlessness and muscular discomfort
- Tardive dyskinesia – rhythmic, involuntary movements of head, limbs and trunk, especially chewing, grimacing of mouth, and protruding, darting movements of tongue.

talking about her lack of self-esteem. After this her posture relaxed, her eye contact improved, and there were moments when she smiled. There were no abnormal movements.

The term "psychomotor" is used to describe a patient's motor activity as a consequence of his or her concurrent mental processes. Psychomotor abnormalities include *retardation* (slow, monotonous speech, slow or absent body movements) and *agitation* (inability to sit still, fidgeting, pacing, or hand-wringing, rubbing or scratching skin or clothes).

Attitude

Note whether you are able to establish a good rapport with patients. What is their attitude towards you? Do they make good eye contact or do they look around the room or at the floor? Patients may be described as cooperative, cordial, uninterested, aggressive, defensive, guarded, suspicious, fearful, perplexed, preoccupied, disinhibited (i.e., a lowering of normal social inhibitions, or being overly familiar or making sexually inappropriate comments), etc.

Speech

Speech should be described in terms of:

- Rate of production (e.g., pressure of speech in mania, long pauses, and poverty of speech in depression)
- Quality and flow of speech: volume, dysarthria (articulation difficulties), dysprosody (unusual speech rhythm, melody, intonation or pitch), stuttering.

Note that disorganized, incoherent, or bizarre speech is usually regarded as a thought disorder and is, therefore, described under the thought section.

Mood and affect

Mood refers to a patient's sustained, subjectively experienced emotional state over a period of time. In the context of the mental status examination, *affect* means the observed, external expression of emotion – as perceived by another person; affect is sometimes called the "objective" assessment of mood.

Mood is assessed by asking patients how they are feeling. So a patient's mood might be depressed, elated, anxious, guilty, frightened, angry, etc. Figure 26.2 lists typical questions that may be used to elicit depressed, elated, or anxious moods.

Affect is assessed by observing patients' posture, facial expression, emotional reactivity, and speech. There are two components to consider when assessing affect:

1. The appropriateness or congruity of the observed affect to the patient's subjectively reported mood. For example, a schizophrenic woman who reports feeling suicidal with a happy facial expression would be described as having an *incongruous* affect.
2. The range of affect or range of emotional expressivity. In this sense affect may be:
   a. Within the normal range
   b. Blunted: a noticeable reduction in the normal intensity of emotional expression as evidenced by a monotonous voice and minimal facial expression
   c. Flat: very little or no emotional expression.

Note that a *labile* mood refers to a fluctuating mood state that alternates between extremes. For example, a young man with a mixed affective episode alternates between feeling overjoyed, with pressured speech, and miserable, with suicidal ideation.

Perception

At this stage of the assessment, the interviewer will probably have elicited hallucinations following the patient's presenting complaint. However, this is not always the case, so it is important that you specifically inquire about abnormal perceptual experiences. (Perceptual abnormalities are defined and classified in Ch. 4.) If patients admit to problems with perception, it is important to ascertain:

- Whether the abnormal perceptions are genuine hallucinations, pseudohallucinations, illusions, or just intrusive thoughts.
- From which sensory organ the hallucinations appear to arise, that is, are they auditory, visual, olfactory, gustatory, or somatic hallucinations – see Chapter 4.
- Whether auditory hallucinations are elementary or complex. If complex, are they experienced in the first person (audible thoughts, thought echo), second person (critical, persecutory, complimentary, or command hallucinations), or

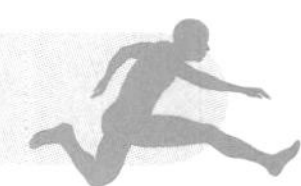

Typical questions used to elicit psychiatric symptoms	
Symptom	**Typical questions**
Depressive symptoms (Ch. 1)	Have you been cheerful or quite low in mood or spirits lately? Do you find that you no longer enjoy things the way you used to? Do you find yourself often feeling very tired or worn out? How do you see things turning out in the future? Sometimes when people are depressed they have a poor sex drive. Has this happened to you?
Mania/hypomania (Ch. 2)	Have you been feeling particularly happy or on top of the world lately? Do you sometimes feel as though you have too much energy compared to people around you? Do you find yourself needing less sleep but not getting tired? Have you had any new interests or exciting ideas lately? Have you noticed your thoughts racing in your head? Do you have any special abilities or powers?
Suicidal ideation (Ch. 3)	Have you been feeling that life isn't worth living? Do you sometimes feel like you would like to end it all? Have you actually given some thought as to how you might do it? How close do you think you are to going through with your plans? Do you currently have the means (rope, gun, pills) to carry out this plan? Is there anything that might stop you from attempting suicide?
Delusions(Ch. 4)	Are you afraid that someone is trying to harm or poison you? (*persecutory delusions*) Have you noticed that people are doing or saying things that have a special meaning for you? (*delusions of reference*) Do you have any special abilities or powers? (*grandiose delusions*) Does it seem as though you are being controlled or influenced by some external force? (*delusions of control*) Are thoughts that don't belong to you being put into your head? (*thought insertion*)
Hallucinations (Ch. 4)	Do you ever hear strange noises or voices when there is no one else about? Do you ever hear your own thoughts spoken aloud such that someone standing next to you might possibly hear them? Do you ever hear your thoughts echoed just after you have thought them? (*thought echo*) Do these voices talk directly to you or give you commands? Do these voices ever talk about you with each other or make comments about what you are doing?
Symptoms of anxiety (Ch. 5)	Do you sometimes wake up feeling anxious and dreading the day ahead? (*any form of anxiety*) Do you worry excessively about minor matters on most days of the week? (*generalized anxiety*) Have you ever been so frightened that your heart was pounding and you thought you might die? (*panic attack*) Do you avoid leaving the house alone because you are afraid of having a panic attack or being in situation (like being in a crowded shop or on a train) from which escape will be difficult or embarrassing? (*panic disorder with agoraphobia*) Do you get anxious in social situations, like speaking in front of people or making conversation? (*social phobia*) Do some things or situations make you very scared? Do you avoid them? (*specific phobia*)

Fig. 26.2 Typical questions used to elicit specific psychiatric symptoms.

Continued over

Typical questions used to elicit psychiatric symptoms	
Symptom	**Typical questions**
Obsessions and compulsions (Ch. 7)	Do you worry about contamination with dirt even when you have already washed? Do you have awful thoughts entering your mind despite trying hard to keep them out? Do you repeatedly have to check things that you have already done (stoves, lights, faucets, etc.)? Do you find that you have to arrange, touch, or count things many times over?
Somatoform disorders (Ch. 8)	Do you often worry about your health? Are you bothered by many different symptoms? Are you concerned that you might have a serious illness? Are you concerned about your facial or bodily appearance? Do you find it hard to believe doctors when they tell you that there is nothing wrong with you?
Memory and cognition (Ch. 9)	Mini Mental Status Examination (Table 9.10)
Problem drinking (Ch. 10)	**CAGE** questionnaire: Have you ever felt you ought to **C**ut down on your drinking? Have people ever **A**nnoyed you by criticizing your drinking? Have you ever felt **G**uilty about your drinking? Have you ever needed a drink first thing in the morning to steady your nerves or get rid of a hangover ("**E**ye-opener")?
Eating disorders (Ch. 12)	*Anorexic symptoms* Body weight and shape can be very important to some people. Do you find that you are quite concerned about your weight? A common way of losing weight is to eat less or to exercise a lot. Are these things that you do? Sometimes when women lose weight, their periods can become irregular or stop. Has this happened to you? *Bulimic symptoms* Are there times when you feel that your eating seems excessive or out of control? During these times, do you ever try to make yourself sick so that you feel better? Sometimes people might use pharmaceutical or street drugs to help control their weight. Have you ever had to do this?
Symptoms of insomnia	Do you fall asleep quickly or do you find yourself tossing and turning for some time before dropping off? Do you wake up repeatedly in the night, or can you sleep through once you have managed to get to sleep? Do you sometimes awaken too early in the morning and then find that you are unable to get back to sleep? Is your sleep refreshing, or do you still feel tired in the morning?

Fig. 26.2, cont'd.

third person (voices arguing or discussing the patient, or giving a running commentary)?

It is also important to note whether patients seem to be responding to hallucinations during the interview, as evidenced by them laughing inappropriately as though they are sharing a private joke, or suddenly tilting their head as though listening, or quizzically looking at hallucinatory objects around the room.

Figure 26.2 lists typical questions that may be used to elicit hallucinations.

Thought process and content

Thought process can be described by the following terms:

- Linear, logical, and goal-directed
- Circumstantiality
- Tangentiality
- Loosening of associations

- Racing thoughts
- Word salad
- Thought blocking
- Neologisms

Thought content can be described by the following terms:
- Hallucinations
- Delusions
- Obsessions
- Suicidal and homicidal ideation
- Ideas of reference
- Poverty of content.

In Chapter 4, thought disorders were simply classified by dividing them into two broad groups: abnormal beliefs and disorganized thinking.

Abnormal beliefs: delusions and overvalued ideas

It is diagnostically significant to classify delusions as:
- Primary or secondary
- Mood congruent or mood incongruent
- Bizarre or nonbizarre
- According to the content of the delusion (summarized in Fig. 4.2).

See Chapter 4 for a detailed discussion.

Disorganized thinking

Disorganized thinking includes circumstantial and tangential thinking, loosening of association (derailment), neologisms and idiosyncratic word use, flight of ideas, thought blocking, perseveration, echolalia, and irrelevant answers (see Ch. 4 for the definitions of these terms). Whenever possible, record patients' disorganized speech word for word, as it can be very difficult to label disorganized thinking with a single technical term and written language may be easier to evaluate than spoken language.

Figure 26.2 lists typical questions that may be used to elicit delusions.

Sensorium and cognition

Cognitive tests were discussed fully in Chapter 9, including tests of memory function and the Mini-Mental State Examination (MMSE), which tests orientation, registration, attention, calculation, language, executive functioning, and visuospatial skills. Figures 9.2 and 9.10 illustrate these memory function tests and the MMSE.

Insight and judgment

Insight describes patients' understanding of the nature and degree of their mental illness as well as the recognition of the need for treatment. Insight may range from a complete denial of mental illness with the refusal to accept any form of treatment to a genuine understanding, and acceptance, of the course, nature, and impact of the illness on oneself and others.

Risk assessment

Although it is extremely difficult to make an accurate assessment of risk based on a single assessment, clinicians are expected, as far as is possible, to establish some idea of a patient's risk to:
- Self: through self-harm, suicide or self-neglect. Chapter 3 explains the assessment of suicide risk in detail.
- Others: includes violent or sexual crime, stalking, and harassment. Chapter 25 discusses key principles in assessing dangerousness.
- Children: includes physical, sexual, or emotional abuse as well as neglect or deprivation. Child abuse is discussed in more detail in Chapter 23.
- Property: includes arson and physical destruction of property.

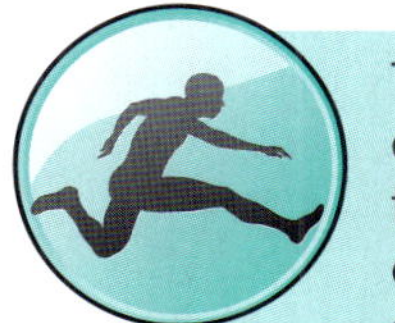

The risk assessment is an extremely important part of the mental state examination, especially the risk of harm to self, as many patients with depression will have had suicidal thoughts or intent. Make a special point of mentioning your assessment of risk to examiners, admitting that your opinion is based on only one assessment.

Physical examination

The psychiatric examination includes a general physical examination, with special focus on the neurological and endocrine system. Always remember to look for signs relevant to the psychiatric history, such as signs of liver disease in patients who abuse alcohol, signs of self-mutilation in patients with a personality disorder, or signs of intravenous drug use (track marks) in patients who use drugs. Also, examine for side effects of psychiatric medication (e.g., parkinsonism, tardive dyskinesia, dystonia, and hypotension). In an exam situation, although only a short, focused physical may be practical, it should always be done. And always make a point of mentioning your positive findings when summarizing the case.

The formulation: presenting the case

The "formulation" is the term psychiatrists use to describe the integrated summary and understanding of a particular patient's problems. It usually includes:

- Description of the patient
- Differential diagnosis
- Etiology
- Management
- Prognosis.

Description of the patient

The patient may be described: (1) in detail by recounting all of the information obtained under the various headings in the psychiatric history and mental state examination; or (2) in the form of a case summary. The case summary consists of one or two paragraphs and contains only the salient features of a case, specifically:

- Identifying information
- Main features of the presenting complaint
- Relevant background details (e.g., past psychiatric history, positive family history)
- Positive findings in the mental state examination and physical examination.

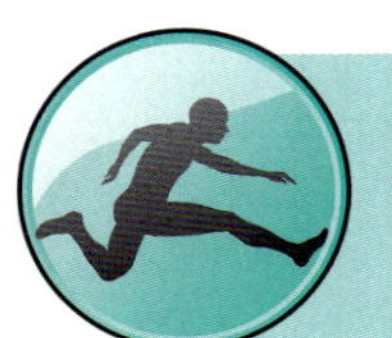

When presenting your differential diagnosis, remember that two or more psychiatric disorders can coexist (e.g., depression and alcohol abuse). In this event, it is important to ascertain whether the conditions are independent or related (e.g., alcohol abuse that has developed secondary to the depressive symptoms of emptiness and difficulty sleeping).

Differential diagnosis

The differential diagnosis is mentioned in order of decreasing probability. Only mention conditions that you have obtained evidence for in your assessment, as you should be able to provide reasons for and against all the alternatives on your list. Figure 26.3 provides an example of a typical differential diagnosis.

Differential diagnosis

Diagnosis	Comments
1. Schizophrenia	For: symptoms present for more than 1 month For: DSM-IV-TR symptoms of delusions of control or persecution (thought insertion; delusional perception; running commentary hallucinations) For: clear and marked deterioration in social and work functioning
2. Schizoaffective disorder	For: typical symptoms of schizophrenia Against: no prominent mood symptoms
3. Mood disorder: either manic or depressive episode with psychotic features	Against: on mental status examination, mood was mainly suspicious as opposed to lowered or elevated and appeared secondary to delusional beliefs Against: no other prominent features of mania or depression Against: mood-incongruent delusions and hallucinations
4. Substance-induced psychotic disorder	For: long duration of symptoms Against: no evidence of illicit substance or alcohol use
5. Psychotic disorder secondary to a medical condition	Against: no signs of medical illness or abnormalities on physical examination

Fig. 26.3 Differential diagnosis.

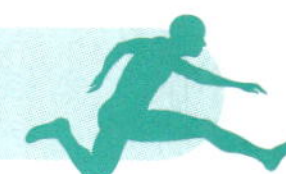

Biopsychosocial assessment

The exact cause of most psychiatric disorders is very often unknown, and most cases seem to involve a complex interplay of biologic, social, and psychological factors. In clinical practice, psychiatrists are especially concerned with the question: "What factors led to this particular patient presenting with this specific problem at this specific point in time?" That is, what factors predisposed to the problem, what factors precipitated the problem, and what factors are perpetuating the problem? Figure 26.4 illustrates an etiology grid that is very helpful in structuring your answers to these questions in terms of biologic, social, and psychological factors. The emphasis should be on *considering* all the blocks in the grid, not necessarily on filling them.

Management

Special investigations

Special investigations are considered part of the management plan and are performed based on findings from the psychiatric assessment. It is useful to divide them into *physical*, *social*, and *psychological* investigations (see Ch. 1 for an example). Appropriate special investigations that are relevant to the specific conditions have

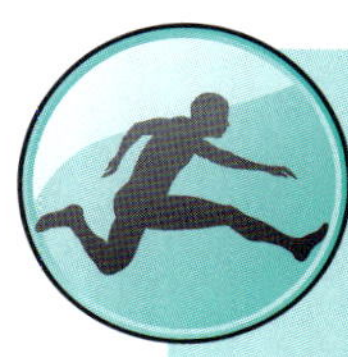

Case summary

Mr PP is a 23-year-old, single, male, full-time student who recently agreed to voluntary hospital admission. He presented with a 6-month history of hearing voices and bizarre beliefs that he was being subjected to government experiments. During this time his college attendance had been uncharacteristically poor, he had terminated his part-time work, and he had become increasingly socially withdrawn. He has no history of past psychiatric illness and denies the use of alcohol or illicit substances; however, he did mention that his maternal uncle suffers from schizophrenia. On mental state examination he appeared unkempt and behaved suspiciously. He had delusions of persecution, reference, and thought control, as well as delusional perception. He also described second person command hallucinations and third person, running commentary hallucinations. He appeared to have no insight into his mental illness as he refused to consider that he might be unwell. There were no abnormalities on physical examination.

Biopsychosocial assessment			
	Biologic	**Psychological**	**Social**
Predisposing (what made the patient prone to this problem?)	Family history of schizophrenia	–	–
Precipitating (what made this problem start now?)	The peak age of onset for schizophrenia in men is 18–25 years	–	Break-up of relationship Recently started college
Perpetuating (what is maintaining this problem?)	Poor compliance with medication due to lack of insight	High expressed emotion family	Lack of social support

Fig. 26.4 Biopsychosocial assessment.

Management and prognosis

1. Special investigations: social, psychological, and physical
2. Management plan below

Term	Biologic	Psychological	Social
Immediate to short term	Antipsychotic medication, with benzodiazepine if necessary	Establish therapeutic relationship Support for family caregivers	Admission to hospital Help with financial, housing, and social problems
Medium to long term	Review progress in outpatient clinic Consider another antipsychotic for nonresponse Consider depot medications for compliance problems	Relapse prevention work Consider cognitive-behavioral and family therapy	Consider day hospital Vocational training

Prognosis
Assuming Mr PP ha a diagnosis of schizophrenia, it is likely that his illness will run a chronic course, showing a relapsing and remitting pattern. Being a young man with a high level of education, Mr PP is particularly at risk for suicide, especially following discharge from the hospital. Good prognostic factors include a high level of premorbid functioning and the absence of negative symptoms.

Fig. 26.5 Management and prognosis.

been given in the chapters in Part I. Familiarize yourself with these, as you should be able to give reasons for any special investigation you propose.

Specific management plan

It may help to structure your management plan by considering biologic, social, and psychological aspects of treatment – *the biopsychosocial approach* – in terms of immediate to short-term and medium- to long-term management. See Figure 26.5 for an example of this method.

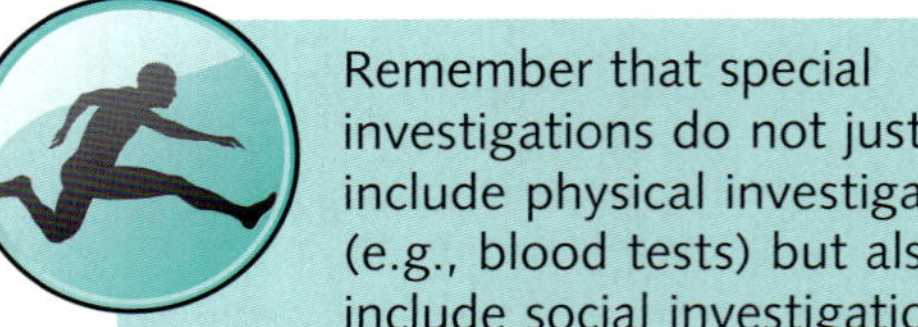

Remember that special investigations do not just include physical investigations (e.g., blood tests) but also include social investigations (e.g., obtaining collateral information from the patient's family doctor or family, obtaining social worker reports); and psychological investigations (e.g., psychometric testing, mood rating scales).

Prognosis

The prognosis is dependent on two factors:

1. The natural course of the condition, which is based on studies of patient populations; these are discussed for each disorder in Part II, Diseases and Disorders
2. Individual patient factors, including social support, compliance with treatment, comorbid substance abuse.

See Figure 26.5 for an example.

Classification in psychiatry

There are two main categorical classification systems in psychiatry:

1. DSM-IV: the fourth edition of the Diagnostic and Statistical Manual of Mental Disorders (published by the American Psychiatric Association), revised edition published in 2000 – DSM-IV-TR (TR, Text Revision)
2. ICD-10: the tenth revision of the International Classification of Diseases, Chapter V (F) – Mental and behavioral disorders (published by the World Health Organization).

In the US, the DSM-IV-TR classification is commonly used in clinical practice. The ICD-10 classification is not commonly used in the US except occasionally in research or for billing purposes.

Both the DSM-IV-TR and ICD-10 make use of a *categorical classification* system, which refers to the process of dividing mental disorders into discrete entities by means of accurate descriptions of specific categories. In contrast, a *dimensional approach* rejects the idea of separate categories, hypothesizing that mental conditions exist on a continuum that merges into normality.

The DSM-IV-TR categorizes mental disorders according to *operational definitions*, which means that mental disorders are defined by a series of precise inclusion and exclusion criteria. The ICD-10 categorizes mental disorders according to descriptive statements and diagnostic guidelines. Note that the research version of the ICD-10 (Diagnostic criteria for research) also makes use of operational definitions.

In general, both the DSM-IV-TR and the ICD-10 propose a *hierarchical* diagnostic system, whereby disorders higher on the hierarchical ladder tend to be given precedence. As a broad rule, organic and substance-related conditions take precedence over conditions such as schizophrenia and mood disorders, which take precedence over anxiety disorders. This does not mean that patients may not have more than one diagnosis; they may. It means that clinicians should:

- Always consider a medical, or substance-related, cause of psychological symptoms, before any other
- Remember that certain conditions have some psychological symptoms in common. For example, schizophrenia commonly presents with features of depression and anxiety, and depression commonly presents with features of anxiety. In both cases, the treatment of the primary condition results in resolution of the symptoms – a separate diagnosis for every symptom is not needed.

The DSM-IV-TR and the ICD-10 share similar diagnostic categories and are, for the most part, technically compatible. The DSM-IV uses a multiaxial diagnostic system with five axes. Axes I and II comprise the entire spectrum of mental disorders:

- Axis I includes all mental disorders except personality disorders and mental retardation, which fall under axis II.
- Axis III includes any concurrent physical disorder or medical condition, whether causative of the mental condition or not.
- Axis IV includes any social or environmental problems that contribute to the mental condition.
- Axis V consists of a score from 0 to 100, obtained from a global assessment of functioning (GAF) scale (Fig. 26.6). The GAF scale considers psychological, social, and occupational functioning on a hypothetical continuum. It does not include functional impairment due to physical or environmental limitations.

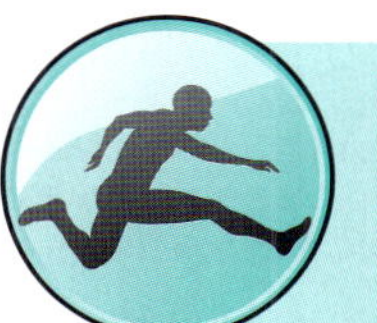

The term "neurosis" is no longer used in the DSM-IV-TR, although it is retained in the ICD-10 as the group heading title for the anxiety disorders: *F4 – Neurotic, stress-related, and somatoform disorders*. When first introduced, "neurosis" was the label given to all "diseases of the nerves."

Global assessment of functioning (GAF) scale	
Consider psychological, social, and occupational functioning on a hypothetical continuum of mental health–illness. Do not include impairment in functioning due to physical (or environmental) limitations.	
Code (Note: Use intermediate codes when appropriate, e.g., 45, 68, 72.)	
100 | 91	**Superior functioning in a wide range of activities, life's problems never seem to get out of hand, is sought out by others because of his or her many positive qualities. No symptoms.**
90 | 81	**Absent or minimal symptoms** (e.g., mild anxiety before an exam), **good functioning in all areas, interested and involved in a wide range of activities, socially effective, generally satisfied with life, no more than everyday problems or concerns** (e.g., an occasional argument with family members).
80 | 71	**If symptoms are present, they are transient and expectable reactions to psychosocial stressors** (e.g., difficulty concentrating after family argument); **no more than slight impairment in social, occupational, or school functioning** (e.g., temporarily falling behind in schoolwork).
70 | 61	**Some mild symptoms** (e.g., depressed mood and mild insomnia) **OR some diffi culty in social, occupational, or school functioning** (e.g., occasional truancy, or theft within the household), **but generally functioning pretty well, has some meaningful interpersonal relationships.**
60 | 51	**Moderate symptoms** (e.g., flat affect and circumstantial speech, occasional panic attacks) **OR moderate difficulty in social, occupational, or school functioning** (e.g., few friends, conflicts with peers or co-workers).
50 | 41	**Serious symptoms** (e.g., suicidal ideation, severe obsessional rituals, frequent shoplifting) **OR any serious impairment in social, occupational, or school functioning** (e.g., no friends, unable to keep a job).
40 | 31	**Some impairment in reality testing or communication** (e.g., speech is at times illogical, obscure, or irrelevant) **OR major impairment in several areas, such as work or school, family relations, judgment, thinking, or mood** (e.g., depressed man avoids friends, neglects family, and is unable to work; child frequently beats up younger children, is defiant at home, and is failing at school).
30 | 21	**Behavior is considerably influenced by delusions or hallucinations OR serious impairment in communication or judgment** (e.g., sometimes incoherent, acts grossly inappropriately, suicidal preoccupation) **OR inability to function in almost all areas** (e.g., stays in bed all day; no job, home, or friends).
20 | 11	**Some danger of hurting self or others** (e.g., suicide attempts without clear expectation of death; frequently violent; manic excitement) **OR occasionally fails to maintain minimal personal hygiene** (e.g., smears feces) **OR gross impairment in communication** (e.g., largely incoherent or mute).
10 | 1	**Persistent danger of severely hurting self or others** (e.g., recurrent violence) **OR persistent inability to maintain minimal personal hygiene OR serious suicidal act with clear expectation of death.**
0	Inadequate information.

Fig. 26.6 Global assessment of functioning (GAF) scale. (Reproduced with permission from DSM-IV-TR. American Psychiatric Association, Washington, DC, 2005, p 34.)

27. Pharmacologic Therapy and ECT

Psychotropic (mind-altering) medication can be divided into the following groups:

- Antidepressants
- Mood stabilizers
- Antipsychotics
- Anxiolytics and hypnotics
- Other.

Unfortunately, this method of grouping drugs is overly simplistic because many drugs from one class are now used to treat disorders in another class. For example, antidepressants are first-line therapies for many anxiety disorders.

Antidepressants

History

Antidepressants were first used in the late 1950s, with the appearance of the tricyclic antidepressant (TCA) imipramine and the monoamine oxidase inhibitor (MAOI) phenelzine. Research into TCAs throughout the 1960s and 1970s developed many more tricyclic agents and related compounds. A major development in the late 1980s was the arrival of the first selective serotonin reuptake inhibitor (SSRI), fluoxetine (Prozac). There has since been considerable expansion of the SSRI class.

Classification and mechanism of action

At present we classify antidepressants according to their pharmacologic actions, as we do not as yet have an adequate explanation as to what exactly makes the antidepressants work. Although there are at least eight different types of antidepressants, the collective action of all antidepressants is to boost the levels of one or more monoamine neurotransmitters in the synaptic cleft. Figure 27.1 illustrates the mechanism of action of antidepressants at the synaptic cleft. The latest research has focused on monoamine neurotransmitter activation of "second messenger" signal transduction mechanisms. This results in the production of transcription factors that lead to the activation of genes controlling the expression of "brain-derived neurotrophic factor" (BDNF). BDNF is neuroprotective and could be the "final common pathway" of antidepressant action. Figure 27.2 summarizes the classification and pharmacodynamics of the important antidepressants.

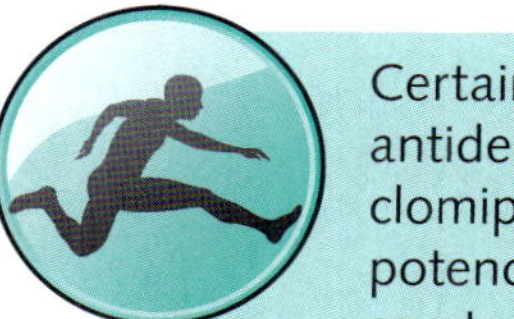

Certain tricyclic antidepressants, such as clomipramine, have more potency for blocking the serotonin reuptake pump, whereas others are more selective for norepinephrine over serotonin (e.g., desipramine, nortriptyline, maprotiline). Most, however, block both norepinephrine and serotonin reuptake.

Indications for antidepressants

Tricyclic antidepressants are used in the treatment of:

- Depression (see Ch. 13)
- Anxiety disorders (see Ch. 15)
- Obsessive-compulsive disorder (clomipramine) (see Ch. 15)
- Other: chronic pain, nocturnal enuresis (see Ch. 23), narcolepsy (see Ch. 21), eating disorders.

SSRIs are used in the treatment of:

- Depression (see Ch. 13)
- Anxiety disorders (see Ch. 15)
- Obsessive-compulsive disorder (see Ch. 15)
- Bulimia nervosa (fluoxetine) (see Ch. 19).

MAOIs are used in the treatment of:

- Depression (especially atypical depression, i.e., hypersomnia, overeating, anxiety) (see Ch. 13)
- Anxiety disorders (see Ch. 15)
- Other: eating disorders, chronic pain.

Side effects and contraindications

Tricyclic antidepressants

Side effects

Figure 27.3 summarizes the common side effects of the TCAs, most of which are related to the

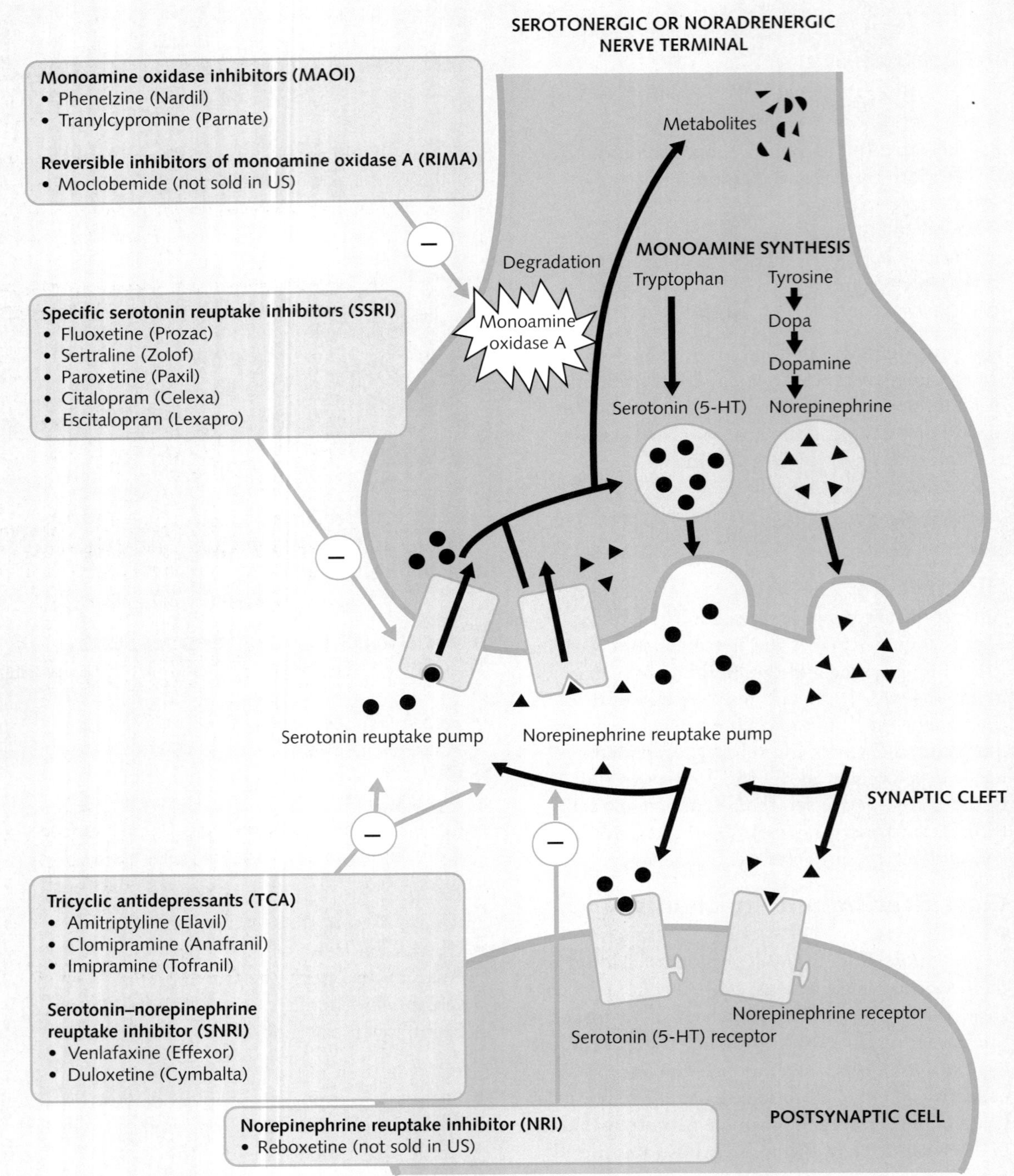

Fig. 27.1 Mechanism of action of antidepressants at the synaptic cleft.

Classification and pharmacodynamics of the antidepressants		
Class of antidepressant	**Examples**	**Mechanism of action**
Tricyclic antidepressant (TCA)	Amitriptyline, nortriptyline, clomipramine, imipramine	Presynaptic blockade of both norepinephrine and serotonin reuptake pumps (to a lesser extent – dopamine) Also blockade of muscarinic, histaminergic, and α-adrenergic pumps
Selective serotonin reuptake inhibitor (SSRI)	Fluoxetine, sertraline, paroxetine, citalopram, fluvoxamine, escitalopram	Selective presynaptic blockade of serotonin reuptake pump
Serotonin–norepinephrine reuptake inhibitor (SNRI)	Venlafaxine, duloxetine	Presynaptic blockade of both norepinephrine and serotonin reuptake pumps (also dopamine in high doses) but with negligible effects on muscarinic, histaminergic, or α-adrenergic receptors (in contrast to TCAs)
Monoamine oxidase inhibitor (MAOI)	Phenelzine, tranylcypromine, isocarboxazid	Nonselective and irreversible inhibition of monoamine oxidase A
Reversible inhibitor of monoamine oxidase A (RIMA)	Moclobemide (UK)	Selective and reversible inhibition of monoamine oxidase A
Noradrenergic and specific serotonergic antidepressant (NaSSA)	Mirtazapine	Presynaptic alpha 2 receptor blockade (results in increased release of norepinephrine and serotonin from presynaptic neurons)
Norepinephrine reuptake inhibitor (NRI)	Reboxetine	Selective presynaptic blockade of norepinephrine reuptake pumps
Norepinephrine, dopamine, and serotonin reuptake inhibitor	Bupropion	Weak inhibitor of neuronal uptake of norepinephrine, dopamine, and serotonin

Fig. 27.2 Classification and pharmacodynamics of the antidepressants.

Common side effects of tricyclic antidepressants	
Mechanism	**Side effect**
Anticholinergic: muscarinic receptor blockade	Dry mouth Constipation Urinary retention Blurred vision
Alpha-adrenergic receptor blockade	Postural hypotension (dizziness, syncope)
Histaminergic receptor blockade	Weight gain Sedation
Cardiotoxic effects	QT interval prolongation, ST segment elevation, heart block, arrhythmias

Fig. 27.3 Common side effects of tricyclic antidepressants.

multireceptor-blocking effects of these drugs. Some patients benefit from the sedative properties of TCAs. Those with prominent sedative effects include amitriptyline, clomipramine, and trazodone (tricyclic-related compound). Those with less sedative effects include imipramine. Because of their cardiotoxic effects, some TCAs, especially amitriptyline, are dangerous in overdose; trazodone is relatively safer, though male patients need to be advised of the risk of priapism (persistent abnormal erection of penis) when using trazodones.

Contraindications

- Recent myocardial infarction
- Arrhythmias
- Severe liver disease
- Mania.

SSRIs

Side effects

SSRIs have fewer anticholinergic effects than the TCAs and are less sedating. Because of the absence of cardiotoxic effects, they are the antidepressant of choice in patients with cardiac disease and in those who are at risk of taking an overdose. However, they do have their own side effects, which may be unacceptable to some patients. These are summarized in Figure 27.4.

Concerns have been expressed that SSRIs might be associated with an increased risk of completed suicide. There is no convincing evidence to support this claim. However, some data suggests that patients may be at an increased risk for suicidal ideation and/or attempted suicide shortly after beginning an SSRI or SNRI. The FDA has placed a black box warning about the increased risk of suicidal thoughts and behavior in children and adolescents taking antidepressants (see section on child psychiatry for details). The bottom line is that the patient must be carefully evaluated prior to beginning a medication for depression and closely monitored, particularly in the first month after starting the medication.

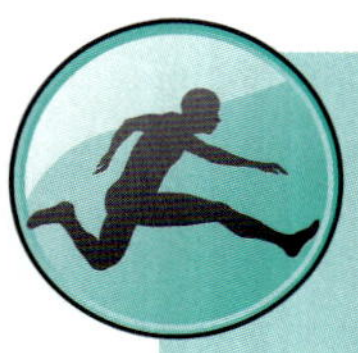

Antidepressants should be used with caution in patients with epilepsy, as they tend to lower the seizure threshold.

Contraindications

The main contraindication to SSRIs is mania.

MAOIs/RIMA

Side effects

Because of the risk of serious interactions with certain foods and other drugs, the MAOIs have become second-line antidepressants. Their inhibition of monoamine oxidase A results in the accumulation of amine neurotransmitters and impairs the metabolism of some amines found in certain drugs (e.g., decongestants) and foodstuffs (e.g., tyramine). Because MAOIs bind irreversibly to monoamine oxidase A, amines may accumulate to dangerously high levels, which may precipitate a life-threatening hypertensive crisis. An example of this occurs when the ingestion of dietary tyramine results in a massive release of norepinephrine from endogenous stores. This is termed the "cheese reaction" because some mature cheeses typically contain high levels of tyramine. Note that an early warning sign is a throbbing headache. Figure 27.5 lists the drugs and foodstuffs that should be avoided in patients taking MAOIs.

The RIMA moclobemide (not currently prescribed in the US) *reversibly* inhibits monoamine oxidase A. Therefore, the drug will be displaced from the enzyme as amines levels start to increase. So, although there is a small risk of developing a hypertensive crisis if high levels of tyramine are ingested, no dietary restrictions are required in general.

When other antidepressants that have a strong serotonergic effect (e.g., SSRIs, clomipramine,

Common side effects of the SSRIs
Gastrointestinal disturbance (nausea, vomiting, diarrhea pain) – early*
Anxiety and agitation – early*
Loss of appetite and weight loss (sometimes weight gain)
Insomnia
Sweating
Sexual dysfunction (anorgasmia, delayed ejaculation)
** Gastrointestinal and anxiety symptoms occur on initiation of treatment and resolve with time.*

Fig. 27.4 Common side effects of the SSRIs.

Drugs and food that may precipitate a hypertensive crisis in combination with MAOIs
Tyramine-rich foods
Cheese – especially mature varieties (e.g., Stilton)
Degraded protein: pickled herring, smoked fish, chicken liver, hung game
Yeast and protein extract: Bovril®, Oxo®, Marmite®
Chianti wine, beer
Broad bean pods
Soya bean extract
Overripe or unfresh food
Drugs
Epinephrine, norepinephrine
Amphetamines
Cocaine
Ephedrine, pseudoephedrine, phenylpropanolamine (cough mixtures, decongestants)
L-dopa, dopamine
Local anesthetics containing epinephrine
Note: the combination of MAOIs and antidepressants or opiates may result in the serotonin syndrome.

Fig. 27.5 Drugs and food that may precipitate a hypertensive crisis in combination with MAOIs.

imipramine) are administered simultaneously with an MAOI, the risk of developing the potentially lethal "serotonin syndrome" is increased. It resembles the neuroleptic malignant syndrome (see later) and is characterized by tremor, hyperreflexia, clonus, muscular rigidity, elevated temperature (>38°C), diaphoresis, and agitation. Therefore, other antidepressants should not be started for 2 weeks after an MAOI has been stopped (3 weeks in the case of clomipramine and imipramine). Conversely, an MAOI should not be started for 1–2 weeks after the termination of another antidepressant (3 weeks in the case of clomipramine and imipramine; 5 weeks in the case of fluoxetine). The coadministration of opiates and an MAOI can also result in the serotonin syndrome. This is because opiates (especially tramadol) have some intrinsic serotonin reuptake inhibitory activity.

MAOIs may have further side effects similar to the TCAs, including postural hypotension and anticholinergic effects.

Contraindications to MAOIs

- Pheochromocytoma
- Cerebrovascular disease
- Hepatic impairment
- Mania.

> The abrupt withdrawal of any antidepressant may result in a discontinuation syndrome with symptoms such as gastrointestinal disturbance, agitation, dizziness, headache, tremor, and insomnia. SSRIs with short half-lives (e.g., paroxetine, sertraline) and venlafaxine are particular culprits. Therefore, all antidepressants should be gradually tapered downward before being withdrawn completely. Although certain antidepressants may cause a withdrawal syndrome, they do not cause a dependence syndrome or "addiction."

Mood stabilizers

These include lithium and the anticonvulsants, valproate and carbamazepine. Other anticonvulsants such as lamotrigine, gabapentin, topiramate, vigabatrin, and oxcarbazepine are also being investigated for mood-stabilizing properties.

History

In 1949, an Australian, John Cade, discovered that lithium salts caused lethargy when injected into animals and later reported lithium's antimanic properties in humans. Trials in the 1950s and 1960s led to the drug entering mainstream practice in 1970.

Valproate was first recognized as an effective antiepileptic in 1963. Along with carbamazepine, it was later shown to be effective in bipolar affective disorder.

Mechanism of action

The precise mechanism of action remains unclear. Lithium modulates the neurotransmitter-induced activation of second messenger systems. Valproate and carbamazepine exert their effect via the GABA system. They also both possess antiglutamatergic properties. It is also suggested that these medications may have a neuroprotective effect on the brain.

Indications

Lithium is used in the treatment of:

- Acute mania (see Ch. 13)
- Prophylaxis of bipolar affective disorder (prevention of relapse) (see Ch. 13)
- Treatment-resistant depression (lithium augmentation) (see Ch. 13)
- Other: adjunct to antipsychotics in schizoaffective disorder and schizophrenia; and aggression/impulsivity (see Chs 14 and 18).

Valproate is used in the treatment of:

- Epilepsy
- Acute mania (see Ch. 13)
- Prophylaxis of bipolar affective disorder (off-label use) (see Ch. 13).

Carbamazepine is used in the treatment of:

- Epilepsy
- Prophylaxis of bipolar affective disorder (unresponsive to lithium) (see Ch. 13)
- Rapid cycling bipolar disorder (see Ch. 13)
- Other: treatment-resistant mania, depression, or schizophrenia; trigeminal neuralgia; impulse-control disorders (see Ch. 18).

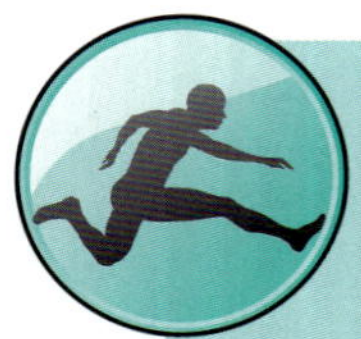

Valproate is available in formulations as sodium valproate, valproic acid, and semisodium valproate (Depakote), which is comprised of equimolar amounts of sodium valproate and valproic acid.

Side effects and contraindications

Lithium

Lithium has a narrow therapeutic window between nontherapeutic and toxic blood levels:

- Therapeutic levels: 0.5–1.0 mmol/L
- Toxic levels: > 1.5 mmol/L
- Dangerously toxic levels: > 2 mmol/L.

Lithium is only taken orally and is excreted almost entirely by the kidneys. Renal clearance of lithium is decreased with renal insufficiency (e.g., in the elderly, dehydration) and sodium depletion. Certain drugs such as diuretics (especially thiazides), nonsteroidal anti-inflammatory drugs (NSAIDs), and ACE-inhibitors can also increase lithium levels and should be prescribed with utmost caution. Furthermore, antipsychotics may synergistically increase lithium-induced neurotoxicity; this is important as lithium and antipsychotics are often coadministered in acute mania. Figure 27.6 summarizes the side effects and signs of toxicity of lithium.

It follows that the following investigations are needed prior to initiating therapy:

- Complete blood count
- Renal function and electrolytes
- Thyroid function
- Pregnancy test
- ECG.

Blood levels are monitored weekly after starting treatment until a therapeutic level has been stable for 4 weeks. Lithium blood levels should then be monitored every 3 months; renal function every 6 months; and thyroid function every 12 months.

Contraindications/cautions

- Pregnancy
- Breast-feeding (see Ch. 20)
- Renal insufficiency
- Thyroid disease
- Cardiac conditions
- Neurologic conditions (e.g., Parkinson's or Huntington's disease).

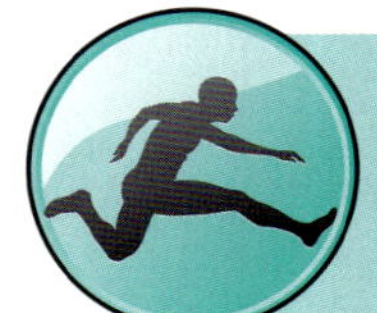

Lithium, carbamazepine, and valproate have potentially serious pharmacokinetic and pharmacodynamic interactions with many other drugs. Therefore, before prescribing new medication for patients on these mood stabilizers, check a drug interactions reference.

Carbamazepine and sodium valproate

Figure 27.7 summarizes the side effects of carbamazepine and valproate. It is important to check liver and hematologic functions prior to, and soon after, starting these drugs because of the risk of serious blood and hepatic disorders.

Side effects and signs of toxicity of lithium	
Side effects	**Signs of toxicity**
Thirst, polydipsia, polyuria, weight gain, edema Fine tremor Precipitates or worsens skin problems/acne Concentration and memory problems Hypothyroidism Impaired renal function Cardiac: T-wave flattening or inversion Leukocytosis Teratogenicity	1.5–2 mmol/L: nausea and vomiting, apathy, coarse tremor, muscle weakness >2 mmol/L: nystagmus, dysarthria, impaired consiousness, hyperactive tendon reflexes, oliguria, hypotension, convulsions, coma Note: the treatment of lithium toxicity is supportive, ensuring adequate hydration, renal function, and electrolyte balance. Anticonvulsants may be necessary for convulsions and hemodialysis may be indicated in cases of renal failure

Fig. 27.6 Side effects and signs of toxicity of lithium.

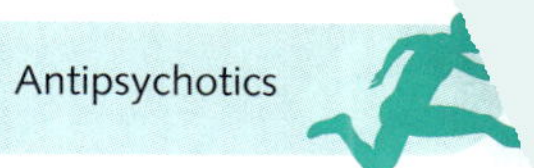

Side effects of carbamazepine and valproate	
Valproate	**Carbamazepine**
Increased appetite and weight gain Sedation and dizziness Ankle swelling Hair loss Nausea and vomiting Tremor Hematologic abnormalities (thrombocytopenia, leukopenia) Elevated liver enzymes (liver damage very uncommon) Pancreatitis *Note: serious blood and liver disorders do occur but are rare*	Nausea and vomiting Skin rashes Blurred or double vision (diplopia) Ataxia, drowsiness, fatigue Hyponatremia and fluid retention Hematologic abnormalities (leukopenia, thrombocytopenia, eosinophilia) Elevated liver enzymes (hepatic or elevated cholestatic jaundice rare) *Note: serious blood and liver disorders do occur but are rare*

Fig. 27.7 Side effects of carbamazepine and valproate.

Blood levels are monitored weekly after starting treatment until a therapeutic level has been reached. Carbamazepine blood levels should be rechecked at 5–6 weeks because of its ability to autoinduce its own metabolism, which can lower blood levels. Blood levels for carbamazepine and valproate should then be monitored every 3 months. Hematologic and pancreatic function should be monitored every 3–6 months.

Antipsychotics

History

Antipsychotics or neuroleptics (originally known as "major tranquilizers") appeared in the early 1950s with the introduction of the phenothiazine, chlorpromazine. Their ability to treat psychotic symptoms had a profound impact on psychiatry, accelerating the movement of patients out of the old mental institutions and into the community. The efficacy of chlorpromazine in treating psychotic symptoms seemed to be related to its blockade of dopamine D_2 receptors in the brain. A number of antipsychotics with a similar pharmacodynamic action soon followed (e.g., the butyrophenone, haloperidol in the 1960s). However, serious side effects (e.g., extrapyramidal side effects), soon became apparent with all these drugs. These side effects were often related to the blockade of dopamine D_2 receptors in other pathways of the brain.

Clozapine, which has comparatively little activity at D_2 receptors (but was able to block 5-HT2 receptors), was the first antipsychotic devoid of extrapyramidal side effects and thus was termed "atypical." It led to the introduction of several other atypical antipsychotics, including risperidone, olanzapine, quetiapine, ziprasidone, and, most recently, aripiprazole. These are currently first-line treatments for schizophrenia. The older antipsychotics such as haloperidol and chlorpromazine became known as the conventional or typical antipsychotics.

The atypical antipsychotics were initially so called because they failed to induce catalepsy (an extrapyramidal syndrome) when given to animals, as the typical antipsychotics were known to do. "Atypicals" thus became antipsychotics that were mostly devoid of extrapyramidal motor effects, the first of which was clozapine. Today, the term atypical has additional meanings. It can also refer to the action of alleviating both negative and positive symptoms as well as to the capacity to block serotonin 2A (5-$HT2_A$) receptors – a property of most of the atypical agents introduced to date.

Indications for antipsychotics

Psychiatric indications

- Schizophrenia, schizoaffective disorder, delusional disorder (see Ch. 14)
- Depression or mania with psychotic features (see Ch. 13)
- Psychotic episodes secondary to a medical condition or psychoactive substance use
- Delirium (see Ch. 16) (use with caution in alcohol withdrawal because it lowers seizure threshold)
- Behavioral disturbance in dementia (see Ch. 16)
- Severe agitation, anxiety, and violent or impulsive behavior (see Ch. 14).

Nonpsychiatric indications

- Motor tics (Gilles de la Tourette's syndrome)
- Nausea and vomiting (e.g., prochlorperazine)
- Intractable hiccups and pruritus (e.g., chlorpromazine, haloperidol).

Classification

Figure 27.8 summarizes the classification of the antipsychotics, which might be useful when trying to understand the side effects that are particular to certain specific types of antipsychotics (see side effects).

Mechanism of action and side effects

Conventional (typical) antipsychotics

The efficacy of the conventional antipsychotics in treating psychotic symptoms is thought to be due to their ability to block dopamine D_2 receptors in the mesolimbic dopamine pathway. Unfortunately, these drugs block all the dopamine D_2 receptors in the entire brain, resulting in their characteristic side effects. In addition, these drugs also cause side effects by blocking muscarinic, histaminergic and α-adrenergic receptors. Figure 27.9 summarizes both the useful and troublesome clinical effects of D_2-receptor antagonism as well as the side effects caused by the blockage of other receptors. Learn this table well; these effects are often asked for in exams. Note that certain types of conventional antipsychotics are associated with specific side effects:

- The phenothiazines with an aliphatic side chain (e.g., chlorpromazine) have strong sedative effects and moderate anticholinergic effects and moderate EPS.
- The phenothiazines with a piperidine side chain (e.g., thioridazine) have strong anticholinergic effects and moderate sedative effects, but weak EPS.

Classification of the antipsychotics	
Chemical class	**Examples**
Conventional/typical antipsychotics	
Phenothiazines	Piperidine side chain: thioridazine (Mellaril®) Piperazine side chain: trifluoperazine (Stelazine®), fluphenazine (Prolixin®), chlorpromazine (Thorazine®)
Butyrophenones	Haloperidol (Haldol®)
Diphenylbutylpiperidines	Pimozide (Orap®)
Atypical antipsychotics	
Dibenzodiazepines	Clozapine (Clozaril®)
Thienobenzodiazepines	Olanzapine (Zyprexa®)
Benzisoxazoles	Risperidone (Risperdal®)
Dibenzothiazepines	Quetiapine (Seroquel®)

Fig. 27.8 Classification of the antipsychotics.

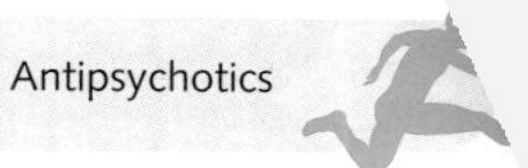

Dopamine D_2-receptor antagonism		
Location of dopamine D_2 receptors	**Function**	**Clinical effect of dopamine D_2-receptor antagonism**
Mesolimbic pathway	Involved in delusions/hallucinations/ thought disorder, euphoria and drug dependence	Treatment of psychotic symptoms
Mesocortical pathway	Mediates cognitive and negative symptoms of schizophrenia	Worsening of negative and cognitive symptoms of schizophrenia
Nigrostriatal pathway (basal ganglia/striatum)	Controls motor movement	Extrapyramidal side effects (EPS) – see Fig. 27.10: • Parkinsonian symptoms • Acute dystonia • Akathisia • Tardive dyskinesia • Neuroleptic malignant syndrome
Tuberoinfindibular pathway	Controls prolactin secretion – dopamine inhibits prolactin release	Hyperprolactinemia • Galactorrhea (breast milk production) • Amenorrhea and infertility • Sexual dysfunction
Chemoreceptor trigger zone	Controls nausea and vomiting	Anti-emetic effect: some phenothiazines, e.g., chlorpromazine (Thorazine®), are very effective in treating nausea and vomiting

Other side effects	
Anticholinergic: muscarinic receptor blockade	Dry mouth, constipation, urinary retention, blurred vision
Alpha-adrenergic receptor blockade	Postural hypotension (dizziness, syncope)
Histaminergic receptor blockade	Sedation, weight gain
Cardiac effects	Prolongation of QT-interval, arrhythmias, myocarditis, sudden death
Dermatologic effects	Photosensitivity, skin rashes (especially chlorpromazine: blue-grey discoloration in the sun)
Other	Lowering of seizure threshold, hepatotoxicity, cholestatic jaundice, pancytopenia, agranulocytosis

Fig. 27.9 The clinical effects and side effects of conventional antipsychotics.

- The phenothiazines with a piperazine side chain (e.g., trifluoperazine, fluphenazine) have strong EPS, but weak sedative and anticholinergic effects.
- The conventional antipsychotics in other classes (e.g., butyrophenones, thioxanthenes) and the depot preparations resemble the phenothiazines with a piperazine side chain, i.e., they have strong EPS and weaker sedative and anticholinergic effects.

The tricyclic antidepressants and the conventional antipsychotics are multireceptor blockers; therefore, both groups of drugs cause anticholinergic (dry mouth, constipation, blurred vision, urinary retention), antiadrenergic (postural hypotension), and antihistaminergic (sedation, weight gain) side effects.

The extrapyramidal side effects (EPS) – parkinson-like motor symptoms, acute dystonia, and akathisia – are due to a relative deficiency of dopamine and an excess of acetylcholine induced by dopamine antagonism in the nigrostriatal pathway. This is why anticholinergic drugs are effective treatments and why piperidine phenothiazines, which inherently have a strong anticholinergic action, do not cause such severe EPS.

Figure 27.10 summarizes the antipsychotic-induced extrapyramidal side effects and treatment. Note that atypical antipsychotics may also be associated with EPS, especially in high doses.

Certain antipsychotics are available in a slow-release form, as an intramuscular depot preparation that can be administered every 2–4 weeks. Examples include fluphenazine decanoate (Prolixin) and haloperidol decanoate (Haldol). They are used for patients who are poorly compliant with oral therapy.

Atypical antipsychotics

Although the pharmacodynamic actions of the atypical antipsychotics are diverse, most of the atypical antipsychotics block both serotonin 2A receptors (5-HT2_A) and dopamine D_2 receptors. Atypicals also have differing affinities for other receptors including muscarinic, histaminergic, and α-adrenergic receptors, which accounts for their varied side-effect profiles. Figure 27.11 summarizes some of the important side effects associated with the atypical antipsychotics.

The atypical antipsychotic clozapine is a very effective antipsychotic but, because of the life-threatening risk of bone marrow suppression with agranulocytosis (1% of patients), is used only in treatment-resistant schizophrenia. Patients should be registered with a clozapine-monitoring service and have a complete blood count (CBC) with differential prior to starting treatment. This is followed by regular CBCs in an outpatient clinic.

Anxiolytic and hypnotic drugs

A hypnotic drug is one that induces sleep. An anxiolytic or sedative drug is one that reduces anxiety. This differentiation is not particularly helpful, as anxiolytic drugs can induce sleep when given in higher doses and hypnotics can have a calming effect when given in lower doses (e.g., the benzodiazepines, which are anxiolytic in low doses and hypnotic in high doses). All these drugs can result in tolerance, dependence, and withdrawal symptoms. Furthermore, their effects, when used in combination or with alcohol, are additive. The benzodiazepines are the most important drugs in this group.

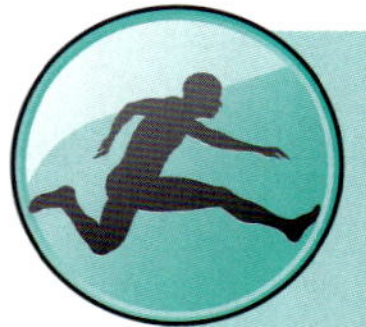

In the past, the antipsychotics have been referred to as the "major tranquilizers" and the anxiolytics as the "minor tranquilizers." This is misleading because (1) these drugs are not pharmacologically related; (2) the antipsychotics do far more than just tranquilize; and (3) the effect and use of anxiolytics are in no way minor.

History

In the 1960s the benzodiazepines replaced the often-abused barbiturates as the drugs of choice for the treatment of anxiety and insomnia. However, this initial enthusiasm was tempered by the observation that they were associated with serious dependence and withdrawal syndromes. Today, benzodiazepines are recognized as highly effective and relatively safe drugs when prescribed judiciously with good patient education.

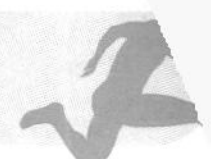

Extrapyramidal side effect	Description	Treatment
Parkinsonian motor symptoms	Muscular rigidity, bradykinesia (lack of, or slowing, of movement), resting tremor Generally occurs within a month of starting antipsychotic	Anticholinergics, (e.g., benzotropine) Consider reducing dose of antipsychotic or switching to antipsychotic with fewer EPS (e.g., atypical)
Acute dystonia	Involuntary sustained muscular contractions or spasms, e.g., neck (spasmodic torticollis), clenched jaw (trismus), protruding tongue, eyes roll upwards (oculogyric crisis) More common in young men Usually occurs within 72 hours of treatment	
Akathisia	Subjective feeling of inner restlessness and muscular discomfort Occurs within 6–60 days	Propranolol or short-term benzodiazepines Consider reducing dose of antipsychotic or switching to antipsychotic with fewer EPS (e.g., atypical)
Tardive dyskinesia (TD)	Rhythmic, involuntary movements of head, limbs, and trunk, especially chewing, grimacing of mouth, and protruding, darting movements of tongue Develops in up to 20% of patients who receive long-term treatment with conventional antipsychotics	No effective treatment Withdraw antipsychotic if possible Clozapine might be helpful Consider benzodiazepines Do not give anticholinergics (may worsen TD)
Neuroleptic malignant syndrome	Life-threatening condition characterized by: *Motor signs*: severe muscular rigidity *Mental signs*: fluctuating consciousness *Autonomic disturbance*: hyperthermia, unstable blood pressure, rapid pulse, sweating *Blood tests*: high creatinine kinase levels Usually occurs within 4–11 days of initiation of treatment or change of dosage	Stop antipsychotic Supportive treatment: • Cool patient • Monitor vital signs • Monitor renal function • Monitor electrolytes Consider dantrolene (may reduce muscle rigidity but has risk of hepatotoxicity) Consider bromocriptine (a beta-2 agonist but may worsen underlying psychosis)

Fig. 27.10 Antipsychotic-induced extrapyramidal side effects and treatment.

Classification

From a clinical perspective, it is important to classify benzodiazepines according to their strength, their length of action, and their route of administration. Figure 27.12 summarizes these qualities in some common benzodiazepines.

Mechanism of action

Benzodiazepines potentiate the action of gamma-aminobutyric acid (GABA), the main inhibitory neurotransmitter in the brain. They bind to specific benzodiazepine receptors on the $GABA_A$ receptor complex, which results in an increased affinity of the complex for GABA. This results in increased activity of chloride ion channels with the flow of chloride into the neuron, thereby hyperpolarizing the postsynaptic membrane. Benzodiazepines are effective hypnotics, anxiolytics, anticonvulsants, and muscle relaxants.

Indications for benzodiazepines

- Insomnia, especially short-acting benzodiazepines (see Ch. 21)
- Anxiety disorders (see Ch. 15)

Important side effects of the atypical antipsychotics

Drug	Side effect
Clozapine	Agranulocytosis (regular white blood cell count essential) Risk of seizures in high doses Hypersalivation Weight gain Risk of diabetes
Risperidone	Can cause EPS, especially at higher doses Weight gain Increased prolactin
Olanzapine	Weight gain Sedation High risk of diabetes
Quetiapine	Somnolence Postural hypotension Elevated liver function tests (reversible) Weight gain Decreased T_3 and T_4 Cataracts (potential)
Ziprasidone	Less weight gain Prolongation of QTC Nausea Sedation/activation Dizziness/hypotension
Aripiprazole	Nausea Vomiting Dyspepsia Anxiety Dizziness/hypotension Tachycardia EPS

Fig. 27.11 Important side effects of the atypical antipsychotics.

- Alcohol withdrawal, especially chlordiazepoxide (see Ch. 17)
- Akathisia (see Fig. 27.10)
- Acute mania or psychosis (sedation) (see Ch. 13)
- Other: epilepsy prophylaxis, seizures, muscle spasm (diazepam), anesthetic premedication.

Side effects of benzodiazepines

- Patients should be warned about the potential dangers of driving or operating machinery due to drowsiness, ataxia, and reduced motor coordination.
- Benzodiazepines should be used with caution in patients with chronic respiratory disease (e.g., COPD, sleep apnea) as they may depress respiration.
- Risk of developing dependence, especially with prolonged use and shorter-acting drugs.
- Benzodiazepines are seldom fatal in overdose. Flumazenil, a benzodiazepine receptor antagonist, may be helpful in differentiating benzodiazepine-induced loss of consciousness from other causes.

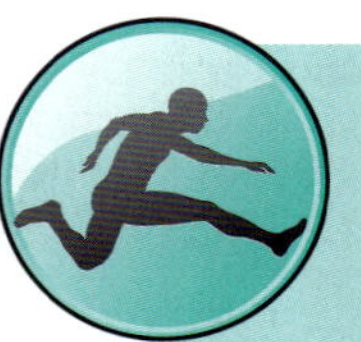

Alcohol, opiates, barbiturates, tricyclic antidepressants, antihistamines, and other sedative-hypnotics may all enhance the effects of benzodiazepines; therefore, moderate doses of benzodiazepines in combination with some of these substances can result in respiratory depression.

Other hypnotic and anxiolytic agents

- The short-acting hypnotics – zolpidem (Ambien) and zaleplon (Sonata) – also act at benzodiazepine receptors, although they are structurally different from the benzodiazepines. Like temazepam, they have a short half-life and do not cause a hangover on the following day.
- Buspirone (BuSpar) is a 5-HT_{1A} receptor agonist that is used to treat generalized anxiety disorder. It is unrelated to the benzodiazepines, does not have hypnotic, anticonvulsant, or muscle relaxant properties, and is not associated with dependence or abuse. Response to treatment may take up to 2 weeks, unlike the benzodiazepines, which have an immediate anxiolytic effect. It is therefore less useful in patients who, having been treated with benzodiazepines in the past, expect rapid relief of anxiety.
- Sedating antihistamines (e.g., diphenhydramine [Benadryl]) are available for insomnia without a prescription. Unfortunately, their long duration of action may lead to drowsiness the following day.
- Meprobamate and chloral hydrate are no longer first-line sedative hypnotics because of their adverse effects (see Ch. 16).

Drug	Dose equivalent to 5 mg diazepam	Length of action	Half-life	Routes of administration
Temazepam	10 mg	Short acting	11 hr	Oral
Oxazepam	15 mg	Short acting	8 hr	Oral
Lorazepam	0.5 mg	Short acting	15 hr	Oral, IM*, IV
Chlordiazepoxide	15 mg	Long acting	100 hr	Oral
Diazepam	5 mg	Long acting	100 hr	Oral, per rectum, IV, IM only if no alternative
Alprazolam	0.5 mg	Short acting	11 hr	Oral
Clonazepam	0.25 mg	Long acting	50 hr	Oral

Classification of the benzodiazepines

* Lorazepam is the only benzodiazepine that has predictable absorption when given IM.

Fig. 27.12 Classification of the benzodiazepines.

Other drugs used in psychiatry

- *Alcohol dependence:* acamprosate, disulfiram, naltrexone (see Ch. 17)
- *Opiate dependence:* methadone, buprenorphine, naltrexone (see Ch. 17)
- *Dementia:* cholinesterase inhibitors (donepezil, rivastigmine, galantamine), memantine (see Ch. 16)
- *Psychostimulants:* methylphenidate, dexamphetamine (see Ch. 23).

Electroconvulsive therapy

History

The idea that seizures could improve psychiatric symptoms arose from the observation that convulsions led to an improvement of psychotic symptoms in patients with both epilepsy and schizophrenia. This led to seizures being induced pharmacologically with intramuscular camphor in the early 1930s. An electric stimulus was later discovered to be a safe and effective way of inducing seizures, although it proved to be a crude and often dangerous procedure without modern-day anesthetic induction agents and muscle relaxants. Today, ECT is a safe and often life-saving treatment for patients with serious mental illness.

Indications

ECT is predominantly used for depression. Although antidepressants are usually the first-line treatment, ECT is considered for the following forms of depression:

- With life-threatening poor fluid intake
- With strong suicidal intent
- With psychotic features or stupor
- When antidepressants are ineffective or not tolerated
- With certain situations during pregnancy.

Although ECT may precipitate a manic episode in patients with bipolar affective disorder, it is an effective treatment for established mania. ECT is also an effective treatment for certain types of schizophrenia, specifically catatonic states, positive psychotic symptoms, and schizoaffective disorder. ECT is also used for postpartum psychosis (see Ch. 20) with prominent mood symptoms in which a rapid improvement is necessary to reunite the mother with her baby.

Administration and mechanism of action

ECT is administered 2–3 times per week. Most patients need between four and 12 treatments. An anesthesiologist administers a short-acting induction agent and muscle relaxant that ensure about 5 minutes of general anesthesia. During this time, a psychiatrist applies two electrodes to the patient's scalp, in a bilateral or unilateral placement, and delivers an electric current of sufficient charge to effect a generalized seizure of at least 15 seconds in duration.

It is still not clear how ECT works. It causes a release of neurotransmitters as well as hypothalamic and pituitary hormones; it also affects neurotransmitter receptors and second-messenger systems and results in a transient increase in blood–brain barrier permeability.

Side effects

The mortality from ECT is the same as that for any minor surgical procedure under general anesthesia. Loss of memory is a common complaint, particularly for events surrounding the ECT. However, some patients may have impairment of some autobiographical memory. Unfortunately, there are few studies that examine the long-term effects of ECT.

Memory impairment might be reduced by unilateral electrode placement (as opposed to bilateral). Minor complaints such as confusion, headache, nausea, and muscle pains, are experienced by 80% of patients. Anesthetic complications (e.g., arrhythmias, aspiration) can be reduced by good preoperative assessment. Prolonged seizures may occur, especially in patients who are on drugs that lower the seizure threshold (e.g., antidepressants and antipsychotics). In contrast, benzodiazepines increase the seizure threshold, making it more difficult to induce a seizure of adequate length.

Contraindications

There are no absolute contraindications to ECT. Relative contraindications include:

- Heart disease (recent myocardial infarction, heart failure, ischemic heart disease)
- Raised intracranial pressure
- Risk of cerebral bleeding (hypertension, recent stroke)
- Poor anesthetic risk.

28. Psychological Therapy

What is it?

Psychological therapy or psychotherapy describes the interaction between a therapist and a patient that leads to beneficial changes in the patient's thoughts, feelings, and behaviors. Psychological therapy, which is sometimes called "talk therapy," may be useful in alleviating specific symptoms (e.g., social phobia) or in helping a patient improve his or her overall sense of well-being.

Who does it?

Members of different professional disciplines, including psychiatrists, clinical psychologists, mental health nurses, clinical social workers, art and drama therapists, and counselors, may all practice psychotherapy, provided they have had adequate training and supervision.

What approaches are there?

There are many different schools of thought and approaches to psychotherapy. Research has shown efficacy for many different types of psychotherapies for many conditions. This has led to the idea that the success of psychotherapy might be due to certain common therapeutic factors as opposed to specific theories or techniques. A comprehensive review of psychotherapy research showed that common factors, operable in any model of therapy, account for 85% of the therapeutic effect, whereas theoretical orientation accounts for only 15% (Lambert 1992). Common therapeutic factors include patient factors (personal strengths, social supports), therapist–patient relationship factors (empathy, acceptance, warmth), and the patient's expectancy of change.

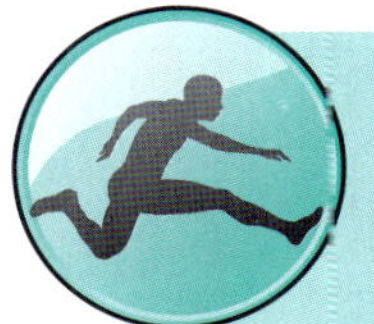

The single factor most commonly associated with a good therapeutic outcome is the strength of the patient–therapist relationship (therapeutic alliance), regardless of the modality of therapy.

Supportive psychotherapy

Psychotherapy exists on a continuum from counseling and supportive psychotherapy, which represent the least complex forms of intervention, to psychodynamic psychotherapy and sophisticated cognitive therapy, which represent the more complex interventions – and which require more specialized training.

Counseling and supportive psychotherapy are often brief in duration and are recommended for patients with minor mental health or interpersonal difficulties, or for those experiencing stressful life circumstances (e.g., grief counseling for bereavement). The emphasis is on helping patients utilize their own strengths, with the therapist being reflective and empathic. It also includes providing information and advice and will therefore be undertaken by all health-care professionals at some time.

In *person-centered counseling* (developed by Carl Rogers), the therapist assumes an empathic and reflective role, allowing patients to discover their own insights, with the basic premise that the patient ultimately knows best (nondirective counseling). *Problem-solving counseling* is more directive and focused as patients are actively assisted in finding solutions to their problems.

There is evidence that counseling confers some benefit for anxiety and depression in primary care settings but not as much for severe presentations and disorders (such as schizophrenia).

Psychodynamic psychotherapy

Sigmund Freud introduced psychoanalytic theory in the late 19th century. Figure 28.1 summarizes

Some of Freud's ideas

The structural model
Freud believed that the psychic apparatus (personality) consisted of three parts:
- Id (the pleasurable): the unconscious part, which is governed by the pleasure principle and demands immediate satisfaction. It is primitive, instinctive, animalistic, and hedonistic.
- Superego (the ideal): the ethical and moral part that sets rigid standards for behavior. It is usually internalized from the parent's moral code and gives rise to feelings of guilt – as a kind of conscience.
- Ego (the actual): the conscious and cognitive part of the mind that is in touch with reality. It mediates between the demands of the id, the superego, and external reality.

Psychosexual development
Freud believed that adult personality types were linked to five stages of development: *oral* (birth to 1 year), *anal* (1–3 years), *phallic* (3–6 years), *latency* (6 years to puberty) and *genital* (maturation). Excessive frustration or gratifi cation in any stage cold lead to an individual becoming *fixated* in that stage, which would present as specifi cneuroses, e.g., so-called oral or anal personality

Fig. 28.1 Some of Freud's ideas.

some of his ideas. Psychoanalysis has changed somewhat since then with the contributions of many other influential theorists (e.g., Carl Jung, Alfred Adle, and Melanie Klein). It is assumed in psychoanalytic theory that it is mainly *unconscious* thoughts, feelings, and fantasies that give rise to distressing symptoms. These are said to arise in childhood, if an individual does not progress adequately through the various stages of psychological development.

The essential aim of psychoanalysis or psychodynamic psychotherapy is to make symptom-causing, unconscious processes conscious. It is the therapist's role to identify and interpret these repressed processes, of which patients are unaware, and then to help them understand these in the context of a safe, caring relationship. The methods used to access these repressed processes include:
- Free association: with prompting, the patient reports the first thoughts that come to mind.
- Hypnosis.
- The interpretation of dreams and fantasy material.
- The analysis of defense mechanisms: individuals are said to employ defenses when anxiety-producing aspects of the self that are unconscious threaten to break through to the conscious mind, potentially giving rise to intolerable feelings. Examples include. repression (anxiety-provoking feelings, thoughts, or fantasies are pushed into the unconscious) and projection (one's own unacknowledged feelings are attributed to someone else).
- The analysis of transference and countertransference: *transference* occurs when the patient transfers feelings or attitudes experienced in an earlier significant relationship onto the therapist. For example, a male patient becomes angry with his therapist, whom he sees as cold and uncaring, unconsciously reminding him of his mother. *Countertransference* occurs when the therapist transfers feelings or attitudes experienced in an earlier significant relationship onto the patient.

Although the terms *psychoanalytic and psychodynamic* are often used interchangeably, the following therapeutic techniques are distinguished:
- The term *psychoanalysis* is traditionally used to describe the therapy in which patients see their analyst up to five times per week for a nonspecified, but usually very long (on the order of years) period of time; therapy is conducted with patients on a couch in the recumbent position with the analyst out of view. The analyst hardly says anything except to make an "interpretation."
- The term *psychodynamic psychotherapy* usually describes the therapy in which (although it is based on psychoanalytic theory), patient and therapist sit face-to-face for about one session per week. Therapy tends to be more interactive than psychoanalysis. *Brief insight-oriented psychotherapy* (also called *focused psychotherapy*) is a shorter version of psychodynamic therapy (6–9 months) and tends to focus only on problems affecting current functioning. Psychodynamic psychotherapy may be conducted on an individual basis or in a group setting (group therapy will be discussed later in the chapter).

Transference and countertransference often occur in settings outside of psychotherapy. Patients may inappropriately react to health-care professionals as if they were some significant figure from the past. An example is when patients express unwarranted anger toward doctors or nurses when they do not receive immediate attention; this may be anger that was initially experienced toward neglectful parents. Similarly, health workers may misplace feelings from their own earlier relationships onto patients.

Behavior therapy

Behavior therapists are concerned with changing maladaptive behavior patterns that have arisen through inappropriate learning (classical or operant conditioning). They are not concerned with the patient's inner experience or conflicts, and treatment aims only to replace unhelpful behavior with more adaptive behavior. Figure 28.2 summarizes some of the techniques used in behavior therapy. See Chapter 22 for the specific techniques used in the psychosexual disorders.

Cognitive-behavioral therapy

Cognitive-behavioral therapy (CBT), which is also referred to as cognitive therapy, was developed by Aaron T. Beck and is based on the assumption that how individuals think about or interpret things (i.e., their *cognitions*) subsequently determines how they feel and behave. Cognitive techniques include eliciting *automatic thoughts* and *dysfunctional assumptions* and then testing their validity.

Some techniques used in behavior therapy

Behavioral technique	Clinical uses	Description
Exposure	Phobias and avoidance, posttraumatic stress disorder	Systematic desensitization: a hierarchy of increasingly threatening situations is created, e.g., spider in another room → spider in the same room → spider near the patient → spider on the patient's hand. Patients imagine, or are exposed to, the least threatening situation while practising relaxation techniques. When anxiety relief has been achieved, patients are then exposed to increasingly threatening situations. There is evidence that real-life exposure; rather than visualization, is more effective, although sometimes impractical. Flooding: patients are instantly exposed to the highest level of their anxiety hierarchy (i.e., flooded) until their anxiety diminishes, e.g., putting a patient in a room filled with spiders (flooding by imagination is termed implosion therapy)
Exposure with response prevention	OCD	Patients are encouraged to resist carrying out compulsions until the urge diminishes. They are then exposed to more severe compulsion-evoking situations
Relaxation	Anxiety	Progressive relaxation of muscle groups; breathing exercises; visualizing relaxing images and situations (*guided imagery*)
Modeling	Phobias and avoidance, OCD	Patients observe the therapist being exposed to the phobic stimulus, then attempt the same
Activity scheduling and target setting	Depression	Patients are encouraged to structure their day with certain activities, as depression-induced reduced activity can lead to a further lowering of mood due to reduced stimulation and opportunity for positive experiences

OCD, obsessive-compulsive disorder

Fig. 28.2 Some techniques used in behavior therapy.

Automatic thoughts. Automatic thoughts are the many thoughts that involuntarily enter an individual's mind in response to specific situations. Examples include: "He doesn't like me," "I'm such an idiot," "I'm so boring."

Dysfunctional assumptions. Dysfunctional assumptions are the faulty "rules" that individuals live by, which, when broken, as they inevitably are, lead to psychological distress. Examples include: "If I don't come first, then I am completely useless," "If I hurt someone, then I am evil."

Using an example, Figure 28.3 summarizes some important aspects of the cognitive model.

CBT also draws on principles from behavioral theory. For example, dysfunctional assumptions may be challenged by behavioral experiments (testing irrational thoughts against reality).

Note that CBT differs from psychodynamic psychotherapy in the following ways:

- CBT tends to be time-limited (12–25 sessions).
- CBT is goal-oriented and focuses predominantly on present problems. It is less concerned with the details of how problems developed or unconscious drives.
- The patient and CBT therapist are strongly collaborative, deciding together on the session's agenda and case formulation.
- CBT involves patients doing "homework assignments."
- Because of its structured format, CBT is more amenable to efficacy studies.

The other forms of therapy that incorporate elements of CBT are summarized in Figure 28.4.

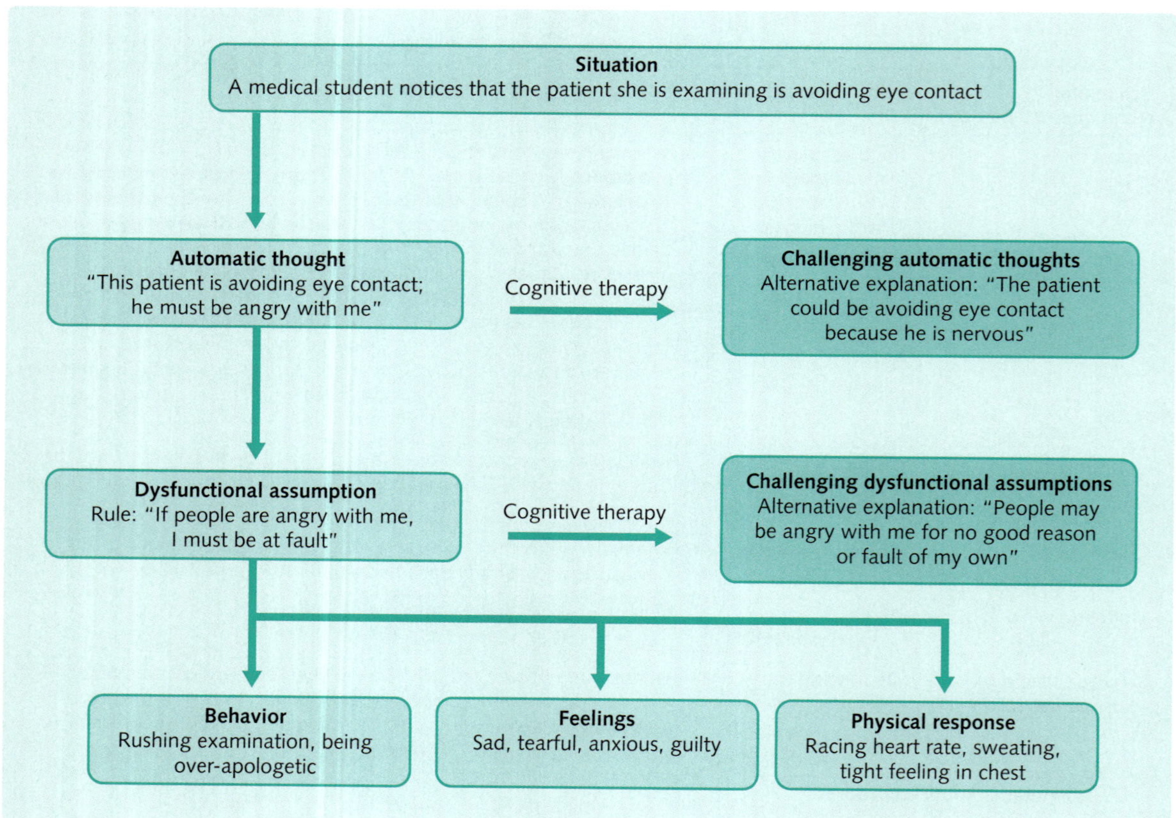

Fig. 28.3 Illustration of some aspects of the cognitive model.

Some therapies incorporating elements of cognitive-behavioral therapy (CBT)		
Therapy type	**Description**	**Developer**
Dialectical behaviour therapy (DBT)	An intensive and demanding form of therapy that has shown promising results in the treatment of borderline personality disorder and self-harm	Marsha Linehan
Cognitive analytic therapy (CAT)	A brief integrative therapy combining elements of both cognitive behavior and psychoanalytic theories	Anthony Ryle
Rational emotive behavior therapy (REBT)	Consists of encouraging patients to challenge and dispel "irrational thoughts"	Albert Ellis

Fig. 28.4 Some therapies incorporating elements of cognitive-behavioral therapy (CBT).

Beck classically described how depressed patients suffered from a *cognitive triad* of symptoms:

- Negative view of oneself (e.g., "I am a worthless failure")
- Negative view of one's environment (e.g., "The world is harsh and pointless")
- Negative view of the future (e.g., "There is nothing for me to live for.")

Interpersonal therapy

Interpersonal therapy (IPT) is based on the assumption that problems with interpersonal relationships and social functioning are significant contributors to the development of mental illness, as well as being a consequence of mental illness, particularly depression. IPT attempts to enable patients to evaluate their social interactions and improve their interpersonal skills in all social roles, from close family and friendships to community and work-related roles. Main areas of focus include (1) role disputes, (2) role transitions, (3) interpersonal deficits, and (4) loss or grief. IPT is similar to CBT in that it tends to focus on current problems and is brief in duration (12–16 sessions). It was developed by Weissman and Klerman and was largely influenced by Harry Stack Sullivan's *Interpersonal Psychiatry*.

Group therapy

Group therapy may be practiced according to different theoretical orientations, from supportive to cognitive-behavioral to psychodynamic approaches. Most groups meet once weekly for an hour and consist of one or two therapists and a selection of about 8–10 patients. Therapy can run from months (CBT orientation) to years (psychodynamic orientation). Group therapy allows patients (and therapists) the opportunity to observe and analyze their psychological and behavioral responses to other individuals in the group in a "safe" social setting. It is thought that group therapy owes its effectiveness to a number of "curative factors," such as universality, which describes the process of patients realizing that they are not alone in having particular problems.

Family therapy

Instead of focusing on the individual patient, this form of therapy treats the family as a whole. It may include just parents and siblings or extended family. It is hoped that improved family communication and conflict resolution will result in an improvement of the "identified patient." Similarly to group therapy, there are many different orientations, most notably the psychodynamic, structural, and systems approach.

The term *eclectic therapy* refers to the practice of using a mixture of psychotherapeutic theories and techniques (e.g., psychodynamic, interpersonal, and cognitive-behavioral therapy) in understanding and treating the same patient. Many therapists use it to create a therapy package uniquely tailored to the individual.

Main indications of psychological treatments	
Psychiatric condition	**Main psychological treatment used**
Stressful life events, illnesses, bereavements	Supportive therapy
Depression	Cognitive-behavior therapy, interpersonal therapy Other: psychodynamic therapy, group therapy
Anxiety disorders (including OCD)	Cognitive-behavioral therapy
Posttraumatic stress disorder	Systematic desensitization Eye movement desensitization Other: psychodynamic therapy, hypnotherapy
Schizophrenia	Cognitive-behavioral therapy Family therapy
Eating disorders	Cognitive-behavioral therapy Interpersonal therapy Family therapy
Borderline personality disorder	Dialectical behavior therapy Psychodynamic therapy Cognitive analytic therapy Therapeutic communities
Alcohol dependence	Cognitive-behavioral therapy Group therapy
OCD, obsessive-compulsive disorder	Cognitive-behavioral therapy Other: exposure with response prevention, modeling

Fig. 28.5 Main indications of psychological treatments.

What is it used for?

The psychological treatment options for specific conditions have been discussed in each of the relevant chapters on these conditions. The main treatment options with the strongest evidence base, along with relevant cross-references, have been summarized in Figure 28.5. Note, however, that the lack of evidence for certain psychological treatments does not mean that they are not effective.

Index

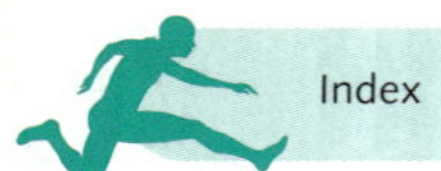